Advanced Practice in Nursing

Under the Auspices of the *International Council of Nurses (ICN)*

Series Editor
Christophe Debout
GIP-IFITS
Health Chair Sciences- Po Paris/IDS UMR Inserm 1145
Paris, France

This series of concise monographs, endorsed by the International Council of Nurses, explores various aspects of advanced practice nursing at the international level.

The ICN International Nurse Practitioner/Advanced Practice Nursing Network definition has been adopted for this series to define advanced practice nursing: "A Nurse Practitioner/Advanced Practice Nurse is a registered nurse who has acquired the expert knowledge base, complex decision-making skills and clinical competencies for expanded practice, the characteristics of which are shaped by the context and/or country in which s/he is credentialed to practice. A master's degree is recommended for entry level."

At the international level, advanced practice nursing encompasses two professional profiles:

Nurse practitioners (NPs) who have mastered advanced practice nursing, and are capable of diagnosing, making prescriptions for and referring patients. Though they mainly work in the community, some also work in hospitals. Clinical nurse specialists (CNSs) are expert nurses who deliver high-quality nursing care to patients and promote quality care and performance in nursing teams.

The duties performed by these two categories of advanced practice nurses on an everyday basis can be divided into five interrelated roles:

Clinical practice

Consultation

Education

Leadership

Research

The series addresses four topics directly related to advanced practice nursing:

APN in practice (NPs and CNSs)

Education and continuous professional development for advanced practice nurses

Managerial issues related to advanced practice nursing

Policy and regulation of advanced practice nursing

The contributing authors are mainly APNs (NPs and CNSs) recruited from the ICN International Nurse Practitioner/Advanced Practice Nursing Network. They include clinicians, educators, researchers, regulators and managers, and are recognized as experts in their respective fields.

Each book within the series reflects the fundamentals of nursing / advanced practice nursing and will promote evidence-based nursing.

More information about this series at http://www.springer.com/series/13871

Melanie Rogers
Editor

Spiritual Dimensions of Advanced Practice Nursing

Stories of Hope

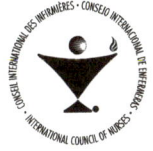

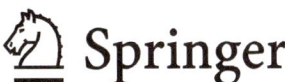

Editor
Melanie Rogers
University of Huddersfield
Huddersfield
UK

ISSN 2511-3917   ISSN 2511-3925   (electronic)
Advanced Practice in Nursing
ISBN 978-3-030-71463-5   ISBN 978-3-030-71464-2   (eBook)
https://doi.org/10.1007/978-3-030-71464-2

This Springer imprint is published by the registered company Springer Nature Switzerland AG
The registered company address is: Gewerbestrasse 11, 6330 Cham, Switzerland

Foreword

There has never been a better moment to publish this book on the spiritual dimensions of advanced nursing practice. As I have been reading the chapters about human connection and spiritual practice, I am reminded constantly of what we have all missed during this pandemic and our times of lockdown: we have missed being with each other to share our lives, our concerns and our joys. This book is about the critical importance of allowing ourselves as nurses to make an authentic human connection with those people we care for, not only because that deep spiritual connection has healing power, but also because it helps us, as nurses, to understand better what matters to the person consulting us.

Talking about spiritual practice has never been easy, but I venture to say that it has, in 2020, become easier. Why? Because we really have been in this pandemic together, deprived of our friends and family, and for many of us working in situations that are stressful beyond our wildest imaginings. We now share a deeper understanding of why loneliness is such a killer, especially for older adults. We feel how stress affects our bodies and, awake and anxious in the dead of night, we know how it is affecting our minds. Enduring 2020 has helped us understand how important it can be for someone to take the time to sit with us and look beyond what we feel comfortable saying to what we really want to talk about. It is this that is at the heart of spiritual practice.

The Nursing Now campaign team which I currently lead has tried to respond to the stress we hear about by offering ways for nurses to connect with each other and these have been enthusiastically taken up. Facebook, WhatsApp, webinars and email have all served to connect us for more than a year now and it is not perfect—but certainly better than nothing. In some ways, despite being locked down, we have become more global than ever and at times I have been deeply moved by the ways that nurses in over 120 countries have sought to support each other by giving positive feedback—cheers and congratulations emoji style—or encouragement and empathy. And I have reflected that, had life been the pre-pandemic 'normal', those nurses might not have made and maintained virtual connections in this way. What lessons we can learn for the future about nurturing each other, even from a distance.

This book is both philosophical and practical. It does not shy away from discussing some of the hardest issues that we have to think about when we are nursing people, but it gives us case studies too and frameworks that will help everyone to consider spirituality in their practice. As nurses, we walk alongside people as they confront challenges to living, and sometimes when they face their death. COVID-19 threw into stark relief the situations that nurses face day by day: too few staff to look after seriously ill people and no families allowed to be with people at their last moments. And it was usually nurses who made themselves available to be present— both physically and spiritually—so that a connection could be made, a hand held, a video call made to a family. It is hard to estimate what those offerings of self by nurses have meant because we so seldom talk about what is hard to express.

During the last year, Nursing Now has run some webinars for nurses on self-compassion and they have been amongst the best attended of all the webinars we have run, precisely because they address the vulnerabilities we all feel when we are open to hearing the most challenging truths and hardest questions. From the first webinar we realised that we were sharing an experience that needed something new from all of us. It went beyond an educational experience to a spiritual one and what we learned was that in order for participants to gain any insights from the webinar, it was essential to bring in a spiritual dimension. As a result, in our lockdown webinars we have hosted chaplains, poets, counsellors, mental health nurses and artists. Together, they have opened minds so that we can find language to share what is deepest in each of us—the sense of despair and the joys as well. I hope that as we return to a world that is more akin to the pre-pandemic normal, we do not lose the good things we have learned and our ability to make connections with each other. This book comes at the right time to remind us all of how important is the spiritual dimension of nursing practice.

Helping nurses understand the deeper meaning in their advanced practice is important for another reason. Research undertaken by Dan Pink[1] shows that there are three critical drivers that motivate all of us to perform well and these are autonomy, mastery and purpose. Pink's work has always seemed to me to be an unassailable argument in support of advanced nursing practice because it results in autonomy as a practitioner and mastery of clinical practice. The spiritual dimension to practice completes the trilogy: it shows us that there is a greater purpose to what we do than can be captured in tasks and performance indicators. What Pink found was that when people were reminded of the higher purpose inherent in their jobs—what he calls 'a cause larger than themselves' (p. 131)—they became more productive and performed better.

This book is important for many reasons: because of the moment it is arriving when we have such a need to reconnect with each other at a deep level; because it shows the clinical value in spiritual practice—being open to hearing what is troubling people beyond what they present; and because it reinforces the need to describe competence in spiritual practice for nurses and that, I would argue, begins to help us meet the challenge of showing value in spiritually competent practice. Policy makers have not been renowned for acting on the strong evidence of nursing's effectiveness in clinical care and this was one reason why the Nursing Now campaign was established—because nursing work was often invisible. Spiritual care is even less

---

[1] Pink D., *Drive: (2009) The surprising truth about what motivates us.* Riverhead Books. New York. 2009.

visible and yet we know that there are calls for kinder care. Klaber and Bailey, in their 2019 editorial 'Kindness: an underrated currency',[2] identify six types of kindness that improve outcomes for patients with cancer. These include deep listening, empathy and thoughtful support for patients and families—all necessary for spiritually competent practice. Klaber and Bailey argue that the business of health care is in danger of losing the heart of health care—kindness—while we focus purely on the technical.

Our challenge as nurses is to continue to show what a difference our spiritual practice can make and this book is part of that journey because it gives us a framework for describing spiritually competent practice and for researching why it is important. Then we need to get this into language that policy makers, managers and budget holders will understand. That requires data as well as powerful stories that will be remembered when it is time to allocate budgets to nursing time.

We all remember our stories of the time that we had a eureka moment and I thought I would share mine, because it relates so strongly to the importance of connection, deep listening and space for people to explore their own journeys. My story concerns a young Bangladeshi woman, Meena, living with her family in Birmingham, England. Meena had been brought to England by her husband in an arranged marriage. She had no English and relied on her husband and children to interpret for her. She had few friends. Meena started consulting the local GP frequently saying that she had a lump in her throat. This went on for months and eventually Meena was referred to several hospital clinics for investigations, and all came back negative. Desperate to know what to do next the GP asked me to talk with Meena. I arranged a young woman interpreter to be with us. Meena was clearly anxious and I asked about her life in Birmingham and what it was like. She was lonely and reported several times that she had trouble swallowing because of the lump in her throat. I asked Meena what was happening around the time she first began to notice the lump in her throat. Her response was shocking: 'my husband died' she said. We sat quietly for a moment and I told her that in England we had a saying that if you are very sad, you get a lump in your throat. Did she think that might be related to her symptoms? At that point Meena wept, as we all did in that room. Her interpreter, the young woman, told me not to worry that she would look after Meena. They left together and Meena did not consult again for the lump in her throat.

I tell this story to highlight how important it is to help a person tell their story. Training as a Nurse Practitioner I had been told over and over again by my preceptor that if I listened to the patient for long enough they would tell me what was wrong with them. This really stuck and Meena gave me the 'aha moment' when I saw this in action. It took a willingness on my part to take time, to want to hear her story, to connect with her and to make sure she was understood. It is not easy in today's world of performance indicators and 'time is money' to offer deep care but it is important for all the right reasons. Meena could have avoided several hospital

---

[2] Klaber R., Bailey S., (2019) *Kindness: An underrated currency. British Medical Journal* 2019;367:l6099. https://doi.org/10.1136/bmj.l6099.

investigations if we had all built up this picture sooner. The care would—in harsh economic terms—have cost less.

This important book could be transformational as we face a new future, when we have to build cost-effective and resilient health systems that will help us achieve all our health goals. There is no substitute for human connection and kindness and if we are to build a truly effective health system, we need to know what matters to someone, not only what is the matter with them. It is competent spiritual care, which is at the heart of all health care and nursing practice, that will create a different future where we acknowledge that the best medicine for a person is another person. I commend this book to you as an essential companion for your journey.

April, 2021   Barbara Stilwell
                                           Nursing Now Global Campaign
                                                              London, UK

Preface

This book has been one I have wanted to write for many years. The ideas and concepts around spirituality have been percolating and being refined until the right time arrived to put pen to paper. I started the book prior to the global COVID-19 pandemic and finished whilst many of us still face uncertainty and anxiety amid the pandemic. For me there has never been a more necessary time to consider the value of spiritual dimension of practice. Our world is in chaos, and many of us have seen the devastation a global pandemic brings first-hand. We have been starkly reminded of our own mortality and many will have asked themselves deeply existential questions. My hope is that this book will bring to the fore ways of working which bring hope, meaning and purpose to those in our care but also remind us of what brings us hope, meaning and purpose.

It would have been easy for me to fill this book with theoretical discussions, arguments and debate. I have been researching and studying spirituality for many years and have enough evidence and research findings to fill several books. However, I wanted this to be a practical book which will resonate with Advanced Practice Nurses and encourage the implementation of spirituality into practice as part of truly holistic practice.

Whilst writing and bringing the chapters together I have been privileged to work with experts in the field of spirituality and advanced practice nursing, and each has brought their unique contributions to this book. We have offered up alternative ways of thinking about the concept of spirituality by reframing it as spiritually competent practice. In addition, I propose a framework of Availability and Vulnerability which encompasses many key components of spirituality but is immensely practical and easy to integrate into our work.

My hope is that through the chapters you will understand the concept of spirituality further and through the case studies will see the impact that integrating it into your practice can bring. Each one of us can make a difference by seeing those in our care as fellow human beings on this journey together. The need for kindness, compassion and acceptance is universal and bringing these to the heart of care can create a quiet revolution against the reductionist narratives of task and cost-driven health care.

To all who seek to bring hope, meaning and purpose to those in their care and to all who hold a place in my heart.

Huddersfield, UK   Melanie Rogers

Acknowledgements

This book has been completed with the support and encouragement of many friends, family members and colleagues. The contributors to this book have all seen the impact that integrating spiritually competent practice makes to those in their care and I want to thank them for their wonderful contributions. To those patients whom I have been privileged to care for, I honour you for all you have shown me about the value of person-centred care. I also want to thank all of those who have supported me in my journey as a nurse, Nurse Practitioner, educator and researcher, especially those who have encouraged and supported my passion to ensure patients receive truly holistic care. I owe a great debt to colleagues at the University of Huddersfield's Spirituality Special Interest Group, in particular Professor John Wattis and Professor Stephen Curran whom I have had the pleasure of working with, researching with, and journeying together; their ongoing support and mentoring consistently inspire me. I also want to thank Catherine Askew from the Northumbria Community who supported my vision for adapting the concepts of availability and vulnerability into a model for health care, without her and the community this book would never have come to the fore. Additionally, my thanks go to all who are part of the International Council of Nurses Nurse Practitioner/Advanced Practice Network; I have been privileged to Chair this organisation for the past 4 years and I have met many of the contributors through the incredible work the Network does to progress Advance Practice Nursing. Finally, I want to thank my incredible partner, family and long-suffering sausage dogs Minnie and Winnie who have accompanied me on long walks as I have percolated my thoughts and given me the time and space to research and write about spirituality.

Contents

Introduction to Spirituality

1

Melanie Rogers

Abstract

This chapter focuses on the concept of spirituality and evaluates some of the theoretical perspectives related to spirituality in healthcare generally. Challenges around defining spirituality, reasons for integrating spirituality into practice, the relationship of spirituality to religion, how to put spirituality into practice and ethical issues are discussed. The large and diverse literature on the history and meaning of the term spirituality is not explored. The chapter instead seeks to explore how spirituality is generally understood and applied in healthcare.

Keywords

Spirituality · Advanced Practice Nurse · Religion · Spiritual care

1.1 Introduction

This book aims to support the understanding of spirituality and its integration into the work of Advanced Practice Nurses (APNs). There is a lack of clarity about the definition of "spirituality", and relatively little research into spirituality in advanced practice nursing. In research and practice, spirituality is often conflated with religion. The aim of this book is to explore the concept of spirituality in relation to the varied roles APNs have in healthcare settings internationally. APN case studies are provided in Chaps. 6–13 to illustrate how spirituality has been operationalised in diverse settings.

M. Rogers (✉)
University of Huddersfield, Huddersfield, UK
e-mail: m.rogers@hud.ac.uk

© The Author(s), under exclusive license to Springer Nature Switzerland AG 2021
M. Rogers (ed.), *Spiritual Dimensions of Advanced Practice Nursing*,
Advanced Practice in Nursing, https://doi.org/10.1007/978-3-030-71464-2_1

This book starts by exploring the concepts of spirituality, spiritually competent practice and spirituality competencies. Following this, the importance of personal spirituality and self-compassion are discussed. The remaining chapters focus on a framework for integrating spirituality into practice, followed by an introduction to the APN role and spirituality in countries across the world. APN case studies illustrate how spirituality can be integrated into practice.

1.2   Context

My interest in spirituality in nursing has developed throughout many years working as a nurse in a variety of hospital settings for 10 years and as a Primary Care Nurse Practitioner (NP) for over 20 years. Spirituality is an ongoing focus for me as I continue to wrestle with the challenge of providing truly holistic care to patients within, what is often in primary care, a short consultation.

Advanced Practice Nurses are recognised globally as "a generalist or specialised nurse who has acquired, through additional graduate education (minimum of a master's degree), the expert knowledge base, complex decision-making skills and clinical competencies for Advanced Nursing Practice, the characteristics of which are shaped by the context in which they are credentialed to practice. The two most commonly identified APN roles are CNS and NP" (ICN 2020, p. 6).

ICN (2020, p. 14) define a Clinical Nurse Specialist (CNS) as a nurse who has completed a master's degree programme specific to CNS practice. "The CNS provides healthcare services based on advanced specialised expertise when caring for complex and vulnerable patients or populations". NPs are described as generalist nurses who, after additional education (minimum master's degree for entry level), are autonomous clinicians. They are educated to diagnose and treat conditions based on evidence-informed guidelines that include nursing principles that focus on treating the whole person rather than only the condition or disease. The level of practice autonomy and accountability is determined by, and sensitive to, the context of the country or setting and the regulatory policies in which the NP practices (ICN 2020, p. 20).

Although both roles are embedded in nursing there is often an integration of skills previously in the realm of medicine (Royal College of Nursing (RCN) 2008). A challenge for all APNs is to ensure holistic integrated care which does not have a greater focus on the medical model. It is recognised that many APNs routinely adopt the bio-medical approach which can reduce the holistic nature of the role and lead to spiritual care being omitted (Kliewer and Saultz 2006). Even a focus on the bio-psycho-social approach may not fully integrate holistic care, with Sulmasy (2002) identifying that it does not address the totality of the patient's existence. Epstein (2014) suggests that the clinicians often lack self-awareness, resilience and compassion that limits their ability to integrate this approach into their care. To ensure holistic care APNs should aim to integrate the bio-psycho-social-spiritual approach to care embedded in advanced nursing practice which can have a transformational impact on patient care (Saad et al. 2017).

Like many APNs my clinical practice has become increasingly complex with patients attending with multiple presentations and polypharmacy which are often interwoven with mental health and social problems. This has become even more acute during the Covid-19 pandemic which has left many patients struggling to access health services and feeling increasingly isolated (Propper et al. 2020). Historically, more complex presentations would normally lead to more regular contact with patients to support their health needs. This has not been possible this past year as primary care has moved from a predominantly face to face service to a limited virtual service, leaving many patients without care. However, there have still been opportunities to address patients' spiritual needs, albeit remotely.

Normally, in my work as an NP, I am able to maintain regular contact with my patients. I develop effective therapeutic relationships over extended periods of time and patients trust me and open up to me about their concerns. I have noted that some patients express a sense of hopelessness relating to their diagnoses, health needs and life. It is within a therapeutic relationship I can address this hopelessness and explore questions of meaning about their lives, illnesses and experiences. I often find myself supporting patients to explore many of their existential questions relating to these areas. Taking time to listen, support and encourage patients to explore these questions and to make positive changes in their own lives appears to help them to find a sense of hope and peace. I frequently notice that as patients open up to me and share their struggles and concerns, we develop a deeper connection based on respect and trust; this connection I suggest often has a spiritual dimension.

1.3 Spirituality

Puchalski and Ferrell (2011) suggest that it is not uncommon for patients during times of suffering to seek to find meaning in their existence or release from their distress. Patients want someone who is willing to listen to their questioning and help them explore some of their deeper concerns; spirituality is one of the domains where this can happen. APNs need to connect to their patients distress and suffering (Vincensi 2019). It is not complicated, it often requires simple practices which as nurses we are well versed with, for example our willingness to be fully present, listen to and accompany our patients.

Brown (2010) and Beller and Wagner (2020) suggest that many people in society are increasingly isolated, especially in western societies which promote the ethos of individualism. King (2011) asserts that society in general has hit a spiritual crisis leaving individuals isolated and alone as they deal with relationship breakdowns, financial pressures, a hunger for materialism and broken communities. This has been compounded by the Covid-19 pandemic (Ferrell et al. 2020). Rohr (2003) coins the term "affluenza" suggesting that the propensity to an individualistic and materialistic society affects the ability of people to find any sense of peace or purpose. A lack of peace and purpose has dramatically increased for many during the current pandemic and subsequent lock-down restrictions. As APNs we can fight this "affluenza" and our patients' sense of isolation by offering patients time and our presence to explore existential questions not through analysis but through our relationship with them, whether this be time limited or continuous.

There has been much written about the essence of nursing, nurse–patient relationships and intimacy in caring (Benner and Wrubel 1989; Downey 2004; Kirk 2007; Watson and Woodward 2020) which may be relevant to the experience of a spiritual dimension. Holistic care provided by APNs has also been written about (Shuler and Davis 1993; Mezey et al. 2003; Chrash et al. 2011; Rogers 2017; Rogers et al. 2020; Rogers and Wattis 2020) but spirituality as a domain still remains scarcely mentioned in the APN literature.

Spirituality is an important aspect of holistic, person-centred care which is frequently overlooked owing to difficulty conceptualising spirituality and confusion about how to integrate it into care (Wattis et al. 2017). Over the past few decades, spirituality has received heightened interest in the healthcare arena (Pesut and Reimer-Kirkham 2009). Nursing has entered into the many discussions and debates around spirituality. However, the focus often remains on the challenges of both conceptualising and operationalising spirituality (Reinert and Koenig 2013; Wattis et al. 2017). There has been significant criticism of some of the nursing literature on spirituality suggesting it is not robust and lacks critique (Swinton 2006a; Clarke 2009; Koenig 2011). Additionally, the gap in terms of empirical studies has increased criticism aimed at nursing scholars (Sessanna et al. 2010). There are still ongoing debates in the literature about how to define spirituality, with spirituality and religion sometimes viewed as synonymous and often seen as overlapping concepts (Koenig 2009; Hubbell et al. 2006; Chrash et al. 2011).

It is probably an impossible task to arrive at a definition of spirituality that is universally acceptable, especially if it is accepted that spirituality is unique for each individual (Narayanasamy 2006; Chrash et al. 2011). However, there may be aspects of spirituality that are universal and shared regardless of the presence or absence of a specific religious form of belief and expression (Miner-Williams 2005). This view appeals to some, whilst others regard this as secularising spirituality and omitting to include the rich heritage that may be gleaned from religion (Clarke 2009). Despite a lack of clarity around spirituality, research does suggest patients want healthcare practitioners to integrate spirituality into their practice (Puchalski 2001; Ellis and Campbell 2004; Selman et al. 2018; Gardner et al. 2020). However, Tacey (2004) suggests that there seems to be an acute anxiety felt by those in caring professions about spirituality which is often related to the lack of conceptual clarity, concerns about the relationship between spirituality and religion and difficulty understanding how to operationalise spirituality.

Spirituality appears to be becoming more important to individuals and society, especially during the pandemic (Castillo 2020). One possible reason is because many in western society have become impatient with secularisation and modernity and seek alternative ways of living which offer more meaning and purpose. Berger (1969) and Brown (2012) suggest that modernity (with its materialistic worldview) has been swallowed hook, line and sinker. This has now given rise to postmodernism which "views human experience as incoherent, lacking normative approaches for truth and meaning" (Dockery 2001, p. 12).

Clarke (2013, p. 3) suggests that "society is full of people hungry for an acknowledgement of what makes them valuable". Spirituality can be viewed as a way of accepting the complexities of our inner lives and connecting with our very centre (Nouwen 1972). Hinton (1992) proposes that spirituality describes the part of ourselves that lies deepest within, that influences our decisions and the course of our life, hidden yet extremely powerful. The existential and ontological issues of life are important to acknowledge in our search for an understanding of spirituality.

1.4 Defining Spirituality in Healthcare

Extensive reading, research and reflection has helped me to find a definition that feels comfortable and applicable to my practice: Spirituality is simply what gives us hope, meaning and purpose, it is fundamentally human (Rogers 2016). As it will become evident spirituality is further defined and developed through the Rogers' Availability and Vulnerability framework for operationalising spirituality which is presented in Chap. 5. Narayanasamy (2004, p. 1141) identifies a similar definition which defines spirituality as the "essence of being, giving meaning and purpose to our existence". However, even these simple, universal definitions can be controversial since what gives a person meaning and purpose may be contrary to social norms. As Swinton (2006b) reminds us Hitler had meaning and purpose which almost destroyed Europe. Despite my definition being one which I am comfortable with, it is not viewed as an absolute. Throughout my own research my understanding of spirituality has developed and I recognise that spirituality is innately human and influenced by context and emotional engagement. Critical analysis of some of the discourse around spirituality and the inconsistent, differing and contradictory definitions allows exploration of the complexities of defining spirituality. Tacey (2000, p. 38) suggests that we are able to define spirituality less and less "because it includes more and more becoming a veritable baggy monster containing a multitude of activities and experiences". White (2006) echoes this stating that the danger is that spirituality is becoming so broad that it includes everything that brings a feeling of warmth. It is difficult to see how a definition can have meaning yet not become so inclusive that its meaning is lost. Even the simple definition I suggest is so wide and broad that it could end up meaning very little without context.

Spirituality also appears to be an emotive concept polarising opinion. Some see spirituality and religion as synonymous or significantly overlapping (Hubbell et al. 2006; Narayanasamy 2006; Koenig 2009; Cook 2020), this is reflected in a number of case studies included in this book. Whilst others adopt a wider perspective relating spirituality only to concepts of meaning, hope and purpose (Tanyi 2002; Narayanasamy 2004; Pesut and Reimer-Kirkham 2009; Rogers and Wattis 2020). It is difficult to understand how one definition can encompass the multitude of views, opinions and concepts linked with spirituality. For some it is the ethereal attributes of spirituality connected to the transcendent which increase confusion and resistance to spirituality (Milligan 2011), whilst others see this as a way of bringing more clarity to the concept of spirituality (Miner-Williams 2005; Tacey 2004).

Others have recognised literature on the secularisation of spirituality in healthcare (separating it completely from religion) with the aim of finding common ground (Sessana et al. 2007; Pesut et al. 2008). This may result in spirituality "being undistinguishable from psycho-social care" (Clarke 2009, p. 1666; Vermandere et al. 2011). The many definitions and meanings evoked by the term spirituality can create ambiguity and it is been argued that this may lead to reluctance to explore the topic (Agrimson and Toft 2008).

Contemporary APN discussion papers and empirical studies also offer contradictory definitions of spirituality and use a plethora of terms when talking about spirituality, i.e. spiritual care, spiritual dimensions, spiritual behaviour, spiritual needs and spiritual assessment which are often not always defined (Stranahan 2001; Maddox 2001; Hubbell et al. 2006; Helming 2009; Saunders 2017) adding confusion. This is echoed in other health and social care literature with definitions of spirituality varying from the vague to the specific, the diverse to the spurious in an attempt to box in the concept. Cook (2011, p. 1) argues that some of these definitions offer "….no scientific basis and could represent a dangerous crossing of professional boundaries whilst others were too confusing to be useful". Reinert and Koenig (2013) have criticised nursing scholars who attempted to define and discuss spirituality suggesting that there is no rigorous analysis of spirituality in nursing.

The difficulties in defining spirituality and offering rigorous critique may stem from not just the ethereal attributes but also the nebulous nature of the concept (D'Souza 2007; Gilbert 2011). These difficulties include ensuring spirituality is understandable enough to be operationalised in practice. If spirituality is watered down too much it may become vague and over-inclusive (Clarke 2009). Conversely, Swinton and Pattison (2010) suggest that being vague about defining spirituality may be its strength and value in practice, presumably because of the ability to translate spirituality individually. This confusion leads to a paradox; the danger of an over-inclusive definition is that it becomes cumbersome and defies operationalising for research and practice; however, the danger of not embracing spirituality within practice is that we miss the deep interpersonal compassionate connection with our patients which epitomises the heart of nursing care (McSherry 2010).

Sessanna et al. (2010) encourage seeing all our patients as spiritual by virtue of their being human. In Greek "Spirit" is expressed as pneuma meaning breath (Oxford Dictionary 2021). Pneuma is the very part of us which gives life, without it one cannot exist. If this is accepted, then spirituality may simply mean what is at our very being and what makes us human. Miner-Williams (2005, p. 813) suggests that despite spirituality being universal its "depth and profoundness make it beyond the human vocabulary". He also suggests that it is not possible to fully articulate or understand spirituality as it affects individuals so uniquely. What does appear a compelling argument is that as APNs we can determine what is important for our patients individually by listening to them and recognising spirituality as being unique and experienced differently by each individual (Baldacchino 2006; McSherry 2006; Rogers and Wattis 2020).

Spirituality may be expressed in the way we live, relate and perceive the world around us and is often linked with positive attributes (Johnston and Mayers 2004).

Hope, meaning and purpose are common attributes that are often described in literature (Miner-Williams 2005; Reinert and Koenig 2013; Rogers and Wattis 2020). Complexity occurs because for some this may be related to belief in God or a higher power leading to the synergy between religion and spirituality. Nevertheless, those without a belief in God or a higher power may be equally spiritual. They may be more focused upon integration of mind, body and spirit in terms of relationships and connectedness to nature and the world (Johnston and Mayers 2004). These aspects are illustrated throughout the chapters presenting case studies in a number of countries.

Tacey (2004) links spirituality with the sacred which he suggests might or might not be God or a higher power. He views spirituality as a sensitive, contemplative, transformative relationship with the sacred which can sustain uncertainty. Uncertainty is a constant companion for humanity, but an anchor can be provided in terms of how we each embrace spirituality ourselves. Taceys' definition of spirituality focuses upon the mystery of spirituality and a sense of acceptance of an evolving spirituality which is uniquely reflected in each person's journey in life. Tanyi (2002) suggests part of our evolving spirituality is the importance of connectedness. She echoes others by arguing this may not just be with God but could be connectedness with ourselves, others or nature also. She also identifies this connectedness as being what gives meaning to life and what helps people achieve their optimal being.

It is clear that spirituality can evoke deeper connection to existential and ontological questions especially when dealing with uncertainty. Many, when dealing with illness and crisis, will ask themselves why they are suffering, what the suffering means and how can they deal with it (Rogers and Wattis 2015). For some this connects to a desire for transcendence, a desire not to be alone in our struggles. Many definitions include transcendence as a core element of spirituality (Coyle 2002; Pesut et al. 2008). In general, transcendence is linked to a deep connection to God or a higher power (Chrash et al. 2011), whilst others talk of transcendence as escape from the self (Foley 2010). Transcendence is defined as "existence or experience beyond the human experience" (Oxford Dictionary 2021, para 1). For some transcendence appears to increase confusion and at times leads to greater connection of spirituality to religion. In the United Kingdom, the Royal College of Psychiatrists (2011) suggest that it may be more helpful to view the concept of spirituality as individual and more subjective and experiential. This allows for those who view transcendence as being an important aspect of spirituality and those that do not. Key though to the many questions and concerns patients express is the desire for connectedness which provides the human element of spirituality, as APNs we can offer this connection.

Hope, meaning and purpose are recurrent themes when defining spirituality (Reinert and Koenig 2013; Rogers and Wattis 2020). Murrey and Zentner (1989) suggest that the existential debate about life, connection to the universe and understanding of the infinite are often undertaken to understand and discover what brings hope, meaning and purpose. They suggest that these aspects come to the fore when a person is faced with stress, illness and terminal certainty. Helping patients connect to what gives them hope, meaning and purpose is often seen as a motivator when life becomes difficult (Cook 2011; National Center for Continuing Education 2021). Reinert and Koenig (2013) suggest that nearly all definitions of spirituality include elements of positive emotional states when talking about hope, meaning and purpose.

As spirituality is frequently linked to religion and empirical studies often use religious parameters to assess spirituality, it is useful to briefly discuss the concept of religion and some of the research surrounding religion and health.

1.5   Religion

Religion for many is a well-established construct based upon legal, political, societal, historical and sacred values. The Oxford English Dictionary (2021), para 1) gives the primary meaning of religion as "belief in a superhuman controlling power especially in a personal God or gods". This definition implies negativity and belittles the dynamic and individual meaning that can be found with religious belief and relationship to the sacred (however the individual defines this). It has been suggested that religion is a construct which is both individual and institutional (Hill and Pargament 2003). Religion may be viewed as the politics of spirituality and in the midst of current world issues it could be argued that atrocities in the name of religion have added to negativity around religion (Rausch 2015), even though personal belief may see many of these acts as misinterpretations of religious doctrine. Pesut et al. (2008, p. 2806) suggest that religion is a "narrow band construct concerned with institutionalised beliefs and rituals whilst spirituality is seen as a broad band experiential journey". This implication could lead to religion being viewed less positively than spirituality. Viewing religion in this way may be unfair as many with religious beliefs identify this as integral to their expression of spirituality (Kilpatrick et al. 2005). Others, though, seek differentiation as noted by Clarke (2006) and Hill and Pargament (2003) with spirituality often seen in more positive terms than religion. A differentiation between the two concepts may not be possible due to the many interpretations and definitions of religion which often reflect those of spirituality.

Clarke (2006) argues that reductive and functional definitions of religion may lead to increased negativity and are limiting. One of these reductive definitions recognised by Hill and Pargament (2003, p. 64) is the view that religion is a "fixed system of ideas of ideological commitments". They suggest that this view negates the deep spiritual expression that can transpire for those with religious belief. In the United Kingdom (UK), sociological factors have impacted the move away from widespread Christian beliefs. This includes the impact on how communities interacted, even as recently as the Victorian era, to the more individualised, driven, materialistic culture of today (Rohr 2003; James 2007). Many seem drawn to something which appears more universal and encompassing than religion but the decline in religious belief and expression may leave some floundering for meaning and purpose in their life (Rohr 2003). Others see religion as much more vibrant, flexible and expansive, for example religion could be seen as that which incites passion and interest and builds community. Rose describes religion as "the human quest to relate to an immaterial dimension of beatitude……" (Rose 2013, p. 12).

Historically, religion has been viewed as a community and societal practice where those without belief may be seen as heretical. In recent history, religion appears to have become a more individual practice and those in some countries with religious belief viewed as almost heretical or deluded (Dawkins 2006). Recent polls suggest the UK population is more aligned to secularism than Christianity, with 41% not aligned to any religion and only 27% believing in a god (You Gov 2021). Statistics in China identify 31.8% of the population align to no faith (Council for Foreign Relations 2021). In comparison 29% of those polled in the United States aligned themselves to no faith with three quarters identifying themselves as Christian (Gallup 2021). However, in Chile only 11.5% of the population align to no religion at all (Index Mundi 2021). Some of these cultural differences may partially explain why the synergy with religion that some writers make with spirituality is viewed from a religious perspective and other not. In a multicultural and increasingly secularised society, it may be helpful to view spirituality and religion as distinct concepts whilst acknowledging that for some religion may be a means of expressing their spirituality. Chapter 2 explores cultural aspects of spirituality further.

As APNs, recognising that faith in God or a higher power may be integral to someone's spirituality is important, as for some patients spirituality and religion may not be differentiated. Religion normally equates to a concept of God; however, this is viewed, whether as sacred and transcendent, or as part of self. It is equally important to recognise that one can be religious without being spiritual and vice versa and that some people may follow a religion purely for "social, political or cultural reasons without deriving much spiritual value from it" (Stevens Barnum 2011, p. 1).

French sociologist and philosopher Emile Durkheim postulated that "religion is a unified system of beliefs and practices relative to sacred things…..beliefs and practices which unite into one single moral community called a church and all who adhere to them" (Durkheim 1912, p. 44). The frequently quoted definition by Karl Marx proposes that "religion is the sigh of the oppressed creature, the heart of a heartless world and the soul of soulless conditions. It is the opium of the people" (Marx and Engels 2008, p. 255). This definition is often viewed negatively due to the parallel drawn between religion and opium. However, Marx can be regarded as at least partly sympathetic to religion by recognising the need for solace in an oppressed society (Cline 2021). A more comprehensive and balanced view of religion offered from sociology proposes that religion includes personal beliefs and actions, in addition to those of institutions. These beliefs and actions assume the existence of a supreme being (Bruce 2009). This definition is valid for most religions and assumes a moral purpose of belief in this being. What is clear is that in the midst of multicultural society a definition needs to firstly have meaning but more importantly be substantive and inclusive enough to warrant acceptance. Definitions may stem from a particular religious tradition emphasising a core belief for example in an eternal God or it may be functional describing the attributes associated with religion. Harrison (2006) suggests that, like spirituality, religion is impossible to define because of its varied meaning and potential to cause division and contention. She proposes that it might be simpler to describe religious tradition as this may be a more sensitive approach to the diversity of belief in a multicultural society.

McSherry et al. (2004) prompt us to remember that religious factors led to the historical heritage in nursing. There is a rich heritage in nursing passed down the generations from religious orders who founded the first hospitals. Traditionally spirituality was rooted in religious experience and relationship with God (Pesut et al. 2008) yet, in the struggle to make spirituality more secular some have stepped away from its religious roots. Florence Nightingale held deeply religious beliefs which guided her vocationally. She was the first nurse to advocate holistic care and suggested that spiritual needs are at the heart of nursing (O'Brien 2008: Young and Koopsen 2011). Nightingale (2009) reminds us that the spiritual needs of a patient are as vital to health as the bodily organs. Distancing spirituality from its historical roots for wider usage in a multicultural and secular society may be causing too much dilution.

Clarke (2006), in a literature review, found that religion is often seen as being about comfort and ritual, it includes expression of spirituality and it can be seen as a social activity. Some of the literature suggests a narrower and more restrictive view of religion compared to spirituality. Clarke suggests that these views are reductive and often defined without reference to expert sources such as theology, anthropology and sociology. Clarke (2006, p. 782) reminds us of the heritage of religion stemming from "spiritual longings of cultures" who have formed many practices to "talk about God, usher God into everyday life and prepare the ground for his entering". Clarke (2006) goes on to cite definition: "religion is the human enterprise by which a sacred cosmos is established......" which she suggests is more meaningful.

The need to present more inclusive and positive definitions of religion and spirituality is argued in view of changes in society and research identifying the positive impact (in the main) of religion and/or spirituality. Pesut et al. (2008), writing about spirituality and religion, has attempted this by focusing on what they view as a healthy outworking of religion. They describe this as being transcendent through acts of compassion, focusing on the suffering of others, by acting as an individual and society. Finally, Pesut et al. (2008) suggest that recognising commonality as humans whilst accepting difference is paramount within religion. This description of religion could be widely accepted.

1.6   Religion and Spirituality in Health Research

Religion and spirituality have been shown in research to positively impact people's perceived health and well-being. The impact of health and illness in connection to religion and spirituality has been widely researched. Koenig et al. (2011) undertook a comprehensive review of the international literature. From their extensive work, it is clear that religion, religious practices and beliefs have a significant influence on the aetiology of illness, the ability for a patient to heal and the ability of the patient to endure serious debilitating illness with a sense of hope and purpose. Out of the 1200 studies and 400 reviews they examined, the majority suggest a positive correlation between health, religion and spirituality despite many of the trials not setting out to show whether religion and spirituality affected health. Some showed a negative correlation between religion, spirituality and health but these were minimal when compared to the vast number showing positive correlations. Hill and Pargament (2003) also reviewed earlier studies into religion and spirituality with similar outcomes but identified that the reasons for these correlations are unclear. Many of these positive findings could only be indirectly linked to religion and spirituality. For instance, those with religious and spiritual beliefs might have healthier lifestyles (not smoking, not drinking, monogamous, etc.). They might have a tight community of friends from their place of worship supporting them leading to a greater sense of connectedness. They might positively rate mood in questionnaires as they believe not to do so might be seen as lacking faith. It is clear that some of the findings are anecdotal and tenuous when subjected to more rigorous study. However, the authors conclude there is enough strong empirical data to support the importance of religion and spirituality for many patients and its positive impact on illness and recovery. Koenig et al. (2011) concludes that patients with a religious belief remain generally healthier and more resilient to managing and living with health issues. Koenig et al.'s (2011) review mainly focused on religious belief and religious practice (largely Christianity) as being more measurable than spirituality. The concepts of religion and spirituality were viewed by the authors as largely interchangeable in this context.

It is difficult to measure spirituality. The studies reviewed by Koenig et al. (2011) show that many attempts to do so use religious practice as an indirect indicator of spirituality. Hill and Pargament (2003) suggest that attempting to use religious and spiritual indices misjudges the complexities of these concepts including the plethora of definitions and interpretations.

Empirical research to date has mainly examined religious practice and health outcomes; this is often located in the prevailing culture studied. Many have utilised measures to do so focusing on global indices for example religious affiliation, belief and practice (Hill and Pargament 2003). Attempts have also been made to measure spirituality directly using various rating scales. Monod et al. (2011) conducted a systematic review which identified 35 such scales. These were characterised as measuring general spirituality ($N = 22$), spiritual well-being ($N = 5$), spiritual coping ($N = 4$), and spiritual needs ($N = 4$). In healthcare research, the two measures most commonly used included FACIT-Sp (Peterman et al. 2002) and the Spiritual Well-Being Scale (SWBS) (Paloutzian and Ellison 1982). Both of these scales include subscales relating to religious and existential dimensions. For example, the SWBS has two subscales, one for religious well-being (RWB) and the other for existential well-being (EWB). This may have more value than focusing on religious affiliation, belief and practice alone (Hill and Pargament 2003). The scores when summated give the overall SWBS score which gives a general indicator of perceived well-being (including spiritual well-being and spiritual quality of life as well as relationship with God and life's purpose and satisfaction). The SWBS was developed in North America and reflects the researchers' perceptions of spirituality influenced by the predominant culture. It could be argued that the inclusion of the EWB improves applicability for those without a religious belief. Face validity is present for items which score in a positive direction in both subscales, for example "I believe that God loves me and cares about me" (RWB) and "I feel that life is a positive experience" (EWB). The RWB scale (which relates to God or a higher power rather than a specific set of religious beliefs) tends to have a ceiling effect in communities with strong religious beliefs. Moberg (2010, p. 107) criticised some of the scales used because they only gave a snapshot of information at a set time. He also suggested that statistical analysis "waters down complex feelings".

Spiritual measurement scales may be helpful for specific research in specific groups. However, these will always have limitations as they are dependent on how spirituality is understood by researchers and participants. At the practical level in healthcare, as Gordon et al. (2011) assert it is more important when considering spirituality and spiritual care to understand what it means to the person being cared for.

1.7   Rationale and Challenges for Spirituality

Despite the International Council of Nursing (ICN 2012) identifying that spirituality should be embedded into practice many nursing and advanced practice code of conducts do not clearly identify spirituality as a domain. For example, in the UK spirituality was previously embedded clearly in the Nursing and Midwifery Council (NMC) Code of Conduct (NMC 2010). They stated that holistic care "considers physical, social, economic, psychological, spiritual and other factors when assessing, planning and delivering care" (NMC 2010, p. 148). However, the most recent NMC code of conduct does not mention spirituality. The code of conduct now states that nurses should "make sure that people's physical, social and psychological needs are assessed and responded to" (NMC 2015, p. 5). At first glance this omits spirituality which could lead to some nurses viewing spirituality as unimportant or being more confused about the place of spirituality within nursing care. However, it could be argued that spirituality is integral to all aspects of care and flows through the bio-psycho-social-spiritual model to make it truly holistic. Several national nursing associations and boards do recognise that spirituality is an integral dimension of health and suggest that prejudicial attitudes to individuals spirituality need to be eliminated by nurses (Canadian Nurses Association 2014; Nursing and Midwifery Board of Australia 2008); however, like the UK most codes refer to holistic, culturally sensitive or person-centred care rather than spirituality. Not referring directly to spirituality and omitting spiritual care could be seen as negligent (Tanyi et al. 2009). Code of conducts should clearly articulate the importance of spiritualty to ensure this important domain is not omitted. However, this is not the only issue. Policymakers must also highlight the importance of spirituality to help nurses (and the wider healthcare team) understand and integrate spirituality into their practice.

The UK has made some inroads into supporting healthcare staff to consider spirituality through policy. Policymakers acknowledge that spirituality plays a significant role during illness and in the healing process (Department of Health 2008; National Health Service (NHS) Scotland 2009) and have published a resource for all health and social care staff in the UK entitled Spiritual Care Matters (NHS Scotland 2009). NHS Scotland (2009, p. 6) suggests that spiritual care is:

> "care which recognises and responds to the needs of the human spirit when faced with trauma, ill health or sadness and can include the need for meaning, for self-worth, to express oneself, for faith support, perhaps for rites or prayer or sacrament, or simply to be a sensitive listener. Spiritual care begins with encouraging human contact in compassionate relationship, and moves in whatever direction need requires."

This definition for spiritual care has recently been adopted across Europe by the Enhancing Nurses and Midwives Competence in Providing Spiritual Care through Innovative Education and Compassionate Care project (see Chap. 3).

Within this Spiritual Care Matters resource, spiritual care and compassionate care are seen as going hand in hand and are highlighted as integral to holistic care, alongside psychological, social and physical care. Nolan (2011) sees spiritual care and psychological care as sharing many of the same attributes and skill sets. He suggests that good spiritual care focuses on the soul which seems to connect with the essence of a person as described by Narayanasamy (2004). Compassion is integral to holistic care and can be viewed as an operational way of demonstrating care for a patient's suffering in all its manifestations. Compassionate approaches to care ensure the relationship between patient and clinician is based upon respect and dignity with an empathic stance maintained (Cummings and Bennett 2012). Working in this way allows opportunities to be aware of patients' holistic needs and not to focus purely upon the initial presenting problem.

1.8   Barriers to Integrating Spirituality

Evidence suggests that many nurses find discussing spiritual dimensions of care with patients, family members and fellow clinicians challenging. Potential barriers to embedding spirituality into practice include time constraints, lack of education and understanding of what spirituality is, lack of confidence, personal discomfort, not wanting to intrude on something seen as private, fear of proselytising and belief it is not the clinician's role (Stranahan 2001; Maddox 2001; Hubbell et al. 2006; McSherry and Jamieson 2013; Tanyi et al. 2009 Lewinson et al. 2015; DeKoninck et al. 2016).

A large survey of 4054 nurses' perceptions of spirituality and spiritual care discovered that although there is a struggle for many nurses to conceptualise spirituality (McSherry and Jamieson 2011) 92.6% of the nurses surveyed felt that spiritual care should be offered to patients. However, only 5.3% felt they could meet spiritual needs of patients all the time. Despite this 92.2% of the nurses identified that they could sometimes address spiritual needs. There was no information about how they would do this and lack of training in this area was highlighted as a barrier to operationalising spiritual care (McSherry and Jamieson 2013). The findings suggest that nurses need more education and specific guidance about spirituality and spiritual care, clarification about boundaries and help to pick up the clues that might indicate a spiritual need.

In light of the need for nurse education to integrate spirituality into the curriculum, a study of nurse educators found that whilst around 90% agreed or agreed strongly that spiritual values were relevant to their subject area and over half thought it was integral to teaching and learning, only 17% agreed it was actually integrated into their curricula (Prentis et al. 2014). It is important that educators embrace spirituality as part of holistic care and integral to the curriculum to support nurses and other healthcare clinicians to be able to understand and offer spiritual care. Ali et al. (2018) in an extensive literature review (1993–2017) of spirituality and education found that there are five major gaps in knowledge and practice in nurse education: lack of ontological integration; lack in phenomenological understanding; lack of support and environmental constraints; curriculum structure and unprepared faculty. Lewinson et al. (2018) echo these findings and identify that curricula should have a consistent approach to teaching spirituality to ensure nurses have the confidence and competence to integrate spirituality into their practice.

There is clearly a drive to integrate spirituality into practice with policymakers, clinicians and educators viewing this as important. The challenge is how we do this in a way which meets patients' needs. Being clear about what spirituality means can make addressing this subject with patients much easier. Including spirituality within the nursing and APN curricula is an important way of ensuring nurses have the opportunity to explore what spirituality is and how to address it in practice.

1.9 Spiritual Care in Practice

Many robust studies show that spirituality is fundamental for patients (Koenig 2004; Ellis and Campbell 2004; Burkhart 2008; D'Souza 2007) in helping them regain hope, meaning and purpose in the midst of illness. There is growing evidence to show that addressing spirituality improves comfort levels (emotionally and physically) and has a positive effect on patients' responses to illness and treatments (Koenig 2004). Thus failing to address these issues may be exposing patients to more suffering.

Spiritual care is how spirituality is operationalised in practice. Pfeiffer et al. (2014) propose that spiritual care is fundamentally compassionate care which is deeply respectful and needs intentional connection between nurses and patients. McSherry (2006, p. 917) suggests that "spiritual care permeates and integrates all aspects of care provision just as spirituality integrates and unites all dimensions of the individual". Nursing has engaged partly with the debate about how to provide care which is not just physical and emotional but also spiritual. Nevertheless, this may have been reduced to asking about whether a patient has a faith rather than what are their spiritual needs (Eagger 2011).

Agrimson and Toft (2008) and Young and Koopsen (2011) suggest that being in touch with our own spirituality is the first step to being able to provide spiritual care for others. This reflects Treloar's (2000) who states that the breadth and depth of the spiritual care offered reflects the APNs own spiritual maturity. In order to be a spiritually competent practitioner, it appears necessary to explore one's own spirituality. As you will read in the next chapter, spiritually competent practice may be an easier concept to understand compared to spiritual care as it integrates aspects of spiritual care, personal qualities and opportunities to develop therapeutic relationships within a supportive work environment.

Addressing spirituality with respect for patients' values and dignity is vital. An individualised, holistic approach emphasises that one of the main aspects of integrating spirituality into practice is to understand what spirituality means for the patient being cared for (Gordon et al. 2011). Some patients want to talk about spirituality with clinicians (Ellis et al. 2002; Ellis and Campbell 2004). Listening attentively to patient cues may lead naturally to discussions about spirituality (Ellis and Campbell 2004; Helming 2009). As APNs when we are open, accepting and compassionate patients may find it easier to open up to us about their deepest concerns. As APNs continue to strive to offer holistic care we need to be aware that when patients are faced with illness, pain, vulnerability and distress they often need us to address issues related to spirituality (Rogers and Wattis 2015). APNs are in the ideal place to listen to patients as they ask often deeply spiritual questions and invite us into their questioning. A number of spiritual assessment tools have been developed for practice including "FICA" (Puchalski and Romer 2000) and "HOPE" (Anandarajah and Hight 2001). However, in an individualised approach to spiritual care a formal tool is not necessarily the best way to approach the issue and may not be helpful in many APN consultations.

Leathard and Cook (2008) suggest spiritual care is about being with a patient and simply listening attentively to these cues, taking time and presencing. Listening has been shown to be a common feature of spiritual care (McSherry and Jamieson 2013; Pfeiffer et al. 2014). Simply allowing a patient to tell their own story and to listen empathetically with suitable prompts to give the patient an opportunity to discuss what illness means for them and to understand how it may be disrupting their sense of purpose in life may be the most important aspect of spiritual care. These fundamentals of nursing practice lead APNs towards spiritual care if they take time to recognise it as such.

To operationalise spirituality in practice, it is necessary for APNs to adopt a positive attitude. A key starting point is recognising that patients do want to talk about spirituality and that it is important in their recovery. Ellis and Campbell (2004) in a study of patients and spirituality found that patients will not begin to talk about their spiritual needs unless they felt honoured and respected. APNs therefore need to value patients and spend time building up a good rapport. If spirituality is not addressed, some patients believe that it will adversely impact the healing process. APNs who already integrate spirituality into their own practice appear to be those who are aware of their own spirituality and listen to patient cues (Treloar 2000; Stranahan 2001; Hubbell et al. 2006; Rogers 2017).

Spiritual care is fundamental to holistic practice. It includes the core skills of compassion, presencing, individual care, listening and respect. It is integrated in the way we as APNs interact with patients and it requires a level of maturity and recognition of the importance of spirituality to patients.

1.10 Ethical Issues in Operationalising Spiritual Care

The autonomous nature of the APN role makes ethical issues and appropriate boundaries particularly relevant when addressing spirituality. Fundamentally all practitioners work within a code of conduct and are accountable for their own practice. Integrating spirituality into practice is no different to any other area of healthcare and demands the same levels of professionalism. APNs should be aware of, and practice within, the International Council of Nurses Code of Ethics (ICN 2021).

Tacitly, a level of trust must be present in all patient consultations with the expectation that nurses are committed to, and work within, the code of conduct laid out by their professional bodies. It is important to practise in a way which is validating of the patient and non-judgmental, with the core aim of altruism rather than professional status.

Patients may ask directly about your personal beliefs. Even when initiated by the patient, there is a need to be prudent to share appropriately and not to proselytise. Personal beliefs should not be expressed to a patient in an inappropriate way (NMC 2015). Many patients draw comfort and support from their spirituality and some by shared religious values and beliefs.

Spirituality is an area where nurses appear to be concerned about crossing boundaries and ethical issues (McSherry and Jamieson 2013). Studies confirm concern about not imposing one's own values and relate to a fear of projecting one's own belief onto a patient which is seen as an abuse of the relationship (Ellis et al. 2002; Monroe et al. 2003; Ellis and Campbell 2004). There have been cases of nurses being suspended or sacked for crossing ethical boundaries for example offering to pray for a patient (BBC News 2021), in some countries this may have increased reticence to explore spirituality for fear of being accused of proselytising. Conversely, in the United States of America it is more common for APNs to offer prayer for their patients with consent (Taylor et al. 2014). These cultural differences need to be understood and navigated to ensure professional practice is always maintained. Cook (2011) suggests that, when discussing religious beliefs or spirituality, consent should be elicited from patients before entering into discussions. Patients should never be put under pressure to share their own beliefs and never be put under any pressure to adopt practitioners' beliefs.

In order to act in the best interests of patients in judging how much to say about spirituality, it is worth bearing in mind fundamental ethical principle of beneficence. Clarke (2013, p. 43) states that "being aware of the other person and recognising their worth and value"….is the basis of spiritual care. This she suggests is simply "being human…..built on the desire for the welfare of the other" (Clarke 2013, p. 43).

1.11 Conclusion

This chapter presents an introduction to the theoretical perspectives of spirituality in relation to healthcare. It engages with some of the contemporary discussions around how to define spirituality and why it is often conflated with religion. A brief overview of the research into religion and health has been presented in order to balance the argument regarding lack of empirical studies on spirituality. Consideration has been given to the rationale for spirituality in healthcare in addition to operationalising spirituality in practice. Despite the many challenges surrounding spirituality APNs should offer spiritual care as part of their holistic practice. For clarity spirituality is fundamentally human and connects with what gives us hope, meaning and purpose. Religion for some may connect to spirituality but it is also a separate construct which relates an organised set of belief(s).

References

Agrimson L, Toft L (2008) Spiritual crisis-a concept analysis. J Adv Nurs 65(2):454–461

Ali G, Snowden M, Wattis J, Rogers M (2018) Spirituality in nursing education: knowledge and practice gaps. Int J Multidiscipl Comparat Stud 5(1–3):27–49

Anandarajah G, Hight E (2001) Spirituality and medical practice- using the HOPE questions as a practical tool for spiritual assessment. Am Fam Physician 63(1):81–89

Baldacchino D (2006) Nursing competencies for spiritual care. J Clin Nurs 15:885–896

BBC News. (2021). Prayer row nurse remains defiant (online). http://news.bbc.co.uk/1/hi/england/somerset/7874892.stm. Accessed 7 Jan 2021

Beller J, Wagner A (2020) Loneliness and health: the moderating effect of cross-cultural individualism/collectivism. J Age Health. https://doi.org/10.1177/0898264320943336

Benner P, Wrubel J (1989) The primacy of caring: stress and coping in health and illness. Addison-Wesley, Massachusetts

Berger P (1969) A rumour of angels: modern society and the rediscovery of the supernatural. Doubleday, New York

Brown B (2010) The gifts of imperfection. Hazelden, Minnesota

Brown B (2012) Daring greatly- how the courage to be vulnerable transforms the way be live, love, parent and lead. Gotham, New York

Bruce S (2009) Defining religion: a practical approach. Int Rev Sociol 21(1):107–120

Burkhart M (2008) Spirituality and religiousness: differentiating the diagnoses through a review of the nursing literature. Nurs Diagn 12(2):45–54

Canadian Nurses Association (2014) Spiritualty, health and nursing practice- CNA position

Castillo F (2020) Health, spirituality and Covid-19: themes and insights. J Pub Health (Oxf) 43(2):e254–e255

Chrash M, Mulich B, Patton C (2011) The APN role in holistic assessment and integration of spiritual assessment for advanced care planning. J Am Acad Nurse Pract 23:530–536

Clarke J (2006) Religion and spirituality: a discussion paper about negativity, reductionism and differentiation in nursing texts. Int J Nurs Stud 43:775–785

Clarke J (2009) A critical view of how nursing has defined spirituality. J Clin Nurs 18:1666–1673

Clarke J (2013) Spiritual care in everyday nursing practice- a new approach. Palgrave, Hampshire

Cline A (2021) Karl Marx on religion- is religion the opiate of the masses. www.atheism.about.com. Accessed 11 Jan 2021

Cook C (2011) Recommendations for psychiatrists on spirituality and religion. Royal College of Psychiatrists, London

Cook C (2020) Spirituality, religion and mental health: exploring the boundaries. Ment Health Relig Cult 23(5):363–374. https://doi.org/10.1080/13674676.2020.1774525

Council of Foreign Relations (2021) Religions in China. https://www.cfr.org/backgrounder/religion-china. Accesses 16 Jan 2021

Coyle J (2002) Spirituality and health: towards a framework for exploring the relationship between spirituality and health. J Adv Nurs 37(6):589–597

Cummings J, Bennett V (2012) Compassion in practice: nursing, midwifery and care staff- our strategy. Department of Health, Leeds

D'Souza R (2007) The importance of spirituality in medicine and its application to clinical practice. Med J Aust 186(10):57–59

Dawkins R (2006) The god delusion. Bantam Press, London

DeKoninck B, Hawkins LA, Fyke JP, Neal T, Currier K (2016) Spiritual care practices of advanced practice nurses: a multinational study. J Nurse Pract 12(8):536–544

Department of Health (2008) High quality care for all NHS next stage review final report. DOH, London

Dockery D (ed) (2001) The challenges of postmodernism. Bridgepoint Books, Grand Rapids

Downey M (2004) Exploring the relationship between caring, love and intimacy in nursing. Br J Nurs 13(21):1289–1292

Durkheim E (1912) The elementary forms of religious life. Cited in Jones 1986 Emile Durkheim: an introduction to four major works. Sage, Beverly Hills

Eagger S (2011) The challenges of implementing spiritual care. Grasping the Nettle conference, London

Ellis M, Campbell J (2004) Patient's views about discussing spiritual issues with primary care physicians. South Med J 97(12):1158–1163

Ellis M, Campbell J, Detwiller-Breidenbach A, Hubbard D (2002) What do family physicians think about spirituality in clinical practice? J Fam Pract 51(3):249–254

Epstein RM (2014) Realizing Engel's biopsychosocial vision: resilience, compassion and quality of care. Int J Psychiatry Med 47(4):275–287

Ferrell B, Handzo G, Picchi T, Puchalski C, Rosa W (2020) The urgency of spiritual care: Covid 19 and the critical need for whole person palliation. J Pain Manag 60(3):e7–e11. https://doi.org/10.1016/j.jpainsymman.2020.06.034

Foley M (2010) The age of absurdity- why modern life makes it hard to be happy. Simon and Schuster, London

Gallup (2021) Religion considered important to 72% Americans. www.news.gallup.com/poll/245651/religion-considered-important-americans.aspx. Accessed 16 Jan 2021

Gardner F, Tan H, Rumbold B (2020) What spirituality means for patients and families in healthcare. J Relig Health 59(1):195–203

Gilbert P (2011) Spirituality and mental health: a handbook for service users, carers and staff wishing to bring a spiritual dimension to mental health services. Pavilion, Brighton

Gordon T, Kelly E, Mitchell D (2011) Spiritual care for health care practitioners- reflecting on clinical practice. Radcliffe, London

Harrison V (2006) The pragmatics of defining religion in a multi-cultural world. Int J Philos Relig 59:133–152

Helming MA (2009) Integrating spirituality into nurse practitioner practice: the importance of finding the time. J Nurse Pract 5(8):598–8

Hill P, Pargament K (2003) Advanced in the conceptualization and measurement of religion and spirituality. Am Psychol 58(1):64–74

Hinton J (1992) Discover your spirituality everyday spirituality. Hunt and Thorpe, Rydalmere

Hubbell S, Woodard E, Barksdale-Brown D, Parker J (2006) Spiritual care practices of nurse practitioners in federally designated nonmetropolitan areas of North Carolina. J Am Acad Nurse Pract 18(8):379–385

Index Mundi (2021) Chile religions-demographics. https://www.indexmundi.com/chile/religions.html. Accessed 16 Jan 21

International Council of Nurses (2012) The ICN code of ethics for nurses. ICN, Geneva

International Council of Nurses (2020) Guideline's on advanced practice nursing. ICN, Geneva

International Council of Nurses (2021) The ICN code of ethics for nurses. ICN, Geneva

James O (2007) Affluenza. Random House, London

Johnston D, Mayers CA (2004) Response. In Mayers CA (2004) letters page. Br J Occup Ther 67(6):282

Kilpatrick S, Weaver A, McCullouch M, Puchalski C, Larson D, Hays J, Farran C, Flannelly K (2005) A review of spiritual and religious measures in nursing journals: 1995–1999. J Relig Health 44(1):55–66

King U (2011) Can spirituality transform our world? J Study Spirit 1(1):17–34

Kliewer S, Saultz J (2006) Healthcare and spirituality. Radcliffe, Oxford

Koenig H (2004) Religion, spirituality and medicine: research- findings and implications for clinical practice. South Med J 97(12):1194–1200

Koenig H (2009) Research on religion, spirituality and mental health- a review. Can J Psychiatr 54(5):283–291

Koenig H (2011) Spirituality and health research: methods, measurements, statistics, and resources. Templeton Press, Radnor

Koenig H, McCullough ME, Larson DB (2011) Handbook of religion and health. Oxford University Press, Oxford

Kirk TW (2007) Beyond Empathy: Clinical Intimacy in Nursing Practice. Nurs Philos 8(4):233–243

Leathard H, Cook M (2008) Learning for holistic care- addressing practical wisdom (phronesis) and spiritual sphere. J Adv Nurs 65(6):1318–1327

Lewinson L, McSherry W, Kevern P (2015) Spirituality in pre-registration nurse education and practice: a review of the literature. Nurse Educ Today 35(6):806–814

Lewinson LP, McSherry W, Kevern P (2018) Enablement- spirituality engagement in pre-registration nurse education and practice- a grounded theory investigation. Religions 9(11):356–370

Maddox M (2001) Teaching spirituality to nurse practitioner students: the importance of the interconnection of mind, body and spirit. J Am Acad Nurse Pract 13(3):134–139

Marx K, Engels F (2008) On Religion. Dover Publications, Mineola

McSherry W (2006) Making sense of spirituality in nursing and healthcare practice- an integrative approach, 2nd edn. Jessica Kingsley Publishers, London

McSherry W, Jamieson S (2011) An online survey of nurses' perceptions of spirituality and spiritual care. J Clin Nurs 20(11):1757–1767

McSherry W, Jamieson S (2013) The qualitative findings from an online survey investigating nurses' perceptions of spirituality and spiritual care. J Clin Nurs 22(21–22):3170–3182

McSherry W, Cash K, Ross L (2004) Meaning of spirituality: implications for nursing practice. J Clin Nurs 13(8):934–941

McSherry W (2010) RCN Spirituality Survey 2010- A Report by the Royal College of Nursing on Members' Views on Spirituality and Spiritual Care in Nursing Practice. RCN, London

Mezey M, McGivem D, Sullivan-Marx E (2003) Nurse practitioners: evolution of advanced practice, 4th edn. Springer

Milligan S (2011) Addressing the spiritual care needs of people near end of life. Nurs Stand 26(4):47–56

Miner-Williams D (2005) Putting a puzzle together- making spirituality meaningful for nursing using an evolving theoretical framework. J Clin Nurs 15:811–821

Moberg D (2010) Spirituality research: measuring the immeasurable? Perspect Sci Christ Faith 62(2):99–114

Monod S, Brennan M, Rochat E, Martin E, Rochat S, Büla C (2011) Instruments measuring spirituality in clinical research: a systematic review. J Gen Intern Med 26(11):1345–1357

Monroe M, Bynum D, Susi B, Phifer N, Schultz L, Franco M, Maclean C, Cykert S, Garrett J (2003) Primary care physician preference regarding spiritual behaviour in medical practice. Arch Int Med 163:2751–2756

Murrey RB, Zentner JB (1989) Nursing concepts for health promotion. Prentice Hall, London

Narayanasamy A (2004) The puzzle of spirituality for nursing: a guide to practical assessment. Br J Nurs 13(19):1140–1144

Narayanasamy A (2006) The impact of empirical studies of spirituality and culture on nurse education. J Clin Nurs 15:840–851

National Center for Continuing Education (2021) Death and dying-a Christian approach. https://www.nursece.com/courses/9-death-dying-a-christian-approach. Accessed 4 Jan 2021

NHS Scotland (2009) Spiritual care matters. An introduction resource for all NHS staff. NHS Education for Scotland, Edinburgh

Nightingale F (2009) Notes of nursing- what it is and what it is not. Fall River Press, New York

Nolan S (2011) Psychosocial care: new content for old concepts- towards a new paradigm for non-religious spiritual care. J Study Spirit 1(1):50–64

Nouwen H (1972) The wounded healer. Doubleday, New York

Nursing and Midwifery Board of Australia (2008) Code of ethics for nurses in Australia. Nursing and Midwifery Board of Australia

Nursing and Midwifery Council (2010) Standards for pre-registration nursing education. NMC, London

Nursing Midwifery Council (2015) The code professional standards of practice and behaviour for nurses and midwives. NMC, London. http://www.nmc-uk.org/Documents/NMC-Publications/revised-new-NMC-Code.pdf. Accessed 10 Dec 2020

O'Brien M (2008) Spirituality in Nursing- Standing on Holy Ground. Jones and Bartlett, Sudbury

Oxford Dictionary (2021) Oxford dictionaries online. http://www.oxforddictionaries.com/definition/english/religion

Paloutzian R, Ellison C (1982) Loneliness, spiritual Well-being, and quality of life. In: Peplau L, Perlman D (eds) Loneliness: a sourcebook of current theory, research and therapy. Wiley, New York

Pesut B, Reimer-Kirkham S (2009) Situated clinical encounters in the negotiation of religious and spiritual plurality. A critical ethnography. Int J Nurs Stud 47(7):815–825

Pesut B, Fowler M, Taylor EJ, Reimer-Kirkham S, Sawatzky R (2008) Conceptualising spirituality and religion for healthcare. J Clin Nurs 17(21):2803–2810

Peterman A, Fitchett G, Brady M, Hernandez L, Cella D (2002) Measuring spiritual Well-being in people with cancer: the functional assessment of chronic illness therapy--spiritual Well-being scale (FACIT-Sp). Ann Behav Med 24(1):49–58

Pfeiffer J, Gober C, Johnson-Taylor E (2014) How christian nurses converse with patients about spirituality. J Clin Nurs 23:2886–2895

Prentis S, Rogers M, Wattis J, Jones J, Stephenson J (2014) Healthcare lecturers' perceptions of spirituality in education. Nurs Stand 29(3):44–52

Propper C, Stoye G, Zaranko B (2020) The wider impacts of coronavirus pandemic on the NHS. Institute of Fiscal Studies Briefing Note

Puchalski C (2001) The role of spirituality in healthcare. BUMC Proc 14:352–357

Puchalski C, Ferrell B (2011) Making health care whole- integrating spirituality into patient care. Templeton Press

Puchalski C, Romer A (2000) Taking a spiritual history allows clinicians to understand patients more fully. J Palliat Med 3(1):129–137

Rausch C (2015) Fundamentalism and terrorism. J Terror Res 6(2). https://cvir.st-andrews.ac.uk/articles/10.15664/jtr.1153/. Accessed 11 Jan 2021

Reinert K, Koenig H (2013) Re-examining definitions of spirituality in nursing research. J Adv Nurs 69(12):2622–2634

Rogers M (2016) Spiritual dimensions of advanced nurse practitioner consultations in primary care through the lens of availability and vulnerability. A hermeneutic enquiry. PhD, University of Huddersfield

Rogers M (2017) Utilising availability and vulnerability to operationalise spirituality. In: Practising spirituality. Palgrave Macmillan, London, p 145164

Rogers M, Wattis J (2015) Spirituality in nursing. Nurs Stand 29(39):51–57

Rogers M, Wattis J (2020) Understanding the role of spirituality in providing person-centred care. Nurs Stand. https://doi.org/10.7748/ns.2020.e11342

Rogers M, Hargreaves J, Wattis J (2020) Spiritual dimensions of nurse practitioner consultations in family practice. J Holist Nurs 38(1):8–18

Rohr R (2003) Simplicity- the freedom of letting go. Cross Roads Publishing, Wheaton

Rose K (2013) Pluralism: the future of religion. Bloomsbury, New York

Royal College Nursing (2008) RCN spiritual competencies advanced nurse practitioners- a RCN guide to the advanced nurse practitioner role, competencies and programme accreditation. http://www.knowledge.scot.nhs.uk/media/CLT/ResourceUploads/12252/003207.pdf. Accessed 12 Dec 2020

Royal College of Psychiatrists (2011) Recommendations for psychiatrists on spirituality and religion. Royal College of Psychiatrists, London

Saad M, Medeira R, Mosini A (2017) Are we ready for a true biopsychosocial-spiritual model? The many meanings of spiritual. Medicines 4(4):79. https://doi.org/10.3390/medicines4040079

Saunders M (2017) Clinical nurse specialists' perceptions of spiritual care: nurses need support, care falls short. J Christ Nurs 34(3):176–181

Selman L, Bighton L, Sinclair S, Karvinen I, Egan R, Speck P, Powell R, Deskur-Smielecka E, Glajchen M, Adler S, Puchalski C, Hunter J, Gikaara N, Hope J (2018) Patient and caregivers' needs, experiences, preferences and research priorities in spiritual care: a focus group across nine countries. Palliat Med 32(1):216–230. https://doi.org/10.1177/0269216317734954

Sessana L, Finnell D, Jezewski M (2007) Spirituality in nursing- a concept analysis. J Holist Nurs 25(4):252–262

Sessanna L, Finnell D, Underhill M, Chang Y, Peng H (2010) Measures assessing spirituality as more than religiosity- a methodological review of nursing and health related literature. J Adv Nurs 67(8):1677–1694

Shuler P, Davis J (1993) The Shuler nurse practitioner practice model: a theoretical model for nurse practitioner clinicians, educators and researchers. J Am Acad Nurse Pract 5:1–18

Stevens Barnum B (2011) Spirituality in Nursing: The Challenges of Complexity, Third Edition. Springer Publishing, New York

Stranahan S (2001) Spiritual perception, attitudes about spiritual care, and spiritual care practices among nurse practitioners. West J Nurs Res 23(1):90–104

Sulmasy DP (2002) A biopsychosocial-spiritual model for the care of patients at the end of life. The Gerontologist 42(suppl. 3):24–33

Swinton J (2006a) Identity and resistance- why spiritual care needs enemies. J Clin Nurs 15:918–928

Swinton J (2006b) Spirituality and mental health- rediscovering a forgotten dimension. Jessica Kingsley Publishers, London

Swinton J, Pattison S (2010) Moving beyond clarity: towards a thin, vague and useful understanding of spirituality in nursing care. Nurs Philos 11:226–237

Tacey D (2000) Re-enchantment: the new Australian spirituality, Harper Collins, Sydney- cited in Tacey D the rising interest in spirituality today. http://www.austheos.org.au/topics/tacey-website.html.htm. Accessed 22 Feb 2009

Tacey D (2004) The spirituality revolution: the emergence of contemporary spirituality. Brunner Routledge, Sussex

Tanyi R (2002) Towards clarification of the meaning of spirituality. J Adv Nurs 39(5):500–509

Tanyi R, McKenzie M, Chapek C (2009) How family practice physicians, nurse practitioners and physician assistants incorporate spiritual care in practice. J Am Acad Nurse Pract 21:690–697

Taylor EJ, Gober C, Pfeiffer JB (2014) Nurse religiosity and spiritual care. J Adv Nurs 70(11):2612–2621. https://doi.org/10.1111/jan.12446

Treloar L (2000) Integration of spirituality into health care practice by nurse practitioners. J Am Acad Nurse Pract 12(7):280–283

Vermandere M, De Lepeleire J, Smeets S, Hannes K, Van Mechelen W, Warmenhoven F, Van Rijswijk E, Aertgeerts B (2011) Spirituality in general practice: a qualitative evidence synthesis. Br J Gen Pract 13(162):749–760

Vincensi B (2019) Interconnections: spirituality, spiritual care and patient centered care. Asia Pac J Oncol Nurs 6(2):104–110. https://doi.org/10.4103/apjon_48_18

Watson J, Woodward T (2020) Jean Watson's theory of human caring. Sage

Wattis J, Curran S & Rogers M (2017) Spiritually competent practice in health care. CRC Press

White G (2006) Talking about spirituality in health care practice- a resource for the multi professional health care team. Jessica Kingsley, London

You Gov (2021) How religious are British people. www.you.gov.uk/topics/philosophy/articles/reports/2020/12/29/how-religous-are-british-people. Accessed 16 Jan 2021

Young C, Koopsen C (2011) Spirituality, health and healing- an integrated approach. Jones and Bartlett, Sudbury

Spirituality Competent Practice and Cultural Aspects of Spirituality

2

John Wattis, Melanie Rogers, Gulnar Ali, and Stephen Curran

Abstract

In this chapter we introduce the concept of spiritually competent practice as a way of avoiding disputes about the definition of spirituality and avoiding confusion with religion. Spiritually competent practice is described. It involves compassionate engagement, supporting people in sustaining a sense of meaning and purpose even when it is challenged by suffering and illness. It addresses the whole person as a unique individual, in the context of their family and cultural connections. As well as specific competencies it requires personal qualities, including the capacity to form *I-Thou* relationships and a managerial system that enables practitioners to attend to personal as well as technical aspects of healthcare. An ontological model for lifelong learning through reflective practice is presented. Availability and Vulnerability, a framework relating to personal qualities and specifically developed in research with APNs, is described and illuminated by a case study. This can also be understood within the overarching description of spiritually competent practice. We have looked briefly at how to take into account cultural issues without forgetting that individuals within a culture also have their own personal understanding of what spirituality means to them which is not necessarily congruent with their cultural background.

J. Wattis (✉) · M. Rogers
University of Huddersfield, Huddersfield, UK
e-mail: j.wattis@hud.ac.uk; m.rogers@hud.ac.uk

G. Ali
University of Exeter, Exeter, UK
e-mail: g.ali@exeter.ac.uk

S. Curran
University of Huddersfield, Huddersfield, UK

South West Yorkshire Partnership Foundation Trust, Wakefield, UK
e-mail: Steve.curran@swyt.nhs.uk

Keywords

Spirtually competent practice · Cultural competency · Compassionate engagement · Trans-cultural nursing care

2.1 Why Spiritually Competent Practice?

The first chapter explored the difficulties of defining (and measuring) spirituality. The different definitions and the overlap with religion have caused difficulties both for research and practice. Although religion is one way of experiencing and expressing spirituality, *spirituality* is not synonymous with religion (Richardson 2014; Wattis et al. 2017) especially in a multi-cultural, secular society. Because religious practice can be addressed in *quantitative* terms whereas spirituality is more subjective and harder to evaluate, religion is sometimes used as an imperfect surrogate for spirituality in research (Koenig et al. 2012). In practice too, entering a patient's religion on a form may be a substitute for addressing spiritual issues. We developed the concept of spiritually competent practice as a response to these issues. It embraces religious and non-religious manifestations of spirituality and emphasises the pivotal importance of the relationship between practitioner and patient and the practice environment, as well as specific competencies. It arose from an observational study by one of our occupational therapy colleagues (Jones 2016). She elucidated and described the behaviours that were characteristic of good practice in spiritual care. From her description members of our spirituality research group derived a description more generally applicable to all disciplines working in healthcare (Wattis et al. 2017). Subsequent research (Rogers et al. 2020) has caused us to modify the description and, in its latest iteration, we characterise it as follows:

> Spiritually Competent Practice involves compassionate engagement with the whole person as a unique human being in ways which will help them find and sustain their sense of meaning and purpose, where appropriate maintaining or restoring connection with family and community, addressing suffering and promoting wellbeing, this includes the practitioner accepting a person's beliefs and values, whether they are religious in foundation or not, and practising with cultural competency.

2.1.1 The Core: Helping People Sustain a Sense of Meaning and Purpose

When a group of healthcare educators were asked to provide personal definitions of spirituality, several themes emerged (Prentis et al. 2014). Firstly, an understanding of the self, person (or personhood) and being were central to our respondents' understanding spirituality in education and practice. Second, spirituality was that which gave a sense of direction, meaning and purpose to life. Finally, far from being 'other worldly', spirituality in healthcare was practical, affecting people's values and how they lived and acted in relation to others. Sensitivity to a person's sense of direction, meaning and purpose, their connection with other people (as well as the transcendent) and their beliefs and values are fundamental in spiritually competent practice. This is true, whether or not these are linked to religion. That is why, rather than arguing about a precise definition of spirituality, we preferred a brief description of how practitioners operationalise spiritual care in practice.

The importance of finding meaning in life was also at the core of Viktor Frankl's understanding of how people coped with the immense suffering in the concentration camps of the second world war (Frankl 2004). His observations led him to assert that finding meaning, through love, through dedication to a life's work or even through coping with unavoidable suffering was a fundamental part of human nature. All of these are relevant to spiritually competent practice. Compassionate engagement cannot happen without love. Many practitioners can and do find meaning in their work and we are often in contact with people who need to find meaning in unavoidable suffering.

2.1.2 Relationship: Compassionate Engagement with the Whole Person

This issue of compassionate engagement reflects the person-centred care movement, originating in various strands of twentieth-century thinking and practice. The philosophical roots of this can be found in the works of Martin Buber whose seminal work *Ich und Du* was first published in German in 1923 and translated into English as *I and Thou* by R.G. Smith in 1937 (Smith 2013). Buber described two 'basic words' *I-It*, through which we experience other people as objects and *I-Thou* through which we relate to them person-to-person. *I-It* described an attitude in which the other is an object to be understood analytically (corresponding to the neo-Kantian concept of rule-based *nomothetic*, knowledge) (Swinton 2012). Buber argued that we can (and often do) treat other people, as well as inanimate things, as objects; but when we truly *relate to them* as other *subjects*, then this is a person-to-person *I-Thou relationship* (equivalent to Swinton's subjective, experiential *idiographic* knowledge). Both *I-Thou* and *I-It* modalities are necessary in clinical practice. Abramovitch and Schwartz (1996) conceptualised this as a 'three stage dialogue' in which the opening phase is establishing the *I-Thou* relationship, the second stage involves various *I-It* analytical procedures (examination, tests, etc.) designed to identify or exclude specific disease entities and the final stage involves *I-Thou* integration through dialogue or 'healing through meeting'. This over-simplifies the process but reminds us that the both the *I-Thou* relationship and the *I-It* approach of analytical science have important parts to play in the healing encounter.

In the Francophone world Buber's ideas were taken up by Paul Tournier's *Medicine de la Personne* (Cox et al. 2007). Tournier was described by Frankl as the pioneer of person-centred psychotherapy (Pfeifer and Cox 2007). In the USA, Buber's ideas influenced Carl Rogers' development of the concept of client-centred therapy (Rogers 2003; Anderson and Cissna 1997). This developed into the widely applied person-centred approach (McCormack and McCance 2017). In the UK, Kitwood (1997) developed person-centred care in dementia and explicitly acknowledged his debt to Buber, commenting that the *I-It* mode implies 'coolness, detachment, instrumentality' whereas:

> "Daring to relate to another as Thou may involve anxiety or even suffering but Buber sees it as the path to fulfilment and joy" (Kitwood 1997, p. 10).

The Availability and Vulnerability framework which Melanie Rogers presents in this book clearly relates to the *I-Thou* concept, highlighting the importance of holistic person-centred care.

The World Health Organization also endorses a 'people-centred approach' (WHO 2015), the collective noun making room for a public health focus. In everyday practice, we prefer 'person-centred' over the terms 'people-centred', 'client-centred', 'consumer-centred' or even 'patient-centred' because 'person-centred' emphasises the whole person rather than casting them in a role as 'patient' or 'client' or 'consumer'. In England the policymakers who lead and direct the National Health Service (NHS) developed a new concept of 'personalised care' which focuses on the transactional aspects of care and seems to slightly miss the original point that person-centred care is focused on the quality of interpersonal relationship (NHS England 2020).

Person-centred care demands compassionate engagement. The deeper roots of this can be found in many religious traditions. The Hebrew bible uses the concept of *chesed* (חֶסֶד), commonly translated into English as steadfast love or loving kindness, the Greek new testament uses agapē (Ancient Greek ἀγάπη,) for a similar concept; Islam, Buddhism and several other religions have similar words (Templeton 1999). Humanists, too, see the idea of loving kindness (like mindfulness, often borrowed from Buddhist thinking) as foundational to a good life. Educators of health professionals, including nurses have pleaded for humanism (in the sense of human connection) and compassion to balance the technical and corporate aspects of healthcare (Nelson 1995; Gaufberg and Hodges 2016; Younas and Maddigan 2019).

Whole person or *holistic care* emphasises the importance of considering all aspects of the person when planning care: biological, psychological, social *and spiritual* (Sulmasy 2002; Rego and Nunes 2019). The old-fashioned biomedical model of care historically followed by medical colleagues (sometimes referred to simply as the 'medical model') focused on technical issues of diagnosis and treatment. The biopsychosocial model was proposed many years ago as an alternative to the biomedical model, initially in psychiatry, and soon extended to cover the whole of medicine (Engel 1977, 1980, 1992). Borrell-Carrió et al. (2004) reviewed 25 years of the biopsychosocial model and stressed the importance of relationship factors in its realisation. Nurses have often been seen to adopt holistic approaches to care which treat people as complete physical, mental and spiritual persons in a social context (McCormack and McCance 2017; Sulmasy 2002). However, with the continuing emphasis on technology in healthcare, this has sometimes been neglected (Wattis et al. 2017).

2.1.3   Context: Maintaining or Restoring Connection with Family and Community

This part of spiritually competent practice is another aspect of holistic care, important for all but especially important when caring for children, for those with long-term health problems, for those receiving mental healthcare and for those in critical care or end-of-life care. Healthcare problems may disrupt relationships with family and friends so practitioners need to ensure contact is maintained where appropriate. This can be especially important in mental healthcare where family breakdown is common. Further, in some cases of alcohol or drug abuse re-connecting with a community where abuse is common may need to be discouraged and connection with a new community (such as Alcoholics Anonymous) may be better. In some mental health problems, a person's beliefs may be delusional and a sign of illness impacting how a practitioner manages them. Finally, though research shows that in most cases religious practice is helpful to mental health (Koenig et al. 2012), occasionally religious communities may have a negative effect on mental health.

In healthcare for children, the importance of family contact has long been recognised, especially when children are admitted to hospital, though there are issues about its implementation (Shields 2010). In critical care and palliative care (Richardson 2014), maintaining connection between patients and their friends and relatives is seen as an important part of spiritual care. This has been emphasised during the coronavirus pandemic when patients in intensive and critical care have not always been able to have visitors but clinicians, especially nurses, have found ways of maintaining the contacts in difficult circumstances. Beyond any current problems we are helping people through, life will flow on and we need to help maintain links between seriously ill people and their family and friends. If the person survives, this will help them smoothly restore their relational context, in due course. But some of the most important consequences are for friends and relatives of those who die, if they can be assured that their loved one did not die alone and comfortless.

2.1.4   Purpose: Addressing Suffering and Promoting Wellbeing

Suffering can be physical, emotional and/or spiritual. Physical and emotional suffering must be addressed in any holistic approach to care; but it is easy to neglect *spiritual suffering*. This can best be understood by the existential questions people ask (and answers they give themselves) when going through ill health (Wattis et al. 2017). Patients newly diagnosed with cancer may ask themselves 'why me?' or 'why now?' The relatives of people who die unexpectedly in an accident may ask 'why did it happen to them/us?' Family carers for people with serious chronic illnesses may seek meaning for themselves and their loved ones in coping with the problems it brings. Essentially, these 'what's it all about?' questions are about the meaning of an illness or death for the people concerned. People need space to ask these questions and support in finding their own answers. Practitioners who relate to people in an *I-Thou* way can help provide that space by being present, engaged and attentive. As far as possible we need to support people in finding answers that help them to resolve their spiritual distress in a way that helps them move forward positively. This is one way of promoting wellbeing.

2.1.5   Respect: For the Person's Beliefs and Values

Provided they are not pathological, respecting a person's individual beliefs, values and culture are essential in any helping relationship and flow naturally from embracing their status as a person. This respect demands that we are self-aware about our own beliefs and values and aware that the person we are dealing with may be different from us in their way of responding to ill health. This, of course, includes cultural sensitivity and competency which are explored later in this chapter (and throughout much of this book).

2.2   What Is Needed for Spiritually Competent Practice?

Spiritual Care Competencies and Nursing Care
The conditions for spiritually competent practice are threefold. People need to learn *spiritual care competencies* relevant to their area of practice. They need to develop and sustain *personal (ontological) qualities* relevant to their vocation (sometimes known as 'professional formation'; Carlin et al. 2012) such as compassionate motivation. Finally, they need a working environment that it is organised in such a way as to provide *opportunities* for good practice. These three conditions are interdependent and interrelated. For example, when a person is learning to work in a new field their competencies may be gradually developing; but if they have the requisite personal qualities their practice may already exhibit a degree of spiritual competency. However, even a person with well-developed competencies and personal qualities will find it hard to provide spiritually competent care in an environment which does not allow time for developing compassionate engagement with the patient. Sometimes this is difficult to avoid if a practitioner is called away to an emergency when a patient is in the middle of sharing their spiritual needs; but even in this sort of situation a spiritually competent practitioner may be able to find ways of compensating, perhaps by apologising when they are called away and promising and remembering to return to the conversation later. An 'industrialised' task-oriented

approach to nursing, seen by some politicians and managers as a way of increasing productivity, makes it much harder to deliver truly competent care. The 'Tyranny of Metrics' (Muller 2018; especially Chap. 9) with a centralised style of management focused on performance targets can add to this problem. Managers, too, need spiritual competencies and a person-centred approach to *their* work. For a fuller discussion of management and political issues, see Wattis et al. (2021).

2.2.1 Spiritual Care Competencies

Spiritual care competencies have been developed in Europe for undergraduate nurse training (Enhancing Nurses' Competence in Providing Spiritual Care through Innovative Education and Compassionate Care (EPICC), (McSherry et al. 2020). Briefly, competencies include reflective practice and focus on self-awareness, skills in connecting with and addressing spiritual issues with patients and skills in developing a practice environment that enables these skills to be exercised and emphasised in specific areas like critical care. In palliative care in the United Kingdom, specific competencies have been developed on a multidisciplinary basis (Marie Curie Cancer Care 2004). Spiritual care competencies in the context of Advanced Practice Nursing are discussed in Chap. 3 of this book. The important thing to note here is that *spiritual care competencies* are best expressed within the context of person-centred practice and compassionate, trusting, open relationships that demand personal qualities in the nurse to enable compassionate engagement.

2.2.2 Personal (Ontological) Qualities

This refers to who (or what kind of person) we are, rather than what skills or knowledge we possess. The ability to be truly present with a patient, the moment we meet them and throughout a consultation, demands qualities of self-awareness and self-discipline. *Compassionate engagement* flows from a well-developed capacity to connect with the other person through person-centred, *I-Thou* relationships.

Rogers' (2016) Availability and Vulnerability framework for developing this capacity is discussed in detail in Chap. 5 and throughout the chapters from different countries. Here we offer an additional model, based on the philosophy of humanistic psychology to complement the necessary personal qualities needed by healthcare professionals to offer spiritually competent practice. The core of this is *Self-exploration* that focuses on *Ontological, Phenomenological, Humanistic, Ideological and Existential questions* (SOPHIE Fig. 2.1) (Ali 2017; Ali and Snowden 2019; Ali and Lalani 2020). This is a way of developing a mature authentic presence which enables a person-to-person (*I-Thou*) engagement that embraces ethical values. The focus of SOPHIE is on developing the personal qualities that

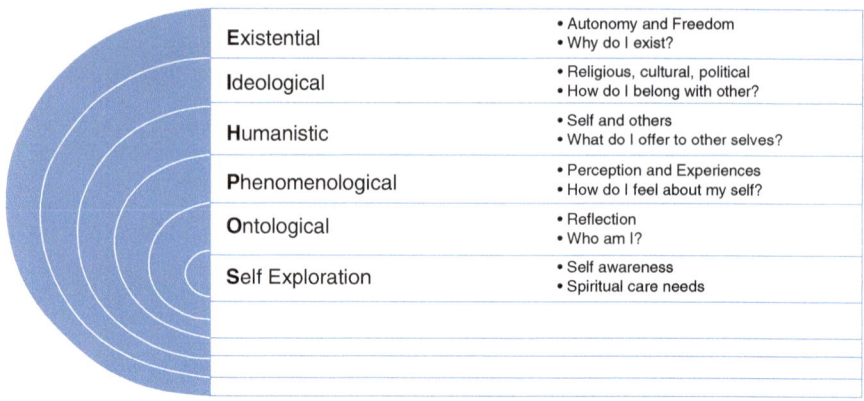

Existential	• Autonomy and Freedom • Why do I exist?
Ideological	• Religious, cultural, political • How do I belong with other?
Humanistic	• Self and others • What do I offer to other selves?
Phenomenological	• Perception and Experiences • How do I feel about my self?
Ontological	• Reflection • Who am I?
Self Exploration	• Self awareness • Spiritual care needs

Fig. 2.1 SOPHIE—Self-exploration through Ontological, Phenomenological, and Humanistic, Ideological, and Existential expressions (Ali 2017)

enable a practitioner to function autonomously to develop and maintain self-efficacy and empowerment (Schneewind 1998; Dworkin 1988).

Self-exploration = I vs Me

Starting from the basic premise that there is a need for continuing *Self-exploration* and reflexivity this model provides a series of questions that can assist in this task to enable congruency, transformation and leadership in trans-cultural nursing practices.

Ontological Aspect: Who am I?

At the *Ontological* level, the questions surround the issues of *who I am* and specifically, in this context: 'Who am I as an Advanced Practice Nurse (APN)?' 'Do I really embrace the nursing values and practise wisdom as my professional conduct?' These questions can be addressed in personal reflection and supervision or professional peer-group discussions to establish professional authenticity and self-determination.

Phenomenological aspect: How am I?

At the *Phenomenological* level of experience and consciousness, the question might be 'How am I (engaging in this situation)?' In the context of clinical work, this might be: 'Am I engaging in *I-Thou* relating with the person or am I just seeing the problems the patient brings'? Or even 'Am I just seeing the patient as a problem?' (*I-It*). We can think of similar questions about how we relate to our colleagues to become aware of our underlying fears, doubts and motivations that could influence our care giving practices.

Humanistic aspect: What can I offer to others?

At the *Humanistic* level, the question might be: 'What do I, as an APN, have to offer to the person I am with right now?' That might be someone who has come to me with a clinical problem or it might be a colleague at work. Reflecting: 'How I can connect with the patient or colleague practising compassionate presence and availability for a therapeutic interaction'.

Ideological aspects: How do I belong to others?

The *Ideological* level asks us to consider *how* we relate to others who may come from a different religious, social, cultural or linguistic background. 'What are the transcultural beliefs or dilemmas, that are required to be acknowledged and addressed during each clinical encounter, to assure equity and fairness'.

Existential Aspect: Why do I exist? What is the meaning of my life?

Finally, at the *Existential* level, we return to questions of meaning for ourselves and others with questions like 'What is the meaning of this experience (for me, for others)?' 'What is the meaning of (my) life and my role as a care provider?', 'Am I honest and genuine in performing my duty of care?', 'What does care means to me?', 'Is it all about task-based interventions'? 'Is it all about symptomatic care?'

This model can be used as a professional developmental tool, as we pause on our journey through a busy clinical life, to ask some basic questions of ourselves. It also can be used educationally coupled with creative ways of teaching appropriate to personal development (Prentis et al. 2014; Ali and Lalani 2020).

2.2.3 Opportunities in the Working Environment

As we have highlighted, the best possible person-centred care can only take place in the context of person-centred management. Management that focuses on tasks rather than people or that denies practitioners opportunity to develop spiritually sensitive relationships with patients or focuses too much on 'targets' and 'performance' indicators is inimical to spiritually competent practice (Muller 2018; Rogers et al. 2020). Even when higher and middle management focus on these approaches, clinical teams often (but not always) provide an environment in which spiritually competent care can flourish; but it is so much better when management recognises the need for person-centred care. Some factors which obstruct or facilitate spiritually competent practice are summarised in Table 2.1.

Table 2.1 Obstructions to and facilitators of spiritually competent practice (Wattis et al. 2019)

Obstructions to spiritually competent practice	Facilitators of spiritually competent practice
Fragmented patterns of working	Good team-working
Time and caseload pressures	Good leadership and supervision/self-care
Bad management systems and cultures	Good management systems

2.2.4   Case Study of Spiritually Competent Practice by an Advanced Practice Nurse

Rogers (2016) research-based Availability and Vulnerability framework for APNs is explained in-depth in Chap. 5. The synergistic relationship between availability and vulnerability is a powerful vehicle for building authentic relationships (Rogers and Beres 2017). Availability relates to simply being present to those in our care, offering care and concern and ensuring we give patients a safe place to be heard and valued. It also encourages the APN to reflect on their own practice and values where the questions suggested by the SOPHIE model may be useful. Vulnerability is often seen negatively in terms of being hurt, in this concept it is a positive attribute which includes being accountable and open to uncertainty, being willing to advocate for those in our care and fundamentally being authentic and honest with our patients, treating them as fellow human beings (see ongoing chapters for more detail).

This anonymised case study is based on the work of a Nurse Practitioner (NP) in primary care in the UK but all identifiable details have been changed. It relates to consultations which took place during the 2020 coronavirus pandemic.

Lydia is a 49-year-old lawyer working for a firm which offers subsidised services to those who are deprived or marginalised. She has been a lawyer for over 25 years and started working in her current practice 10 years ago as she disliked the corporate, money-driven ethos of her previous firm. The consequences of the pandemic were making her workload unmanageable.

She first consulted the NP by phone because the pandemic had severely restricted face-to-face consultations. Lydia had needed to wait for several weeks to get an appointment to talk to the NP. Consultations were still scheduled for 10 min per patient. The NP introduced herself and welcomed Lydia to the call, asking simply 'how can I help' rather than bombarding her with multiple questions. This connects to the availability part of the framework offering a welcome to the patient, giving time and 'space' and being present and listening not just to the words but to the emotional tone and to what was not said.

Lydia told the NP that she had been feeling very tired recently; she was not sleeping and she was feeling anxious most of the day. She explained a little about her working life and about the guilt she felt for letting her clients down during the coronavirus 'lockdown'. Restrictions meant she had to work from home and could not see any of her clients face to face. She still had to meet tight deadlines in her legal work. Several colleagues had already gone off sick or were self-isolating and Lydia was overwhelmed with work.

The NP listened for several minutes and showed her care and concern to Lydia by acknowledging the stress she was under and reassuring her that she was not alone and that the NP wanted to support her through this difficult time. The NP also took the opportunity of trying to build an *I-Thou* relationship which treated Lydia as a fellow human struggling to deal with the demands she was facing.

This necessitated the NP being vulnerable by acknowledging that she also recognised the stress of not being able to see her patients face to face. She apologised to Lydia that this had to be a telephone consultation because face-to-face appointments were no longer available. She also acknowledged that work pressures meant that she had had to wait so long to talk to a clinician and had been left to struggle alone for longer than the NP would have liked. Being honest and open with patients can build rapport and shows patients that they are valued for who they are.

The consultation progressed with some general questions about Lydia's mood and also about her symptoms. The NP recognised the limitations of a phone consultation and made the decision not to overwhelm Lydia on their first consultation with detailed mental health assessments. However, she did tell Lydia that she would like to know more about her mood and offered to send her some questionnaires via email for her to fill out and send back before the next consultation. She also suggested that Lydia had some blood tests at the local phlebotomy service which was still offering face-to-face appointments.

As the NP ended the consultation she took some time to reflect, she felt frustrated that this was a short consultation and that some aspects of her assessment had to be conducted virtually, she thought that she could recognise a loss of hope in some of Lydia's responses. Although she had assessed her for suicidal ideation as part of her brief mental health assessment, she felt she hadn't had the time to try and look at what gives Lydia hope, meaning and purpose. She knew, though, that they had a longer consultation booked a week later.

As with some patients Lydia's consultation stayed with the NP who was very aware of the mental health impact the pandemic was having on her patients and the community as a whole. Mental health problems were common in her clinics but now almost all her patients spoke of the mental health impact self-isolation and lockdown were having on their lives. Part of being available as an APN is being aware of the needs of the community and adapting practice to any changes. This NP had taken time with her colleagues to develop support information which was texted to patients or posted out. Although a small action, it was an important one which patients were grateful for.

The following week the NP reviewed Lydia's blood test results and the mental health assessments. It was clear that she had symptoms of a moderately severe depression with anxiety. However, the NP was more concerned at that moment by severely deranged liver function tests. She met with Lydia again by telephone and asked her how she had been in the last week. Lydia said that she was increasingly tired, she had generalised muscle aches and sometimes struggled to stand up. She felt very weak and was struggling to get through the day. The NP gently but openly asked Lydia if she could tell her if she was using any alcohol or drugs to get her through the day, this was asked without judgement. Lydia started to cry and said she was drinking two bottles of wine every day just to cope with her feelings and her exhaustion. She said she was ashamed and felt a failure. The NP supported her to talk more and reassured her that many people drank alcohol to reduce stress and that she would support her to look at other ways of dealing with her stress. However, it was vital to address the deranged blood results urgently. Lydia was shocked when the NP said she needed to admit Lydia immediately to hospital. She explained why and again told Lydia that she would support her on discharge from the hospital.

The NP had a consultation with Lydia 10 days later. Lydia thanked her profusely for admitting her as she collapsed shortly after admission and was told she might have died if she had not been admitted for urgent treatment. She had been in hospital for 9 days, had gone through detoxification and had received treatment for acute liver failure. She had been home for 1 day. The NP felt overwhelming empathy and care for Lydia as she realised how much stress she must have been under and how alone she had been feeling. She also reflected on how ashamed Lydia had felt. The NP took time to reassure Lydia that they would work together to address her stresses and treat her depression and anxiety alongside the care she was to receive for her alcohol problem.

Over the next few months Lydia opened up to the NP. She said for the first time in a long time she felt able to be open and honest about her own feelings because the NP had provided her a safe place where she felt understood and listened to without judgement. The NP asked open questions during these consultations and was able to explore what had brought Lydia hope, meaning and purpose in the past. It was clear her work was a vocation; but the demands had become overwhelming. She also had struggled in lockdown as she had become more isolated from friends and family. The NP helped her explore using technology to meet those she felt isolated from. Together they addressed her overworking and the demands placed upon her. Lydia, with support, began to address her stressors in a healthier way and reduced her working hours. She also began to be honest about her feelings with friends and found they too felt similar during lockdown. At the time of writing her depression has improved and she has stopped drinking.

In some ways there is nothing unusual about this case study. However, when you look closely you can see how the NP utilised availability and vulnerability throughout the consultations to help Lydia reconnect with her vocation, her friends and family and mostly her meaning and purpose in life. Spiritually competent practice was at the forefront of the NPs approach despite the difficulties with remote consultations.

2.3 Cultural Aspects of Spirituality and Spiritually Competent Practice

2.3.1 Cultural Narratives and Worldviews

APNs work in multicultural societies. In the West the dominant culture is often secular materialism and many people will follow the dominant culture which favours personal autonomy and consumerism. However, many will not adopt the dominant culture and its values for religious, personal or family reasons. Whatever kind of society APNs work in, they need to be aware of cultural factors and how they impinge on people's spirituality, in addition to understanding how their own world views are shaped by the culture they have been brought up in. One way of understanding different cultures is through understanding the (often unconscious) narratives that people use to understand themselves and their place in society. These underpin worldviews which form the substrate of a given culture or society and have to do with matters of ultimate concern. Worldviews have been likened to tinted eyeglasses, habitually worn, that colour the way we see the world without us necessarily being conscious that this is happening. The worldview of people in a traditional monocultural society will be shared by many in the society. However, in multicultural societies the situation will be more complicated. Wright (1992) suggests that worldviews have four components:

- Assumptions about how the world is, expressed through narratives (stories).
- Answers to fundamental questions about existence:
  - who are we?
  - where are we?

- – what is wrong?
- – what is the way to move forward?
- Symbolic expressions through events and artefacts.
- A way of being and behaving derived from the worldview, its associated narratives, questions and symbols.

Today, Monbiot (2017, p. 15) asserts 'the dominant narrative is that of market fundamentalism, widely known in Europe as neoliberalism'. In this worldview, the market is king and is believed to be able to resolve almost all problems in life. The narrative believes the state should be small and interfere with market forces, through regulation and taxation, as little as possible. In answer to the question about *who we are*, the narrative has been that we are autonomous individuals, driven by self-interest and that economic growth is determined as we all compete for our 'share' (or more than our 'share') of the many consumer goods on offer. Relationships are often contractual and people may be treated as commodities whereas APN relationships are based on an ethical commitment and are more covenantal and personal in nature. As to *where we are*—until recently the narrative has been one of confident progress as we make and consume more stuff. Interestingly this reflects the last great period of capitalism in the late Victorian age that was mitigated in the mid-twentieth century by a brief flowering of social democracy. When we get to the question of *what is wrong*, until recently, the neoliberal answer has been 'too much state interference' and so public services have been privatised, public spending and taxes cut and some regulation on industries reduced. The *way to move forward* has been 'more of the same'. The events and artefacts that symbolise this culture include shopping malls, Wall Street, New York; the City of London and an obsession with financial indices like the *Dow-Jones* and the *FTSE*. The *way of being* involves competing in a consumer society and a tendency to treat other people in an *I-It* rather than *an I-Thou* fashion.

Following the 2008 global financial 'crash', the emergence of Covid-19 as a global threat and the looming threat of global climate catastrophe (and many other less immediate problems) this narrative is increasingly questioned (Dyke 2020). Monbiot (2016) refers to it as 'the ideology at the root of all our problems'.

The symbolic events and artefacts of the middle ages in the UK would have been religious festivals, churches and cathedrals. Now January sales, 'black Friday', shopping malls and the towering headquarters of big banks fill the same place. Even Christmas has largely been converted from a religious festival to an orgy of consumerism. Whereas the dominant narratives in Western society in the middle ages would have been based on (Christian) religion, secular neoliberalism is the new normal and religious worldviews are more diverse. Secular neoliberalism has increasingly dominated the political world over the last 50 years or so. But its dominance has been at a largely unconscious level so that, even as we write in the middle of a coronavirus-induced crisis, people are still looking forward to a return to 'normal' when scientific evidence suggests that we would be wiser to aim for a less consumer-oriented recovery. The other problem with neoliberalism as a dominant worldview is that it does not have an intrinsic morality. It needs a morality derived from religion or philosophy to *really* answer the question 'what is wrong?'

However, within the current dominant culture of Western society there are many other groups with different worldviews, chiefly adherents of different religions and/ or members of minority ethnic groups. In the 2011 census of England and Wales

(Office of National Statistics 2011), nearly 60% people classed themselves as 'Christian' and just over a quarter classed themselves as having no religion. Islam at nearly 5% came next, followed by Hinduism, Sikhism, Judaism and Buddhism, smaller but still culturally significant minorities. Even within these broad groupings there are differences in worldview. For example, only a small proportion of those identifying as Christian would be active members of churches and nominal Christians might have an underlying worldview more consonant with secular materialism and neoliberalism. Within religious groupings there will be difference in the emphasis placed on beliefs and ritual behaviours. However, at their root (as discussed above) nearly all have an emphasis on steadfast love expressed through compassion and kindness towards other people. As murdered UK Member of Parliament Jo Cox famously stated (and many of us believe) 'We have more in common than divides us' (British Broadcasting Corporation 2016).

There are broad divisions between European-based cultures, with their emphasis on personal autonomy and individualism, and Eastern and African cultures which still often have a stronger feeling of family or collective responsibility and interdependence. These can affect how people experience illness, disability and ageing. There is a potential for cultural and even ethical conflict when practitioners from an individualistic culture are managing people from a more collective culture and vice versa (Kirschbaum and Rodriguez 2017). During the earlier phases of the coronavirus pandemic the different responses of countries like Japan and South Korea on the one hand, and European-based cultures on the other, may have been based not only on previous experience with the SARS virus but also on these differences in underlying culture. The 'Eastern' cultures quickly took a collective approach to the problem, visible in the normality of wearing face masks to protect others in public places, whereas in the UK, for example, there was an initial reluctance to introduce such measures because of fears about constraining individual autonomy and freedom.

Worldviews are not formed by one single belief, value or view. APN's need to recognise how their own worldview, in addition to nursing worldviews can support or hinder their everyday practice. Maintaining a worldview which connects with the caring and ethical principles of nursing help APNs be clear about what is right or wrong, who they are accountable to, how to care and how to respond to given circumstances. APNs own cultural heritage will have a significant impact on their own worldview and provides the ontological and epistemological foundation that determines their own belief systems. How APNs respond to those in their care with differing worldviews is addressed through cultural competence.

2.3.2 Cultural Competence

Sharifi et al. (2019) conducted a concept analysis of cultural competence in nursing. They briefly defined it as 'the dynamic and evolutionary process of acquiring the ability to provide effective, safe and quality care to individuals from different cultures along with considering the different aspects of their cultures' (Sharifi et al. 2019, pp. 3–4). They found six defining attributes:

1. Cultural awareness
2. Cultural knowledge
3. Cultural sensitivity
4. Cultural skill
5. Cultural proficiency
6. Dynamicity

Cultural awareness means firstly being aware of our own world view or 'cultural spectacles'. We need to understand our own culture which we have probably accepted as 'normal' as we have grown up in our own family and culture (though many challenge family culture in their teenage years). We need to be aware of how this worldview affects our understanding, beliefs and behaviours. Reflection upon our own culture and background is an important part of being able to be aware of other people's culture. This enables understanding of the similarities and differences between our own culture and other cultures and is the basis on which we can learn to recognise and respect these differences.

Cultural knowledge involves continually learning about other people's cultures when we come into contact with them. It means understanding their worldviews and particularly how they affect health-related beliefs and practices. This enables us to better understand and respect how people from a different culture think and behave in relation to illness and health needs. For example, some cultures do not accept a woman receiving healthcare from a male doctor, nurse or midwife. Specific religious cultures may have specific dietary practices which need to be understood and accommodated. Continuing learning is important because we may come across issues we had not anticipated and we need to be sensitive to unexpected reactions from the people we are caring for and their relatives and to seek to understand what is behind these reactions. We also need to recognise that we need to take advice from others when we are uncertain of cultural issues.

Cultural sensitivity is based on the knowledge and respect we have for different cultures. We also need to pay attention to cultural issues and not to make assumptions or unwarranted generalisations about people from different cultures. A culture that appears homogenous from our point of view may in fact be quite diverse to those who know it better (see *ecological fallacy* below). An important aspect of this is listening and clarifying issues in an *I-Thou relationship* with the person we are dealing with. Sometimes there may be language problems and an interpreter may be required and sometimes the interpreter can help interpret the cultural issues as well as the language. Once the cultural issues are understood, any healthcare plans need, as far as possible, to take them into account.

Cultural skill is about effective two-way communication with people from different cultures. People need to realise their concerns are heard, acknowledged and dealt with. Cultural skill enables us to effectively work with people of a different culture, respecting different beliefs, values and customs in partnering with them to provide acceptable healthcare.

Cultural proficiency is developed through the acquisition and transfer of new knowledge about culturally sensitive approaches. This is both an individual *learning from experience* process and a collective *learning from others* through well-conducted and communicated research in this area.

Dynamicity stresses that cultural competence is a lifelong learning experience.

We would add that just as spiritually competent practice requires us to be aware of our own limitations and to seek help when we encounter spiritual issues that we cannot fully understand, so cultural competence requires us to seek help when we are out of our depth. In Western cultures, this usually means seeking help, with the patient's agreement from family members or others from the same cultural or religious background. Always the understanding should proceed from a person-to-person compassionate engagement with the service user.

2.3.3   A Word of Caution (the Ecological Fallacy)

The application of *cultural competence* to nursing encounters with individual patients has been challenged. Dreher and MacNaughton (2002, p. 181) asserted that:

> Although individuals may belong to the same cultural group, the assumption that they are, in fact, the same is an ecologic fallacy

An ecologic/ecological fallacy results from drawing conclusions about the wrong unit of analysis—in this case making generalisations about individuals from data about cultural/subcultural groups. Dreher and McNaughton argued that individual differences were such that cultural generalisations should be applied with great caution at the clinical interface and even that 'cultural competence is really nursing competence'. Their argument is a good one and fits with our description of spiritually competent practice involving compassionate engagement with the whole person as *a unique human being.* It is clearly unreasonable to expect any practitioner to have an encyclopaedic knowledge of all the different religions or cultures. What is required is an awareness that they exist and a willingness to respect how, in a particular patient, a worldview different from that of the practitioner may need to be taken into account in the planning and delivery of healthcare.

2.3.4   Spirituality and Trans-Cultural Nursing Care Perspectives

It is a fundamental aim of nursing and midwifery to promote patients' holistic care needs including mental, physical and spiritual wellbeing (Jubilee Centre for Character and Virtues 2017). Spiritual and existential care competencies are best expressed within the context of person-centred practice and compassionate presence (Ali and Lalani 2020; Benner 1994). A competent nursing care practice necessitates a compassionate-caring presence with authenticity and vulnerability (Ali and Lalani 2020; Wattis et al. 2019). Such nursing care requires embracing spiritual care core values such as availability, active listening, respecting privacy, dignity, providing support and reassurance with empathy (Schwartz et al. 2021; Rogers 2016).

Over the last three decades, spirituality has received special attention in nursing education and practice (Ali et al. 2018). There has been a continuous development around understanding the scope of relating spirituality, spiritual concepts: such as spiritual experiences, spiritual pain, spiritual distress among patients and families in diverse cultural settings (Lalani and Ali 2020). Several nursing theorists have recommended that nurses should embrace transformative care practices that can accelerate the process of developing self-awareness in a patient by expanding subjective consciousness and enabling transcendence on an intuitive level, to promote inclusive and holistic care (Ali 2017). Self-awareness is essential in developing nurse–patient therapeutic relationships and personal reflection in recognising culturally competent, equity-based, existential and spiritual care needs for empowerment (Wattis et al. 2021; Ali and Lalani 2020). However, many nurses have reported lack of preparedness in meeting the spiritual needs of their patients due to '…mismatch between the expectations of education and the reality of practice' (McSherry 2000, p. 40; Ali et al. 2018). Challenges were identified in addressing spirituality in nursing education. These challenges included fear of rejection by offending others due to lack of clarity about diverse cultural values and religious beliefs, confusion related to role expectations of nursing professionals, and the inadequate representation and emphasis on spiritual care in nursing education and practice (Ali 2017). It requires strong nursing standards based on sound philosophical structures, to guide the curriculum and practice environment reflecting the core aspects of spiritual care competencies.

2.4 Conclusion

In this chapter we have introduced the concept of spiritually competent practice as a way of avoiding endless disputes about the definition of spirituality and avoiding confusion with religion. At the core of spiritually competent practice is supporting people in sustaining a sense of meaning and purpose even when it is challenged by suffering and illness. It involves compassionate engagement with the whole person as a unique individual, but also respect for the person's family and cultural connections. As well as specific competencies it requires personal qualities, including the capacity to form *I-Thou* relationships and a managerial system that enables practitioners to attend to personal as well as technical aspects of healthcare. SOPHIE is presented as a model for understanding lifelong learning through reflective practice. The Availability and Vulnerability, framework specifically developed in research with APNs, is illuminated by a case study which can also be understood within the overarching description of spiritually competent practice. Finally, we have briefly considered the importance of taking into account cultural issues without forgetting that individuals within a culture also have their own personal understanding of what spirituality means to them within their culture.

References

Abramovitch H, Schwartz E (1996) Three stages of medical dialogue. Theor Med 17:175–187

Ali G, (2017) Multiple case studies exploring integration of spirituality in undergraduate nursing education in England. Doctoral thesis, University of Huddersfield. http://eprints.hud.ac.uk/id/eprint/34129/

Ali G, Lalani N (2020) Approaching spiritual and existential care needs in health education: applying SOPHIE (self-exploration through ontological, phenomenological, and humanistic, ideological, and existential expressions), as practice methodology. Religions 11:451. https://doi.org/10.3390/rel11090451

Ali G, Snowden M (2019) SOPHIE (self-exploration through ontological, phenomenological, humanistic, ideological and existential expressions): a mentoring framework. In: Snowden M, Halsall J (eds) Mentorship, leadership, and research. International perspectives on social policy, administration, and practice. Springer, pp 107–116

Ali G, Snowden M, Wattis J, Roger M (2018) Spirituality in nursing education: knowledge and practice gaps. Int J Multidiscipl Comparat Stud 5(1–3):27–49. http://www.ijmcs-journal.org/wp-content/uploads/2018/12/Ali.pdf

Anderson R, Cissna KN (1997) The Martin Buber-Carl Rogers dialogue: a new transcript with commentary. State University of New York Press, Albany NY

BBC News (2016) Jo Cox tribute https://www.bbc.co.uk/news/av/uk-36560418/more-in-common-than-that-which-divides-us. Accessed 27 Aug 2020

Benner P (ed) (1994) Interpretative phenomenology: embodiment, care and ethics in health and illness. Sage, Thousand Oaks, CA

Borrell-Carrió F, Suchman AL, Epstein RM (2004) The biopsychosocial model 25 years later: principles, practice, and scientific inquiry. Ann Fam Med 2(6):576–582. https://doi.org/10.1370/afm.245

Carlin N, Cole T, Strobe H (2012) Guidance from the humanities for professional formation. In: Cobb M, Puchalski CM, Rumbold B (eds) Oxford textbook of spirituality in healthcare. Oxford University Press, Oxford, pp 443–449

Cox J, Campbell AV, Fulford BKWM (eds) (2007) Medicine of the person: faith, science and values in health care provision. Jessica Kingsley Publishers, London

Dreher M, MacNaughton N (2002) Cultural competence in nursing: foundation or fallacy. Nurs Outlook 50(5):181–186

Dworkin G (1988) The theory and practice of autonomy (Cambridge studies in philosophy). Cambridge University Press, Cambridge. https://doi.org/10.1017/CBO9780511625206

Dyke J (2020) Coronavirus has paused our environmentally destructive lifestyles – let's do things differently in the future. https://inews.co.uk/opinion/coronavirus-paused-environmentally-destructive-lifestyles-429681. Accessed 24 July 2020

Engel GL (1977) The need for a new medical model: a challenge for biomedicine. Science 196(4286):129–136

Engel GL (1980) The biopsychosocial model. Am J Psychiatr 137(5):535–544

Engel GL (1992) How much longer must medicine's science be bound by a seventeenth century worldview? Psychother Psychosom 57:3–16

Frankl V (2004) Man's search for meaning. Rider Books, London

Gaufberg E, Hodges B (2016) Humanism, compassion and the call to caring. Med Educ 50:264–266. https://doi.org/10.1111/medu.12961

Jones J (2016) A qualitative study exploring how occupational therapists embed spirituality into their practice. Doctoral thesis, University of Huddersfield. Available at: http://eprints.hud.ac.uk

Jubilee Centre for Character and Virtues (2017) Virtuous practice in nursing. Available at: http://www.jubileecentre.ac.uk/1588/projects/current-projects/virtuous-practice-in-nursing. Accessed 20 Dec 2019

Kirschbaum M, Rodriguez A (2017) Spirituality in Western multicultural societies. In: Wattis J, Curran S, Rogers M (eds) Spiritually competent practice in health care. CRC Press, Boca Raton FL

Kitwood T (1997) Dementia reconsidered: the person comes first. Open University Press, Milton Keynes

Koenig H, King D, Carson V (2012) Handbook of religion and health. Oxford University Press, Oxford

Lalani N, Ali G (2020) Methodological and ethical challenges while conducting qualitative research on spirituality and end of life in a Muslim context: a guide to novice researchers. Int J Palliat Nurs 26(7):362–370. https://doi.org/10.12968/ijpn.2020.26.7.362

Marie Curie Cancer Care (2004) Spiritual and religious care competencies for specialist palliative care. http://www.ahpcc.co.uk/wp-content/uploads/2014/07/spiritcomp.pdf. Accessed 27 Aug 2020

McCormack B, McCance T (2017) Person-centred practice in nursing and health care. Wiley, Chichester

McSherry W (2000) Education issues surrounding the teaching of spirituality. Nurs Stand 14:40–43

McSherry W, Ross L, Attard J, van Leeuwen R, Giske T, Kleiven T, Boughey A, the EPICC Network (2020) Preparing undergraduate nurses and midwives for spiritual care: some developments in European education over the last decade. J Study Spiritual 10(1):55–71. https://doi.org/10.1080/20440243.2020.1726053

Monbiot G (2016) Neoliberalism - the ideology at the root of all our problems. The Guardian. Online at: https://www.theguardian.com/books/2016/apr/15/neoliberalism-ideology-problem-george-monbiot. Accessed 25 July 2020

Monbiot G (2017) How did we get into this mess? Verso, London

Muller JZ (2018) The tyranny of metrics. Princeton University Press, Princeton NJ

Nelson S (1995) Humanism in nursing: the emergence of the light. Nurs Inq 2:36–43. https://doi.org/10.1111/j.1440-1800.1995.tb00061.x

NHS England (2020) The comprehensive model of personalised care. Online at: https://www.england.nhs.uk/personalisedcare/comprehensive-model-of-personalised-care/. Accessed 21 July 2020

Office of National Statistics (2011) Religion in England and Wales. Available at: https://www.ons.gov.uk/peoplepopulationandcommunity/culturalidentity/religion/articles/religioninenglandandwales2011/2012-12-11. Accessed 25 July 2020

Pfeifer H-R, Cox J (2007) The man and his message. In: Cox J, Campbell AV, Fulford BKWM (eds) Medicine of the person. Jessica Kingsley, London

Prentis S, Wattis J, Rogers M, Jones J, Stephenson J (2014) Healthcare lecturers' perceptions of spirituality in education. Nurs Stand 29(3):44–52

Rego F, Nunes R (2019) The interface between psychology and spirituality in palliative care. J Health Psychol 24(3):279–287. https://doi.org/10.1177/1359105316664138

Richardson P (2014) Spirituality, religion and palliative care. Ann Palliat Med 3(3):150–159. https://doi.org/10.3978/j.issn.2224-5820.2014.07.05

Rogers CR (2003) Client-centered therapy; its current practice, implications, and theory. Constable, London (original edition published in 1951)

Rogers M (2016) Spiritual dimensions of advanced nurse practitioner consultations in primary care through the lens of availability and vulnerability. A Hermeneutic Enquiry. Doctoral thesis, University of Huddersfield. Available at http://eprints.hud.ac.uk

Rogers M, Beres L (2017) How two practitioners conceptualise spiritually competent practice. In: Wattis J, Curran S, Rogers M (eds) Spiritually competent practice in health care. CRC Press, Boca Raton FL

Rogers M, Wattis J, Moser R, Borthwick R, Walters P, Rickford R (2020) Views of mental health practitioners on spirituality in clinical practice, with special reference to the concepts of spiritually competent practice, availability and vulnerability: a qualitative evaluation. J Study Spiritual. https://doi.org/10.1080/20440243.2021.1857624

Schneewind JB (1998) The invention of autonomy: a history of modern moral philosophy. Cambridge University Press, Cambridge

Schwartz A, Baume K, Snowden A, Patel J, Genders N, Ali G (2021) Self-care. In: McSherry W, Boughey A, Attard J (eds) Enhancing nurses' and midwives' competence in providing spiritual care. Springer, Cham. https://doi.org/10.1007/978-3-030-65888-5_4

Sharifi N, Adib-Hajbaghery M, Najafi M (2019) Cultural competence in nursing: a concept analysis. Int J Nurs Stud 99:103386. https://doi.org/10.1016/j.ijnurstu.2019.103386

Shields L (2010) Questioning family-centred care. J Clin Nurs 19(17–18):2629–2638. https://doi.org/10.1111/j.1365-2702.2010.03214.x

Smith RG (2013) I and thou (translated from Martin Buber (1923) German Ich und Du). Bloomsbury Revelations, London

Sulmasy DP (2002) A biopsychosocial-spiritual model for the care of patients at the end of life. The Gerontologist 42(Suppl. 3):24–33

Swinton J (2012) Healthcare spirituality: a question of knowledge. In: Cobb M, Puchalski CM, Rumbold B (eds) Oxford textbook of spirituality in healthcare. Oxford University Press, Oxford, pp 99–104

Templeton J (1999) Agape love; a tradition found in eight world religions. Templeton Foundation Press, Radnor PA

Wattis J, Curran S, Rogers M (2017) Spiritually competent practice in health care. CRC Press, Boca Raton, FL

Wattis J, Rogers M, Ali G, Curran S (2019) Bringing spirituality and wisdom into practice. In: Practice wisdom: values and interpretations. Brill-Sense Publishers, Rotterdam. https://doi.org/10.1163/9789004410497_014

Wattis J, Rogers M, Curran S, Ali G (2021) In Higgs J, Orrell J, Tasker D, Patton N, (2021) shaping wise futures: shared future possibilities. Brill-Sense Publishers, Rotterdam

World Health Organisation (2015) WHO global strategy on people-centred and integrated health care: Interim Report. Retrieved from: https://www.who.int/servicedeliverysafety/areas/people-centred-care/global-strategy/en/. Accessed 2 June 2020

Wright NT (1992) The new testament and the people of god. SPCK, London

Younas A, Maddigan J (2019) Proposing a policy framework for nursing education for fostering compassion in nursing students: a critical review. J Adv Nurs 75:1621–1636

Spiritual Care Competencies for Advanced Practice Nurses

3

Joanne Pike, Linda A. Ross, and Wilf McSherry

Abstract

This chapter focuses on spiritual care competencies and how Advanced Practice Nurses (APN) can develop these. A framework developed from a recent European project, 'Enhancing Nurses and Midwives Competence in Providing Spiritual Care through Innovative Education and Compassionate Care', provides details of spiritual care competencies and how these can be applied in practice. This chapter also identifies some of the concepts within spiritual care competencies which APNs need to develop and integrate spirituality into practice. A short case study finishes the chapter illustrating aspects of the spiritual care competencies.

Keywords

Spiritual care competencies · Holism · Advanced Practice Nurse · Praxis

J. Pike (✉)
Faculty of Social and Life Sciences, Wrexham Glyndŵr University, Wrexham, North Wales, UK
e-mail: j.pike@glyndwr.ac.uk

L. A. Ross
Faculty of Life Sciences and Education, University of South Wales, Pontypridd, UK
e-mail: linda.ross@southwales.ac.uk

W. McSherry
School of Health and Social Care, Staffordshire University Stoke-on-Trent, Staffordshire, UK
e-mail: w.mcsherry@staffs.ac.uk

3.1   Introduction

This chapter focuses on spiritual care competencies and how Advanced Practice Nurses (APN) can develop these. A framework developed from a recent European project, 'Enhancing Nurses and Midwives Competence in Providing Spiritual Care through Innovative Education and Compassionate Care', provides details of spiritual care competencies and how these can be applied in practice. This chapter also identifies some of the concepts within spiritual care competencies which APNs need to develop and integrate spirituality into practice. A short case study finishes the chapter illustrating aspects of the spiritual care competencies.

3.2   Spiritual Care Competencies

Competence in nursing is fundamental to all practice and has been identified as including core abilities required for fulfilling the nursing role being 'focused on performance or a set of tasks' (Fukada 2018). Hager and Gonczi (1996) in defining competence, note that competency in practice is not only about tasks or attributes, but fundamentally, 'only by taking proper account of the essentially relational nature of the concept of competence can the holistic richness of work be captured ...' (p. 17). Erault (1994) believes that competence in skills performance must exist within a context and purpose, and that possessing a skill is just one facet of knowledge. The context of practice under discussion here is competence in spiritual care through the lens of the ICN and EPICC.

3.2.1   The Art and Science of Advanced Nursing Practice

The role of the APN is undertaken within many settings and contexts involving interactions with individuals from diverse cultures, ethnic backgrounds and worldviews. Irrespective of where this care is provided it requires a blending of both the 'art' and the 'science' of caring (Ross and McSherry 2010). APNs are practising in healthcare situations that are constantly evolving, the horizon of practice continuously shifting especially in this new era of digital and technological innovations. They provide care at the interface of both humanistic and medical practice. This care can be visualised as being on a continuum or spectrum. At the far left is care based on humanistic principles, while at the far right care is based on a purely medical and scientific paradigm.

Advanced practice that relies solely on, or heavily upon, one of these positions becomes problematic and polarised. For example, APNs require a sound scientific and medical knowledge base that will ensure all the treatment and care provided is based upon the most up-to-date evidence. This will ensure that the care provided is competent, and of the highest standards and quality maintaining patient safety. Conversely, care that is lacking human interaction can lead to dehumanisation and depersonalisation of the individual. The danger and pitfalls are that the patient or recipient of any care becomes lost, rendered invisible, because the focus is not upon them as a person but the medical condition or problem that is presented. Adherence to strict and prescriptive algorithms and pathways and formularies can compound this situation. Consequently, the APN must strike a balance walking the tightrope (continuum) between 'art' and 'science' to provide care that is safe, evidence-based and of the highest quality yet sensitive to the humanity of the person.

A further consideration in the relationship between 'art' and 'science' is the notion of holistic and person-centred practice. It could be argued that these matters are dealt with under the 'art' of care. However, to apply this to the totality of advanced practice is to reduce and separate roles, functions and actions into frag-mentary and reductionist models of care. Regarding the 'Art' as separate to the 'sci-ence' sets up a dualist approach to practice. This approach is not holistic or person-centred as it fails to accommodate the relational nature of advanced practice that strives to integrate both treatment and care (McSherry 2007).

3.2.2 Holistic and Person-Centred Care

McEvoy and Duffy (2008, p. 418) provide a useful working definition of holistic nursing care stating:

> 'Holistic nursing care embraces the mind, body and spirit of the patient, in a culture that supports a therapeutic nurse/patient relationship, resulting in wholeness, harmony and heal-ing. Holistic care is patient led and patient focused in order to provide individualised care, thereby, caring for the patient as a whole person rather than in fragmented parts.'

This definition indicates the importance of care embracing the totality of the 'whole' person, body, mind and spirit. McSherry (2006) discusses spirituality within the context of holism highlighting some key issues that explain why the spiritual remains a neglected part of holism. He suggests that ambiguity of definition, lack of attention accredited to this dimension in models of care, theory and practice gaps and finally the need to develop theory that captures the voice of both practitioners and the public whom they serve all contribute to this omission. McSherry (2006, p. 93) concludes that 'some of these issues concerning the place of spirituality within the context of holism will rumble on for many more years'. This statement is prophetic because there has been no real consensus or resolution of these issues in the intervening decades. Jasemi et al.'s (2017) concept analysis suggests that some of these issues still prevail within nursing and healthcare. However, they offer some important insights concluding that a clear definition of holistic care may lead to improvements in clinical performance and thereby enhance the overall quality of nursing care. Perhaps one of the key issues is the interchangeable nature of words used in theories and models of nursing practice. Over recent decades we have used individualised care, holistic care and latterly person-centred care. A resolution seems to be found in the use of person-centred care since this seems to encapsulate and integrate both individualised and holistic attributes. One of the pioneers of this approach McCormack (2003, p. 203) writes 'being person-centred requires the formation of a therapeutic narrative between professional and patient that is built on mutual trust, understanding and a sharing of collective knowledge'. This has significance for those undertaking APN roles since it highlights the key ingredients on which person-centred care is founded.

3.2.3 The Importance of Language

A review of McCormack's work underscores the importance of a truly holistic approach. Despite there being no direct reference to the word spiritual, this may be subsumed under what is termed 'authentic consciousness'. This is described as

> "a consideration of the person's life as a whole in order to help sustain meaning in life. Authentic consciousness is not a hierarchical ordering of possible desires, but a clarification of values to maximise potential for growth and development" (McCormack 2003, p. 204).

Interestingly, the person-centred nursing framework offered by McCormack and McCance (2006) also makes no explicit reference to the spiritual dimension. While this is not problematic, it does raise some interesting observations. For example, is this a deliberate omission or a conscious decision not to refer to the spiritual dimension? Or indeed is this an oversight or do the authors feel that the notion is adequately addressed in other aspects of the framework?

Given the burgeoning literature in nursing and healthcare associated with spirituality and the role this may play in maintaining the health and well-being of individuals a failure to address this adequately within models of holistic and person-centred practice may lead to APNs being hesitant or reluctant to engage with this aspect of their practice. This raises a fundamental question: How do we prepare nurses for spiritual care?

3.2.4 The Gaps in Practice

Before answering the question of how APNs might be prepared for spiritual care, it is necessary to understand how the terms 'spirituality' and 'spiritual care' are understood and what spiritual care competency (SCC) looks like. These were gaps that a three-year (2016–2019) European project, funded by the European Commission, sought to address. The project focused on '*E*nhancing Nurses and Midwives Competence in *P*roviding Spiritual Care through *I*nnovative Education and *C*ompassionate *C*are' (EPICC) (McSherry, et al. 2020).

3.2.5 The EPICC Project

Three groups of people were involved in the project:

Table 3.1 Summary of EPICC project outputs

- *Spiritual Care Education Standard* containing:
  - Consensus on the meaning of 'spirituality' and 'spiritual care'
  - Four core spiritual care competencies
- *Gold Standard Matrix*: a figure depicting what helps/hinders SCC development with accompanying *Narrative*
- *Toolkit* with teaching and learning (T&L) activities to help students to become competent
- *Network* for sharing ideas/experience and best practice
- *Website* to house all of the above
Outputs are available on the website www.epicc-network.org under 'Resources and Tools'

1. Six Partners who developed the bid, obtained the funding, were responsible for running the Project and who participated in all project activities.
2. 31 Participants: pre-registration nursing/midwifery educators from 21 European countries identified through EPICC Partners' networks and an advertisement on ResearchGate in 2016/2017.
3. 60 Participants+: international stakeholders including policymakers (e.g. Welsh Government, Dutch Higher Education Board), professional organisations (e.g. Royal College of Nursing, Norwegian Nursing Association), health organisations (e.g. National Health Service (NHS) England, Public Health England), students, health service users, members of the public.

Over 3 years, Partners, Participants and Participants+ engaged in a number of activities to co-produce 6 important outputs (Table 3.1). Activities were based on the principle of co-production and adopted a consensus approach using Action Learning Cycles and on-line questionnaires (McSherry et al. 2020).

3.2.6 Towards a Shared Understanding of 'Spirituality' and 'Spiritual Care'

Because there was no agreed definition of 'spirituality' and 'spiritual care' within nursing and midwifery, it was considered important to reach a common understanding of these terms for the Project. We selected the European Association of Palliative Care definition of 'spirituality' because of the significant international consensus work underpinning it (Puchalski et al. 2014), and the NHS Education for Scotland (NES) definition of 'spiritual care' which was widely quoted in the literature and seemed a good fit with nursing/midwifery practice (NES 2009). Participants considered these definitions in an on-line survey at the start of the project and reached agreement during the first T&L event in April 2017. The adopted definitions are outlined in Box 3.1, with changes to reflect well-being highlighted in bold. These definitions were added to the Preamble of the EPICC Spiritual Care Education Standard.

Box 3.1 Definitions Adopted for the EPICC Project
Spirituality:

'The dynamic dimension of human life that relates to the way persons (individual and community) experience, express and/or seek meaning, purpose and transcendence, and the way they connect to the moment, to self, to others, to nature, to the significant and/or the sacred'.

The spiritual field is multidimensional:

- 'Existential questions (concerning, for example, identity, meaning, suffering and death, guilt and shame,reconciliation and forgiveness, freedom and responsibility, hope and despair, love and joy).
- Value-based considerations and attitudes (that is, the things most important to each person, such as relations to oneself, family, friends, work, things, nature, art and culture, ethics and morals, and life itself).
- Religious considerations and foundations (faith, beliefs and practices, one's relationship with God or the ultimate)' (Nolan et al. 2011).

Spiritual care

'Care which recognises and responds to the human spirit when faced with *life-changing events (such as birth*, trauma, ill health, *loss*) or sadness, and can include the need for meaning, for self-worth, to express oneself, for faith support, perhaps for rites or prayer or sacrament, or simply for a sensitive listener. Spiritual care begins with encouraging human contact in compassionate relationship and moves in whatever direction need requires' (adapted from NES 2009, p. 6).

3.2.7 What Spiritual Care Competencies Looks Like

Attard et al.'s (2019a, b) 54 item SCC framework was selected as the starting point in thinking about what SCC might look like for nurses/midwives, because it was the most extensive, rigorous and current piece of work in SCC at that time, building on the significant contribution of van Leeuwen et al. (2009). Between April 2017 and September 2018 participants reduced the 54 competencies to 4 through a series of on-line questionnaires, where each competency was rated on importance, and face-to-face group and plenary discussions. The four competencies (Table 3.2) were combined with the preamble to form the EPICC Spiritual Care Education Standard (van Leeuwen et al. 2021). The knowledge, skills and attitudes relating to each competency are briefly discussed throughout this chapter and related to APN praxis. The full Standard can be found on the EPICC website (http://blogs.staffs.ac.uk/epicc/resources-and-tools/epicc-spiritual-care-education-standard/).

Table 3.2 The EPICC spiritual care competencies

1. Intrapersonal spirituality	2. Interpersonal spirituality	3. Spiritual care: assessment and planning	4. Spiritual care: intervention and evaluation
Is aware of the importance of spirituality on health and well-being	Engages with persons' spirituality, acknowledging their unique spiritual and cultural worldviews, beliefs and practices	Assesses spiritual needs and resources using appropriate formal or informal approaches, and plans spiritual care, maintaining confidentiality and obtaining informed consent	Responds to spiritual needs and resources within a caring, compassionate relationship

3.2.8 Preparing APNs for Spiritual Care

3.2.8.1 The Right Ingredients

There is no clear tried and tested 'recipe' for preparing APNs for spiritual care; however, nursing research to date sheds some light on the combination of factors that seem important (Ross et al. 2014, 2016, 2018). To illustrate this, the EPICC Project participants considered the research evidence and co-produced the EPICC Gold Standard Education Matrix, a figure which depicts the complex array and dynamic interaction of factors that may enhance or hinder the development of SCC. It depicts the turbulent cultural, social and political environment, or 'amniotic sac', in which SCC develops (http://blogs.staffs.ac.uk/epicc/resources-and-tools/epicc-gold-standard-matrix-for-spiritual-care-education/), and the accompanying narrative explains it (http://blogs.staffs.ac.uk/epicc/resources-and-tools/epicc-gold-standard-matrix-narrative/). Key points to recognise as an APN are that:

- SCC develops over time—this will be enhanced by education that integrates spirituality into the curriculum from the start.
- Personal qualities should be considered when APNs apply to train in addition to academic qualifications, for example personal warmth, empathy, compassion.
- Key factors which may contribute to development of SCC include:
  - Personal spirituality of the APN, life experiences and perception of spirituality/spiritual care. Being spiritually aware/having high spiritual well-being, having experienced positive or negative life events, and having a broad understanding of spirituality will all support the development of personal spirituality.
  - Academic content threaded throughout pre- and post-registration curricula should provide opportunity for reflection on and discussion of beliefs/values/spirituality, and on experience of caring for patients.
  - Clinical experience of caring for patients in an organisational ethos supportive of person-centred care, which balances 'being' with 'doing', 'art' with 'science' and which has good role models/mentors will enhance SCC.

Spiritual care must therefore be embedded in nursing care at all levels, whether registered nurse, Clinical Nurse Specialist or Nurse Practitioner. This means that even while there is a technical rationality (*dong/science*) inherent in some aspects of APN practice, particularly when medical needs are prioritised, they are always delivered with the holistic (*art/being*) approach of person-centred care.

3.2.8.2 A Toolkit

Exactly how spirituality and spiritual care should be taught has been the focus of many small studies over the years with inconclusive results (Ross et al. 2014). To provide educators with 'tools' to assist with teaching and learning about spiritual care, the EPICC Project took a pragmatic approach. Participants were invited to contribute activities that had worked well for them in their own teaching and learning over the years. Most activities have, therefore, been 'field tested' with different nurse/midwifery student groups in different countries across Europe. Around 25 activities are collected together in the EPICC Toolkit where they are arranged under the four competencies (http://blogs.staffs.ac.uk/epicc/resources-and-tools/epicc-adoption-toolkit/).

The Toolkit provides a useful resource to assist educators seeking to support students in becoming competent in spiritual care, they can easily be adapted to APN education and practice. If you would like to contribute to this toolkit, please contact the authors, as we wish to further develop this resource.

3.2.8.3 A Network

Being able to share ideas, tips, resources and research is crucial to establishing best practice in spiritual care teaching and learning. It was for that very purpose that the EPICC Network was set up supported by the EPICC website where all the resources are housed. You can join the Network by completing and submitting the form located under 'Join us' on the EPICC website.

3.2.9 Advanced Practice Nurse Praxis and Spiritual Care Competencies

Internationally, APNs are recognised as functioning in a role that requires formal education beyond that of a generalist nurse, with a master's degree being the minimum required for the role (International Council of Nurses 2020). The ICN note further that APNs 'are influenced by the global, social, political, economic and technical milieu' (ICN 2020, p. 8). The re-awakening of interest in spirituality across the world, research into APNs perceptions of spirituality and integration to practice, and the work of EPICC are part of the milieu influencing advanced practice nursing. The arguments for integrating spirituality into APN practice are compelling. However, much of the clinical knowledge required by the APN is medical, pharmacological and technical, preparing the APN to work autonomously, admit, refer and discharge patients who may otherwise have been treated by a medical practitioner.

Working largely within a technical rationality and hypothetico-deductive paradigm enables decision-making and clinical reasoning to be underpinned by an evidence-based approach; however, this often omits the spiritual dimension of care.

Seemingly at odds with the evidence-based approach, the ICN state: '… these guidelines emphasise that the APN is fundamentally a nursing role, built on nursing principles' (ICN 2020, p. 11). Therefore, inductive knowledge, supported by *nursing* praxis, would demand any decision-making take into account the *holistic* needs of the patient. Thus, the condition causing the suffering is treated, with the APN's holistic approach attending to the patient's suffering, based on caring, ethical nursing practice (Hoeck and Delmar 2018).

Explaining the concept of praxis and ethics, Cody (2013) notes it is embedded in complex interactions between the nurse and patient, but that the nurse will practice based on their understanding of what will contribute to the patient's well-being. Cody (2013, p. 8) further states:

'Praxis and practical reasoning always unfold in a context that is profoundly interpersonal and relatively unpredictable. The end is not predetermined, and as possible ends evolve situationally, possible means evolve as well. Thus, praxis is creative and dialogical.'

Cody (2013) further explains nursing praxis as intentional and deliberate, guided by nursing science, but also by *other* sources of knowledge. Benner (1984) would add that an important source of knowledge which she terms 'pattern recognition' is part of the reasoning of the advanced or 'expert' practitioner, again, learning from practice in a creative and dialogical way focusing on the patient's needs.

3.3   Developing APN Spiritual Care Competencies

In order to discuss how to prepare APNs for spiritual care, we need to return to the EPICC research discussed at the beginning of the chapter. As spiritual care competence develops over time, and since APNs have significant experience, it could be assumed they would already provide spiritual care as an integral part of their holistic practice. Indeed, spiritual care giving as part of holistic care has been highlighted as being an essential part of advanced nursing care (McMillan et al. 2018; Withers et al. 2017; Arslanian-Engoren et al. 2018), though this requires understanding of spirituality and its expression in the context of caring. Patient-centred or person-centred care is holistic by its very nature, and provides a system of care within which spiritual care can thrive (Vincensi 2019). To achieve person-centred outcomes such as satisfaction with care, involvement with care, well-being, and a therapeutic culture, McCormack and McCance's (2021) model promotes several care processes, including 'sympathetic presence', while Rogers' (2016) Availability and Vulnerability framework (see Chap. 5) ably supports this application in advanced practice.

The four EPICC spiritual care competencies that follow below integrate many aspects of Rogers' (2016) framework as well as the person-centred approach to care.

3.4 Intrapersonal and Interpersonal Competencies

APNs are ideally placed to apply their higher levels of knowledge, skills and attitudes in practice related to intrapersonal and interpersonal spirituality, and indeed, should be acting as mentors in practice, role modelling these actions. Firstly, however, in order to role model these, the APN needs to act on the opportunities as they arise in practice, and to recognise their own availability and vulnerability in order to practice effectively and safely. Developing spiritual care competence in others requires a high level of spiritual care competence oneself.

3.5 Presence, Connectedness and Attachment

Presence is key within SCCs, it is a particular way of being, caring, and relating spiritually to patients that has been discussed in the literature for many years. Being fully present for a patient is a skill that is expressed through the APN's authenticity and unconditional love and has several antecedents: the attention of the APN focused on the patient, receptiveness to the needs of the other and an awareness of a shared humanity (Tavernier 2006). While the technological developments and swift progress of the patient through the healthcare system means patients may spend less time with the APN than ever, being *present* during the nurse-patient encounter has been said to be a powerful resource in care delivery as a therapeutic tool since it provides a sense of meaning, and promotes holistic healing (Covington 2003; Tavernier 2006). Defining presence is difficult however, and without a clear definition, the APN may find discussing and reflecting on the concept challenging. As Wingate (2007, p. 97) notes: 'presence … has unclear boundaries, and has often been combined with other concepts such as caring' and may therefore be problematic to operationalise, let alone teach. Finfgeld-Connett's (2008) conceptual synthesis of the art of nursing, presence and caring helpfully identified similarities that serve to underline the importance of each of the concepts, implying that unclear boundaries of such concepts are not a disadvantage to their understanding of operationalisation in practice. In practical application, Covington (2003, p.313) asserts that 'caring presence offers a context within which spirituality can be expressed, connections can be made with oneself, others, nature, and God/life forces' such that holistic care is given, and a therapeutic environment is provided for physical, emotional, and spiritual healing in a human-to-human way. Being present for a person in the sense of being authentically available for that person, means that a connection can be made that allows growth and an enhancement of spiritual well-being, a true therapeutic, spirit-to-spirit relationship with one another (Burkhardt and Nagai-Jacobsen 2002). As an APN learning to offer caring presence is important, but, as cautioned by McMahon and Christopher (2011), development of competence and skill is needed. The EPICC SCC provide the APN with a framework and context within which to situate this learning.

In order to enable presence, there must be an understanding of how to create this in caring practice. Heidegger (1962) suggested that caring necessitates being with another 'being' and concerning oneself with what the other person is concerned with. This is also connected to *empathy* which is expressed within the EPICC competencies in terms of the ethical attitude supporting spiritual care intervention and evaluation in which the APN will respond to a person's spiritual needs and resources within a caring, compassionate relationship. Rogers (2016) takes this further, stating that the APN must also be available *and* accepting *and* understanding of the other person. Caring for the whole person requires awareness of (or noticing) the interconnectedness of body, mind and spirit, and 'being with' the other person. These are all essential for holistic care. In other words, to care holistically for a person and to demonstrate caring for that person the APN must be fully present and affirm the person in a holistic way taking into account the body, mind and spirit (Potter and Frisch 2007). This is the *skill and attitude* of making oneself available, rather than the *knowledge* of caring alone.

Presence requires connectedness between the APN and the patient. This concept has been part of many nursing theories over the years and has often been said to promote healing and wholeness. The caring occasion according to Watson (2005) is the occurrence, the moment, or the point at which the nurse and patient come together, and during which time caring may occur. Both people in the caring relationship bring their own contexts and come together as human beings with their own vulnerabilities, in what Watson terms a human-to-human transaction. The compassion shown by the APN in these moments, when combined with presence is an important and powerful spiritual care intervention, and requires a clear knowledge of self and personal limitations.

Bowlby's (1967) Attachment Theory describes how being connected to a significant other is important to varying degrees throughout human life, particularly in times of stress. Kaufmann (1981) identifies the tremendous psychological importance of 'secure attachment' in terms of coping when one feels vulnerable. The most common figures for attachments are family and/or a deity, since a person should be loved and feel loved by an attachment figure (Kirkpatrick 2005), but nurses are often seen as attachment figures (Mottram 2009).

Campbell (1984) and Rogers (2016) both suggest that caring is deemed as a form of agape (neighbour love) which is equal regard for human beings, and an altruistic or selfless love for others without reward (Burkhardt and Nagai-Jacobsen 2002). As an APN, recognising the need for attachment and being willing to be available in a connected relationship can have a profound impact on patient care. Buber (1970) contends that to be meaningful there must be relational reciprocity, in that two people must be 'present' and 'connected' in the relationship in a spiritual care encounter. Buber (1970) also proposes the 'I Thou' rather than 'I It' approach to relationship which necessitates a recognition of one another as fellow human beings. More recently, McSherry (2006, p. 156) asserts that spiritual care is underpinned by effective and sensitive communication skills which are the foundation of relationships between patient and nurse, while presence 'means being with the individual in a physical, psychological and spiritual sense'. The APN may therefore offer care and connectedness to the patient, but to transcend to a spiritual competency and connection, mutuality is necessary.

Spiritual competencies are underpinned by the APN's spiritual knowledge, skills and attitude. The EPICC framework demonstrates how spiritual knowledge, skills and attitudes support the APNs intrapersonal and interpersonal spiritual competence, and thus practice holistically. Attitudes are the most difficult to measure, while knowledge and skills development in spiritual care are often visible and are much more easy to test. Attitudes however are reflected in behaviour and are essential in being able to assess spiritual needs, and to implement spiritual care. Learning interpersonal and intrapersonal spiritual competence is important, as the acquisition of knowledge, skills and attitudes through education has been shown to be possible in the classroom as well as via role models in practice (Attard et al. 2014).

3.6 Love and Trust

Trust is fundamental to the SCCs, it is created when relationships are built and nurtured. Carr (2010) notes that this is the foundation of spiritual caregiving. Caring spiritually is a moral imperative and is an unconditional giving of oneself to a relationship, it is the embodiment of spiritual and moral values. Clarke (2013) recognises that the difference between giving care, and giving care spiritually is related to establishing an intentionally caring connectedness that acknowledges the spiritual nature of the interaction.

Carper (2013, p. 28) suggests that it is the act of the therapeutic use of self that 'rejects approaching the patient-client as an object (or as Buber identifies (I-It) and strives instead to actualise an authentic personal relationship between two persons' (I-Thou) thus comprehending more than the technical rationality of advanced practice'.

In order to be truly present for the patient, it has been posited that unconditional regard, or loving presence may be offered (Guenther 2011). Spiritual care based on non-judgemental love can help those in crisis to find meaning and strength through connectedness (Mok et al. 2010). Campbell (1984, p. 85) identifies that in order to connect to the other person, there must be what he terms 'moderate love' which is described as '.... reaching out to another in the desire to enhance the value which is seen'.

Campbell (1984) proposes that professions identify that they not only deal with people fairly, but also that they are governed by an ethic of respect for the people they care for. He argues that moderated love, combined with the ethical commitments of those in the caring profession, are more closely orientated to religious faith (one can substitute *spirituality* here) than to scientific detachment. Developing the ability to offer 'moderated love' requires empathy and integrity. Love, in the sense of care and compassion, is a very powerful healer, and is a manifestation of the human spirit. Scheler (2008, p. 144) identifies that love is extended to those who are suffering in order to relieve their suffering.

3.6.1   Spiritual Care: Assessment and Planning

The first stage of planning care is to undertake some form of assessment, whether this is conducted formally or informally. The challenge when applying either approach to spiritual assessment is to ensure this is conducted with minimal intrusion and great sensitivity. There is a vast amount of literature published in this area advocating a wide range of approaches and spiritual assessment interventions (See McSherry and Ross 2010; Harrad et al. 2019). McSherry et al. (2019) provide a useful overview of the key benefits and challenges of conducting a spiritual assessment.

Interestingly, the evidence from surveys capturing nurses and healthcare professionals' perceptions and practice around spiritual care suggests that formal spiritual assessment tools are very rarely used (McSherry and Jamieson 2011; Austin et al. 2017). Most nurses and practitioners gather this information by asking the patient directly or by observing and listening to them. This is not to say that APNs should not be using these tools in their practice and consultations with patients. Two what can be termed acronym-based models that have been used in spiritual assessment are the FICA (Puchalski and Romer 2000) and HOPE (Anandarajah and Hight 2001). These tools are designed to enquire about the patients personal, religious, and spiritual needs in a non-intrusive, timely and sensitive manner as part of a formal assessment of need.

More recently, Ross and McSherry (2018) recommend taking time to ask two simple questions: 'What's most important to you right now?' and then 'How can I help?' This model is known as the 2QSAM or the 2 Question Spiritual Assessment Model which is a very practical and flexible model of assessment that can be used in the delivery of care in a continuous manner. It is holistic and person-centred and needs led. From the spiritual assessment the APN will be able to liaise with the patient to establish a plan of care that adequately address any specific spiritual/religious needs that they require addressing.

APN Spiritual Care Interventions and Evaluations The context of advanced practice is laid out in detail in the ICN Guidelines (International Council of Nurses 2020) and supports the need for nurses at this level to be able to make complex decisions and to manage a patient throughout a care episode with their advanced assessment, judgement, decision-making and diagnostic reasoning skills. The core of APN practice is based on advanced nursing education and knowledge, meaning that the holistic approach in decision-making is vital. Therefore, spiritual needs must be considered also. While the APN often works at a technically high level, there are times when aspects of spirituality of a patient must take precedence. Working in the cancer unit, Helen, an APN, told me of a patient who profoundly affected her at the time and has affected her approach to practice ever since.

Marge was a young woman in her 30 s with cancer who had two young children with her partner. They lived in a small two-bedroom house with a small yard to the back. Marge was the sort of woman who did not like fuss, she was private, stoical and always seemed to be managing her pain and fatigue very well. However, at one appointment, Marge seemed quieter than usual. Helen reviewed her blood levels and found that Marge was anaemic (which was not unusual as she had been so before) and had a raised white cell count. Helen suspected Marge had an infection. When Helen took a history, Marge told her of some slight urinary urgency which she had been experiencing over the previous 2 or 3 weeks. A urine sample was taken and on analysis there was haematuria. Helen told Marge that although she had not previously had one, it was not unusual for a woman to have a urinary tract infection (UTI), and that she would send the sample off for culture and sensitivity, with a view to commencing antibiotics if Marge agreed.

Helen told me that Marge would not agree to taking antibiotics as she felt that her cancer had got 'into my bladder' and that taking antibiotics would not help, but Helen was convinced that she would benefit from a short course of antibiotics as she felt she had a UTI. However, Helen respected Marge's decision, and said she would still send off her urine sample, giving Marge advice to return if her symptoms worsened and that she would let Marge know the results of the sample as soon as she had them. When Helen asked Marge why she thought her cancer had got into her bladder, Marge replied that she had been dreaming of this and had wakened with a certainty that she would 'be leaving soon'.

Although there is much more to Marge's story in terms of referral for further investigations and results, Helen was always Marge's APN and supported her throughout. Thankfully, Marge was found not to have bladder cancer and all her scans were clear. At a subsequent appointment, Helen reflected back on Marge's feelings and her certainty that cancer had invaded her bladder and asked her why she was so certain. Marge explained that as a young woman, she had not always chosen 'the *right* boyfriend, according to Mum' and she and her mum had often fallen out about it. Now that she no longer had her mum to support her, Marge thought she was being punished for her actions all those years ago and she felt guilty. This resonated with Helen who felt she also could have been kinder to her own parents while she was growing up, feeling empathy and compassion for Marge. And although she did not attempt to compare her feelings with Marge's, Helen understood them, while also recognising her own vulnerabilities in this situation. Helen was therefore able to support Marge to explore her feelings by asking two simple questions:

- What is most important to you now?
- How can I help?

This powerful tool developed by Ross and McSherry (2018) is called the Two Question Spiritual/Holistic Assessment Model or the 2Q-SAM, and can be found in the EPICC Toolkit. It is useful in addressing person-centred care needs and the authors propose it as 'a realistic solution to delivering spiritual care – or care that is spiritual – in a resource-challenged health service' (p. 80). The 2Q-SAM can be used by all APNs whether in acute or community care and helps to balance the art and the science of advanced nursing practice.

As Helen planned her spiritual care intervention, she asked Marge what was important to her now. Marge answered slowly that she wanted to say sorry to her mum somehow. Helen listened with compassion and remained fully present with Marge while she talked it through, gradually beginning to make sense of her guilt. After Marge had finished, Helen asked Marge how she could help her, and was taken aback by Marge simply saying thank you, that she would be okay. Now that it was shared, Marge felt less heavy, less burdened and somehow lifted. There was a change in her posture and she sat a little straighter. Helen accepted Marge's words, and they arranged a date for the next appointment. Helen planned to follow this up with Marge at their next meeting, demonstrating the centrality of her spiritual care knowledge skills and attitude in responding to Marge's spiritual needs.

When Helen evaluated the spiritual care she had given Marge, she felt she had some understanding of Marge's feelings about her mum. Helen thought this had enabled her to connect with Marge, and to respond appropriately to Marge's spiritual needs. In Marge's case, simply sharing her feelings with Helen helped Marge to move beyond the guilt she felt, but Helen also had awareness of her limitations in providing spiritual care, and would have referred Marge to other professionals had she needed more support than Helen was able to provide as an APN.

3.7   Conclusion

This chapter has highlighted the importance of spiritual competencies in supporting the APN to understand and provide spiritually competent practice. We have discussed the importance of holism and spirituality prior to introducing the EPICC spiritual care competencies. A short case study illustrated how the APN assessed spirituality and was able to plan and implement care which addressed the spiritual needs of her patient. The spiritual care competence displayed by Helen was vital in helping Marge to move forwards from her spiritual pain and to begin to cope. Helen's spiritual care competence enabled her to connect with Marge with an open and person-centred attitude, engaging with Marge with compassion and empathy and allowing her to talk through her feelings. Authentic and caring, Helen was aware of her own availability and vulnerability, demonstrating how the EPICC spiritual care competence was applied in practice within a compassionate relationship.

References

Anandarajah G, Hight E (2001) Spirituality and medical practice: using the HOPE questions as a practical tool for spiritual assessment. Am Fam Physician 63(1):81–89

Arslanian-Engoren C, Hicks F, Whall AL, Algase DL (2018) An ontological view of advanced practice nursing. In: Cody WM (ed) Philosophical and theoretical perspectives of advanced practice nursing. Jones & Bartlett Learning, Burlington; MA, pp 361–368

Attard J, Baldacchino D, Camilleri L (2014) Nurses' and midwives' acquisition of competency in spiritual care: a focus on education. Nurse Educ Today 34(12):1406–1466

Attard J, Ross L, Weeks K (2019a) Design and development of a spiritual competency framework for pre-registration nurses and midwives: a modified Delphi study. Nurse Educ Pract 39:96–104

Attard J, Ross L, Weeks K (2019b) Developing a spiritual care competency framework for pre-registration nurses and midwives. Nurse Educ Pract 40:10260. https://doi.org/10.1016/j.nepr.2019.07.010

Austin P, MacLeod R, Siddall P, McSherry W, Egan R (2017) Spiritual care training is needed for clinical and non-clinical staff to manage patients' spiritual needs. J Study Spiritual 7(1):50–53. https://doi.org/10.1080/20440243.2017.1290031

Benner P (1984) From novice to expert: excellence and power in clinical nursing practice. Addison-Wesley Publishing Co, Menlo Park: CA

Bowlby J (1967) Attachment and loss, vol 1. Basic Books, New York

Buber M (1970) I and Thou. Charles Schribner's Sons, New York, NY

Burkhardt MA, Nagai-Jacobsen MG (2002) Sprituality: living our connectedness. Delmar, Albany, NY

Campbell AV (1984) Moderated love: a theology of professional care. SPCK Publishing, London

Carper BA (2013) Fundamental patterns of knowing in nursing. In: Cody WM (ed) Philosophical and theoretical persepctives for advanced nursing practice. Jones & Bartlett Learning, Burlington: MA, pp 23–34

Carr TJ (2010) Facing existential realities: exploring barriers and challenges to spiritual nursing care. Qualitat Health Res 20(10):1379–1392

Clarke J (2013) Spiritual care in everyday nursing practice: a new approach. Palgrave Macmillan, Houndmills

Cody WA (2013) Values-based practice and evidence-based care: pursuing fundamental questions in nursing philosophy and theory. In: Cody WA (ed) Philosiophical and theoretical prespectives for advanced nursing practice. Jones & Bartlett Learning, Burlington: MA, pp 5–14

Covington H (2003) Caring presence: a delineation of a concept for holistic nursing. J Holist Nurs 21(3):301–317

Erault M (1994) Developing professional knowledge and competence. Falmer Press, London

Finfgeld-Connett D (2008) Qualitative convergence of three nursing concepts: art of nursing, presence and caring. J Adv Nurs 63(5):527–534

Fukada F (2018) Nursing competency: definition, structure and development. Yonago Acta Med J Med Sci 61(1):1–7

Guenther MB (2011) Healing: the power of presence. A reflection. J Pain Symptom Manag 41(3):650–654

Hager P, Gonczi A (1996) What is competence? Med Teach 18(1):15–18

Harrad R, Cosentino C, Keasley R, Sulla F (2019) Spiritual care in nursing: an overview of the measures used to assess spiritual care provision and related factors amongst nurses. Acta Bio-Med Atenei Parmen 90(4-S):44–55. https://doi.org/10.23750/abm.v90i4-S.8300

Heidegger M (1962) Being and time. Blackwell Ltd., Oxford

Hoeck B, Delmar C (2018) Theoretical development in the context of nursing - the hidden epistemology of nursing theory. Nurs Philos 19(1)

International Council of Nurses (2020) Guidelines on advanced practice nursing. International Council of Nurses, Geneva

Jasemi M, Valizadeh L, Zamanzadeh V, Keogh B (2017) A concept analysis of holistic care by hybrid model. Indian J Palliat Care 23(1):71–80

Kaufmann GD (1981) The theological imagination: constructing the concept of god. Westminster, Philadelphia, PA

Kirkpatrick LA (2005) Attachment, evolution and the psychology of religion. Guildford Press, London

McCormack B (2003) A conceptual framework for person-centred practice with older people. Int J Nurs Pract 9(3):202–209

McCormack B, McCance TV (2006) Development of a framework for person-centred nursing. J Adv Nurs 56(5):472–479

McCormack B, McCance T (2021) Person-centred healthcare practice: a guide for healthcare students. Wiley, Newark, CA
McEvoy L, Duffy A (2008) Holistic practice – a concept analysis. Nurse Educ Pract 8:412–219
McMahon MA, Christopher KA (2011) Toward a mid-range theory of nursing presence. Nurs Forum 46(2):71–82
McMillan E, Stanga N, Van Sell S (2018) Holism: a concept analysis. Int J Nurs Clin Pract 5(282):1–6
McSherry W (2006) Making sense of spirituality in nursing and health care practice: an interactive approach, 2nd edn. Jessica Kingsley, London
McSherry W (2007) The meaning of spirituality and spiritual care within nursing and health care practice. Qusy Books, Wiltshire
McSherry W, Jamieson S (2011) An online survey of nurses perceptions of spirituality and spiritual care. J Clin Nurs 20(7–8). https://doi.org/10.1111/j.1365-2702.2010.03547.x
McSherry W, Ross L (2010) Spiritual assessment in health care practice. M&K Publishing, Keswick
McSherry W, Ross L, Balthip K, Ross N, Young S (2019) Spiritual assessment in healthcare: an overview of comprehensive, sensitive approaches to spiritual assessment for use within the interdisciplinary healthcare team. In: Timmins F, Caldeira S (eds) Spirituality in healthcare: perspectives for innovative practice. Springer Nature Quality and Performance, Switzerland, pp 39–54
McSherry W, Ross L, Attard J, van Leeuwen R, Giske T, Kleiven T, Boughey A, The EPICC Network (2020) Preparing undergraduate nurses and midwives for spiritual care: some developments in education over the last decade. J Study Spirit 10(1):55–71
Mok E, Wong F, Wong D (2010) The meaning of spirituality and spiritual care among the Hong Kong Chinese terminally ill. J Adv Nurs 66(2):360–370
Mottram A (2009) Therapeutic relationships in day surgery: a grounded theory study. Int J Nurs Stud 18(20):165–174
NHS Education Scotland (2009) Spiritual care matters: an introductory resource for all NHS Scotland staff. NES, Edinburgh
Nolan S, Saltmarsh P, Leget C (2011) Spiritual care in palliative care: working towards and EAPC task force. Eur J Palliat Care 18:86–89
Potter PJ, Frisch N (2007) Holistic assessment and care: presence in the process. Nurs Clin N Am 42(2):213–228
Puchalski C, Romer AL (2000) Taking a spiritual history allows clinicians to understand patients more fully. J Palliat Med 3(1):129–137
Puchalski CM, Vitillo R, Hull SK, Reller N (2014) Improving the spiritual dimension of whole person care: reaching national and international consensus. J Palliat Med 17(6):642–656
Rogers M (2016) Spiritual dimensions of advanced nurse practitioner consultations in primary care through the lens of availability and vulnerability. Unpublished PhD thesis, University of Huddersfield, Huddersfield
Ross L, McSherry W (2010) Considerations for the future of spiritual assessment features. In: Ross L, McSherry W (eds) Spiritual assessment in health care practice. M&K Publishing, Keswick, pp 161–171
Ross L, McSherry W (2018) The power of two simple questions. Nurs Stand 33(9):78–80
Ross L et al (2014) Student nurses perceptions of spirituality and competence in delivering spiritual care: a European pilot study. Nurse Educ Today 34(5):697–702
Ross L et al (2016) Factors contributing to student nurses'/midwives' perceived competency in spiritual care. Nurse Educ Today 36:445–451
Ross L et al (2018) Nursing and midwifery students' perceptions of spirituality, spiritual care, and spiritual care competency: a prospective, longitududinal, correlational European study. Nurse Educ Today 67:64–71
Scheler M (2008) The nature of sympathy, 5th edn. Transaction Publishers, Brunswick,NJ
Tavernier SS (2006) An evidence-based conceptual analysis of presence. Holist Nurs Pract 20(3):152–156

van Leeuwen R et al (2009) The validity and reliability of an instrument to assess nursing competences in spiritual care. J Clin Nurs 18:2857–2869

van Leeuwen R et al (2021) The development of a European consensus based standard in spiritual care competencies for undergraduate nurses and midwives. J Advan Nurs 77:973–986

Vincensi BB (2019) Interconnections: spirituality, spiritual care and patient-centred care. Asia-Pacific J Onclol Nurs 6(2):104–110

Watson J (2005) Caring science as sacred science. FA Davies CompNY, Philadelphia, PA

Wingate S (2007) Commentary on the impact of nursing presence in the community heart failure program. J Cardiovasc Nurs 22(2):97–98

Withers A, Zuniga K, Van Sell S (2017) Spirituality: concept analysis. Int J Nurs Clin Pact 4(234):1–5

Personal Spirituality and Self-Compassion in Advanced Practice Nursing

4

Wendy Showell Nicholas

Abstract

This chapter focuses on caring for the carer. It examines why personal spirituality and self-compassion are necessary components of an Advanced Practice Nurse's (APN) ability to maintain good levels of personal health and wellbeing and of their ability to work in a spiritually competent way. Practical examples of self-compassion and personal spirituality in practice are drawn from the author's experience as a psychotherapist working with APNs and suggestions are offered for self-development in both areas.

Like all healthcare practitioners the APN does not operate in isolation. The organisational values, professional training and standards practiced all impact on the APN's capacity for self-compassion and personal spirituality.

I argue for a change in the approach to research in health and social care settings which focuses on the qualitative and, values-based approaches, that are more likely to consider the need for a focus on personal spirituality and self-compassion in all healthcare training and competency standards. I also call for all of us working in health and social care settings to personify and promote the practice of self-compassion and personal spirituality through reflective practice, role modelling, mentoring and advocacy.

Keywords

Self-compassion · Personal spirituality · Learning organisations · Reflective practice · Compassionate practice · Psychotherapy · Self-care · Training Mentoring

W. Showell Nicholas (✉)
Psychotherapy and Workplace Wellbeing, Huddersfield, West Yorkshire, UK
e-mail: w.nicholas@mac.com

This chapter is written from my perspective as a psychotherapist. Much of my work is specifically focused on burnout in Health and Social Care professionals. Spirituality and self-compassion are often key factors in their recovery. This chapter is an attempt to provide a practical, straight-forward approach to understanding the role that personal spirituality and self-compassion play in ensuring nurses remain effective caregivers. It provides practical examples of how personal spirituality and self-compassion can be built and sustained.

In an attempt to reduce any power imbalance that the hierarchical language of "professional" and "patient", "client ", or "service user" brings (White and Epston 1990) and for my own authenticity, I will use the term "person", where possible and write in the first person in parts.

The short anonymised illustrative examples, given to support certain points of practice are taken from my work as a psychotherapist supporting nurses and others who work in health, care, education and law who are required to work compassionately with others in challenging circumstances.

It may be that as you read, some of these case examples resonate with you. I hope that if you are experiencing the kind of problems I associate with lack of personal spiritual practice and self-compassion, these illustrative examples will provide you with ideas for replenishing your own reserves. There is a point, however, where the problems can become chronic, when our physical, mental and spiritual resources are sapped on a daily basis. This can result in significant health problems. If, like many people, you find yourself feeling something like despair, exhaustion, isolation, fear and anxiety much of the time, please know that you cannot and should not carry this alone. You need to access the professionals who are there to support you, speak to the people who love you and allow them to help.

4.1   Introduction

Personal spirituality and self-compassion do not feature highly in the training and development of APNs, yet they are essential elements in the delivery of spiritually competent, holistic healthcare. Healthcare is about relationship as much as technical competency. The subjective, interpersonal experiences of compassion, empathy, warmth and genuineness which are intentionally cultivated and offered by the nurse and received by the person being cared for, are core to good quality person-centred care (Rogers 1957). Indeed, in the field of psychotherapy, research highlights the quality of relationship between therapist and person attending therapy as *the* most significant indicator that a person will get well; more so, in fact, than the specific approach or techniques used (Norcross 2002).

Despite the evidence that good care is a subjective, relational experience, health and social care often prioritise the development and operationalising of techniques rather than the nurse's capacity for intrapersonal and interpersonal encounters (Wattis et al. 2017). Policy frameworks, targets and measures for good practice within the National Health Service (NHS) in the United Kingdom maintain a persistent focus on objective, numerical values as outcomes, often at the detriment of patient experience of care. This is often mirrored globally in healthcare settings. Ali et al. (2015) identified that many nursing standards and competencies in training tend to evidence technical competency over human impact which can result in target driven interventions at the expense of good quality, spiritually competent health care. Wattis et al. (2017) noted that despite spiritually competent practice being a key factor in helping people to get well, it is rarely factored into the scientific process and evidence base in health care. Rather than being central factors, the inter- and intrapersonal connections, through which compassion and spirituality are expressed, are commonly considered under the "catch all" of "non-specific variables".

In a climate where the measurement of successful nursing is dependent on the ability to take a mechanised approach to the people cared for, the nurses' own capacity for sustaining positive, healing human connection cannot thrive (Seager and Bush 2017). There is little wonder that many nurses who continuously attempt to draw from their own personal reserves of compassion, spirituality and care risk burnout. Nurses' reserves are not limitless and need to be replenished by self-nourishing practices and behaviours and spiritually aware working environments where colleagues respect and support one another and engage in reflective practice (Zohar and Marshall 2004; Wattis et al. 2017). In this context, a key element of reflective practice is an examination of the personal values, biases, stress levels and life experience the APN brings to the situation on which they are reflecting (Nicholas and Kerr 2017). This is especially important when we consider the impact of wider factors that increase pressure and stress on healthcare, for example, we know that the Covid-19 Virus Pandemic caused APNs resilience levels to plummet and APNs struggled to maintain their emotional and spiritual wellbeing (M. Rogers 2021, personal communication, 10 March).

4.2 Personal Spirituality

As with the term "spirituality", there is some confusion about the term "personal spirituality". In our secular society, many people find the term problematic because they equate spirituality with religion and may be suspicious of the latter (Hay 1985). This lack of understanding in wider society is reflected in professional concepts of spirituality and personal spirituality. My own experience of working in a hospital was that there was a belief amongst some people that, as an organisation, we had "ticked the box" for spiritually competent practice because we had a chapel and prayer room, or a person had been asked their religion or dietary needs. This conflation with religion and the focus on ticking boxes that address religious and cultural needs, may be one reason that nurses often feel ill-equipped to address spirituality in their work (Timmins and Caldeira 2017). Sadly, a focus on nursing care without the integration of spirituality may also mean that nurses do not nurture their own spiritual needs either.

Spirituality in the context of providing care to others as well as nurturing one's own wellbeing should be thought of as those things that bring hope, meaning and purpose to our lives (Narayanasamy 2004). More specifically, spirituality is "the expression of a person's humanity, whatever it is that helps to shape that person, and the well of inner strength from which that person draws support at times of crisis" (Slay 2007, p. 26). For some people this may include a religious belief or practice, but it is not restricted to that (Rogers and Wattis 2020). In essence, in a work context, personal spirituality is the very human, existential concern for hope, meaning and purpose in our professional lives (Zohar and Marshall 2004). It is what we are concerned with when we follow a vocation, show humility and when we learn from our mistakes. It is also apparent when we ask "what difference am I making?", "why do I do this job?" or "what did I get into this career for?". It is what we question when we only half-jokingly, cry "that's it! I'm going to work in a supermarket! The pay is as good!" and it is what we feel when we not at all jokingly say, "I'm tired of caring for everyone else and not having energy left for own family" or "I feel empty and exhausted. I just can't go on".

These are the questions and statements that I often hear in my psychotherapy practice and which I help people to address in an effort to improve their quality of life. These spiritual concerns are key factors to be addressed if I am to support people in improving their wellbeing at work and in their wider lives. For me, psychotherapy, like nursing, is a practice of holistic care. It includes but surpasses competencies and involves tending to the whole person and their physical, mental, emotional and spiritual needs. This requires a purposeful intention to replenish my own capacity for compassionate and spiritually competent practice by tending to my own personal spirituality and practicing self-compassion. It is from this position of lived experience, as well as from a professional understanding, that I hope I bring authenticity and genuineness to my work and support others to do the same in theirs.

Working towards spiritually competent practice and caring for ourselves is not easy when healthcare tends to focus on the biomedical model. A holistic model that incorporates the spiritual aspects of practice can be challenging. Attempts have been made to create tools that measure spiritual competence in nursing but spirituality is fundamentally subjective and therefore not easily falsifiable, replicable and generalisable using positivistic methods of inquiry (Swinton 2012). This, in turn, leads to difficulties in the provision of support, training, supervision and mentoring pertaining to the development of personal spirituality, a quality that cannot be "known" in the nomothetic sense. (Wattis et al. 2017). Despite this, it is understood that embedding spirituality into health care practice involves "developing a personal understanding of spirituality" (Jones et al. 2017).

As with my practice, the resource of an APN's personal spirituality is not limitless. It must be sustained and replenished, especially when signs of reaching burnout are emerging. When making a choice to sustain and replenish one's own resources, you support your ability to connect with other people, including those we care for, but it also boosts resilience to face challenges in practice, in particular, when caring for very ill patients (McSherry and Smith 2012). In addition, Upton (2018) suggests that if we address our personal spirituality it can help us to better care for patients who we find challenging and reduces the potential for burnout or compassion fatigue. However, if our resources are depleted, both the carer and the person being cared for will suffer. Ultimately, so too, will the organisation in which they are engaged. Whilst as an APN you should bear some responsibility for self-care and maintenance of your own spirituality, it is the organisation which bears the responsibility for providing a working environment in which you can practice that self-care and flourish. In the same way that the APN should hold the patient in a spiritually competent way, the workplace is the environment that can optimise or hinder the APN's ability to practice in a spiritually competent, holistic and person-centred way.

When considering personal spirituality in professional practice, then, we turn our attention from the spiritual needs of the person being cared for and examine the needs of the person who is doing the caring. The personal spirituality of the APN will underpin their interpersonal abilities with what Rogers (1957) described as the core competencies of empathy, congruence and unconditional positive regard. Brown (2010) states that we cannot give to others to a greater extent than we can give to ourselves. As an APN there are several things you can do to support your personal spirituality:

Provide Empathy As Brown (2010) suggests this is different to sympathy. As an APN you use this daily in that you have a sense of how another person feels and you are able to express empathy in a way that makes them feel seen and understood. To do this you must have a degree of self-knowledge and awareness, and a sense of yourself being known, seen and understood. You need to have empathy for yourself. Linked to Rogers (2016) concept of availability, it requires your openness and avail-ability to your own feelings, and a willingness to reflect with others on them in a way that allows for another to understand. Many of the nurses I work with who are experiencing burnout, report that if reflective conversations happen with their seniors, they focus on clinical and task-related decision-making. This is a missed opportunity. To include how the nurse was feeling, what emotional responses were present when working with certain scenarios, increases the APN's own emotional intelligence and therefore ability to provide empathetic care.

Have Congruence As an APN, you strive for your patients to know that the care you offer is genuine. There is a true relational connection within professional boundaries. You are not "acting a part" but are engaging wholeheartedly and genu-inely in your work. This means that the values and beliefs that are important to you are explicitly drawn upon and practiced in the workplace. You are not "playing a role" in signing up to professional standards and codes of conduct, rather these should be fully aligned with your own personal values and beliefs. Again, I encour-age regular reflective practice as a means of holding one's values and beliefs at the forefront of your practice, ensuring you work in a congruent way. This is part of sustaining your personal spirituality through authenticity. This will ensure there is a genuine authenticity in your interpersonal exchanges. You can make a choice to genuinely care for another—not doing so risks inauthenticity which will often be perceived by the person being looked after (Mearns and Cooper 2017). It can also be a sign that you are reaching compassion fatigue.

Finally, *unconditional positive regard*. As an APN showing genuine non-judgmental, positive regard in a way that allows the person being cared for to be vulnerable and to share feelings in a way that feels safe is paramount. This is often not possible unless you practice self-compassion, non-judgmental, positive regard and sense of self-worth for yourself. You need to have the capacity to accept your own feelings (including feelings of shame or inadequacy) as a human, and to share them in a way that feels safe and "held" within professional boundaries. This requires what Rogers (2016) in her Availability and Vulnerability framework, includes as emotional vulnerability. Here, she challenges the idea of vulnerability being a weakness but rather presents it as a capacity for humility, accountability, and the ability to reflect on one's mistakes. Evident in the APNs ability to receive feedback from colleagues and patients and learn from training, practice and mistakes shows a willingness to be humble and be teachable. An APN needs to be always aware that they do not know everything, this is a great protector against unsafe practice (Syed 2015). Vulnerability in the case of the APN also includes the ability to advocate for the people being cared for. This can be an act of bravery; involving putting one's head above the parapet and occasionally (potentially, even) risking professional criticism for the sake of promoting the needs of the people who are being cared for (Rogers 2016). However, to maintain personal spirituality you must learn to advocate for yourself and ask for the help you may need when life and work are tough.

My hope is that you can see how personal spirituality is a fundamental prerequisite of spiritually competent practice, but it also has other benefits. If you can exercise your own personal spirituality you will engage more wholeheartedly in your work. If you continually develop your own personal spirituality practices you will be less likely to experience compassion fatigue and/or burnout. Wright (2010) conceptualises burnout as a spiritual crisis that manifests in numbness, detachment and disengagement. This defensive shutdown due to spiritual depletion that he describes is a common experience in health and social care practitioners, can be mitigated by embedding the requirement for an awareness of, and commitment to, personal spirituality in practice and ensuring an environment and culture where personal spirituality is valued and nurtured.

4.2.1   Illustrative Example, Jane

Jane came to me as a 50-year-old Nurse Practitioner, with a 23-year career in nursing. Neatly presented both in her dress and in her manner, she calmly and quietly explained that she had begun to be very tearful after work and often felt a rising anger in her day-to-day dealings with colleagues. She described herself as having fallen out of love with the job and, in fact, she had little enthusiasm for anything in her life. She could muster no motivation for her work or her relationship with her husband, nor for any of the social activities she used to engage in. She described feeling like she was watching the world happening around her rather than living in it.

In further sessions, I discovered that nursing was a path that Jane's mother had wanted her to take. She was always a studious girl and attended to others needs. Her parents, she recalled, discouraged anything that they didn't see as "academic", or that meant she would get "messy or sweaty"!

In her homelife now, Jane reported being constantly engaged in boring unrewarding activities that, like her work seemed to fill her day and leave her exhausted. She only cooked and cleaned, she said, because her husband expected it. If it were down to her, she would just eat toast and live in one room. It was important at this stage to validate how Jane felt and acknowledge her lack of interest in and motivation for life, commenting that it must feel very tiring.

As therapy progressed, this lack of motivation became a focus, but Jane did not find the idea of trying anything new appealing—she felt no hope for the future. Accepting this, I took it a step back, asking Jane to not pressure herself to find new activities but instead, to simply notice her experience of the day-to-day activities that she already undertook and to notice if any of them felt more bearable than others.

The next week, Jane reported having felt generally no better apart from one morning, where she had become engrossed in potting some flowers in her window boxes. She described herself as having lost track of time and spent hours out there until a neighbour passed and began chatting, at which point Jane noticed her unkempt appearance and felt concern that they may ask her about a medical condition she knew they had, so she quickly made her excuses and retreated back indoors.

Over the weeks, I encouraged Jane, outside of the core activities she absolutely needed to do, to let go of any activities that she felt were expected of her but which she didn't find nourishing. To her surprise, her husband was very encouraging, saying he welcomed the opportunity to do more cooking, which he found enjoyable. He also commented he had enjoyed spending more time in her company rather than her always doing housework. Gradually, Jane began to feel a little less exhausted and began to arrive looking a little more dishevelled but a little happier. She had begun to think about our conversation about her childhood and how certain activities had been discouraged. She commented on their maybe being something out there that she might enjoy that she hadn't tried. To my surprise, Jane arrived at our next session telling me she had signed up for a last-minute place on a bushcraft course! We both laughed at how incongruent this seemed at first given the pressure she had felt growing up not to get "messy". Jane reflected on this and told me that she had loved the course. Her whole demeanour changed as she described exploring woodland, looking for materials and learning new skills. She described the group and how she was fascinated by a few people who, as they sat around a campfire, whittling spoons, had talked openly about their love of nature and its impact on their wellbeing. Jane attended every session, revelling in getting dirty and being connected with nature and other people who shared her joy for the outdoors. She talked about how making mess and mistakes didn't matter outdoors. She also described an accident that had happened that resulted in a minor cut to one of the group's fingers. Jane had been able to help by treating the wound but also really enjoyed showing the others how to do basic first aid so that they would be equipped to help themselves and others if need be. Over the weeks, Jane was able to share her frustrations with the procedural nature of her work and her experience of what she now perceived to be burnout, with some of the group. Simultaneously, Jane, with my encouragement, sought out a mentor at work whom she met with regularly for reflective conversations about her work. In these conversations, they explored the personal skills, values and beliefs that Jane held around the importance of outdoor space as an aid to healing. Through these discussions, together with the group, they hatched a plan. Over the next 18 months, Jane, supported by the group and group leader, approached the hospital and raised funding to overhaul an unused piece of land. The group, Jane included, volunteered to make the land into a peace garden, a place that patients and staff could go to be in touch with nature as a means to improve recovery and wellbeing. Jane had found hope, meaning and purpose in her newly found connection with the outdoors and through this, she found new enthusiasm for her work. Feeling nourished herself, she was able to make time to connect with patients and colleagues and she is a great advocate for helping others find their own sense of hope, meaning and purpose.

4.3   Self-Compassion

The word compassion is rooted in ecclesiastical Latin (Goetz et al. 2010), from "com" (with) and "pati" (to suffer). Lazarus (1991, p. 289) states that compassion means "being moved by another's suffering and wanting to help". The emphasis on the desire to relieve another's suffering as well as being emotionally engaged in it, is what distinguishes it from "empathy". It is a concept emphasised in all main world religions and in the wider concept of spirituality. Compassion is our emotional capacity to be with another's suffering and be moved to help, it is part of our humanity and contributes to us living full and meaningful lives (Fox 2010).

Nursing and other health and social care disciplines, have always held compassion as a core value (Armstrong 2011). It remains one of the six core values in the United Kingdom's National Health Service (Department of Health 2012a, b). Additionally, compassion is embedded in the "6 C's of Nursing Practice" (Department of Health 2012a, b). Unsurprisingly, compassionate practice improves patient satisfaction and provides numerous benefits, including to clinical outcomes (Epstein et al. 2005) Why then, have there been a number of well documented failures in compassionate care in many hospitals and care settings globally?

As with spirituality, there is a paucity of robust measurement tools for the actual measurement of compassionate practice and it is therefore difficult to quantify and assess. Studies are more likely to measure it by its absence than by qualifiable presence and this contributes to the challenges inherent in the development of training and assessment packages (McSherry and Draper 1997). On an individual level, two frequently cited reasons for poor practice in this area are compassion fatigue and burnout. Both when exacerbated by organisational failings to support the spiritual needs of staff and too heavy a focus on financial and activity-based targets over spiritually competent practice, may contribute to poor quality of care and scandals in the health and care system (Najjar et al. 2009).

When we are faced with others suffering, this can cause a reaction in us that is emotionally overwhelming. Unless we have a level of "distress tolerance", we risk becoming overwhelmed by our own reaction and subconsciously reduce our awareness of and compassion for, another's distress in an act of self-protection (Gilbert 2010).

Self-compassion, however, promotes individual wellbeing, and mental health and is a protective factor against compassion fatigue and burnout (Cosley et al. 2010). In other words, when our own suffering becomes too uncomfortable, we can become less able to connect with others, including the person who's suffering has prompted our discomfort, but the ability to practice self-compassion is a protective factor against this.

Whilst the link between the capacity to show compassion and the capacity for self- compassion is still an area for further research (Strauss et al. 2016), there is empirical evidence that we cannot give to others to a greater extent than we can give to ourselves (Brown 2010). Put simply, we cannot sit with others suffering if we cannot respond compassionately to our own. We can revisit the ideas of "non-judgement" (Gilbert 2010), "availability" and "vulnerability" to self and others here (Rogers 2016). These areas are at the core of remaining accepting of, and tolerant towards another person. We can be aware that their suffering is giving rise to difficult emotions in ourselves, including on occasion anger, sadness, shame, fear and disgust but we can choose to face these emotions with self-compassion, rather than supress them. Reflective practice, a supportive working environment or supervisory relationship and indeed, therapy can all be helpful in supporting and developing this skill (Seager and Bush 2017).

4.3.1 How to Nurture Self-Compassion

Self-compassion can be viewed as the active practice of taking the capacity for compassion we have for others and directing it inward to ourselves (Neff 2003). She describes three main practices that together create self-compassion:

- Kindness—being kind and non-judgmental towards oneself can be difficult, and self-criticism can easily set in. Mindfulness practices can be very helpful in building a daily practice of kindness and non-judgement towards oneself. Therapy can be a great help if self-criticism or perfectionism are deep rooted. Therapists can take a number of approaches and it is worth thinking about which might best suit you before you commit to one. For issues relating to self-criticism and perfectionism, a relational approach can be helpful. (Please do ensure your therapist is registered with a reputable professional body such as the UK's BACP Counselling Directory). I always offer a short session at no cost to see if the person looking for therapy and myself are a good fit, and I would expect any good practitioner to do the same.

  At work, a spiritually competent mentor and reflective supervision can further strengthen this practice. People can worry about kindness at work; perhaps perceiving it as un-boundaried, or even un-professional. But rather than being a fixed set of rules, experienced practitioners will tell you that boundaried practice, in fact, requires the ability to be flexible and to work reflectively in a way which requires continual self-awareness, self-compassion and reflective conversations in supervision. (Wright 2010).

- Mindfulness—though not the panacea it can be held up to be, a regular mindfulness practice can be very effective in building "distress tolerance", described earlier. To be able to hold awareness of painful feelings, without over-identifying with them, is not an academic exercise, but rather requires a *regular practice* to build the capacity to respond, rather than react to our feelings (Kabat-Zinn 2013). I recommend being taught this practice rather than attempting to just try it yourself. The "Headspace" app is a very good introduction and teaches the basic principles well. For a more in-depth experience, I strongly recommend an 8-week Mindfulness-Based Stress Reduction (MBSR) or Mindfulness-Based Cognitive Therapy (MBCT) course and you can find qualified, registered teachers at www. mindfulnessnetwork.com.

- Common humanity is the ability to see one's own suffering as part of the human condition rather than a flaw in oneself. This is aided by the two practices of kindness and mindfulness discussed above but many people also find this capacity is boosted through collective connection (Murthy 2020) with others, with a focus on spirituality. This could be a religious practice, but could equally be a shared passion for music, art, nature or the reading of books that express the human condition with all its beauty and flaws. The social science researcher, Brene Brown, has produced some wonderful books and web resources to this effect.

I would add to these three principles a capacity for retreat. The Benedictines hold the concept of welcoming dear to their hearts. To welcome a stranger, is, for them, akin to welcoming Christ (Christian History Institute 2017). In this principle, they capture the idea of seeing the sacred in all of humanity. But making oneself available to this extent can be a drain on resources in the same way that, for an APN to be emotionally available in the face of suffering can be a drain on their own spiritual reserves. For the Benedictines, this existential threat can be guarded against by the idea of retreat. The generous reception to guests is balanced by a drawing back, in order to focus on, and replenish the needs and spiritual resources of the monastic community (Swan 2005). As an APN you can learn to mirror this approach whilst tending to your work. This might include awareness of boundaries in practice, engaged use of reflective supervision, attending to one's own basic needs at work and practicing a healthy work/life balance. In this way, you can be fully available and compassionate towards the people being cared for, and balance that with ensuring full availability to oneself and one's homelife, in order to nourish and preserve the resources which make caring possible.

4.3.2   Illustrative Example, Jamal

Jamal was a Nurse Practitioner who worked in a busy inner-city General Practice (the UK term for Primary Care/Family Practice). He had been living alone since splitting from his partner who he met when he was student. The demands of his job and paying the mortgage for his flat on his own meant he had little time or money to see friends and he described himself as not very close to his family, who he said were "not touchy, feely people", and with whom he felt he had quite an emotionally distant relationship.

At work, he felt people had always seen him as being capable and professional, but perhaps a little "old school", in that he had what he described as a "backbone", he wouldn't be pushed around and also wouldn't be found chatting about his love life or what sports he'd played at the weekend, like some of his peers, when he was on shift.

Jamal came to me initially saying he felt overloaded and had begun to feel impatient with people using services. He reported feeling numb at work and dreading going in, but he also hating being at home on his own in the flat. He was experiencing severe tension headaches and often felt exhausted and unwell.

A few sessions in, Jamal confided he often felt real anger and disgust at patients, who he just wanted to "get well and get out". He reported "I just can't listen to their problems anymore. I can feel myself switching off and even being irritated with them—what do they want from me? I have my own problems too. Sometimes I want to scream".

Jamal felt great shame in describing this to me and when his "confession" was met with an understanding and a non-judgmental response, he went on. He had recently had a number of complaints made about him by patients, often relating to him being rude and dismissive in his manner and behaviour.

Jamal described subsequent conversations with the practice manager, who he described as "letting him off easy" by asking him to write cursory letters of apology to the people complaining. He felt uncomfortable, as he had allowed the practice manager to put the incidents down to being busy and pressured to meet targets, when in fact he knew he had treated the people badly because he felt angry and frustrated with them. Rather than feeling relief about his practice manager not seeing this, it added to his distress. He had, he realised, almost hoped that the practice manager would notice that he just wasn't coping and offer him support. He also reported that there had been no acknowledgment of the emotional impact having complaints made about him had had. He felt people just thought, perhaps because he was male, he was "tough" and "thick skinned" and could cope, but he felt extreme anxiety about the situation which led to further feelings of inadequacy and shame. Exhausted and isolated, Jamal had turned to therapy in despair.

Over the course of the first few sessions, it became evident that Jamal did not share his feelings with anyone. In fact, when I asked him about feelings, Jamal was often confused and would describe behaviours rather than emotions. He struggled to connect with his emotions on a day-to-day basis and when we explored them in therapy he found it deeply uncomfortable, brushing them away and making judgements about himself being "weak" and "needy". Jamal noted my sadness at hearing this harshness towards himself and justified it with "evidence". He reported having a hard time with stress and putting pressure on himself to get the best marks at university and, after a few too many drinks at a family gathering, he had told his parents, brother and sister in law, how much he struggled with his emotions, resulting in a long awkward silence in which everyone, including Jamal, had felt embarrassed. Jamal knew his father did not feel comfortable with the idea of a man working as a nurse but on this occasion, his father made a comment that perhaps he "didn't have what it takes" to work in medicine, and Jamal felt shame and anger.

With some encouragement we were able to allow Jamal a route to his emotions through therapy, he found them overwhelming and often cried through much of the sessions when he felt he was getting close to the emotional sources of his discomfort. Initially he felt shame at his tears, apologising for crying. I assured him that his tears were welcome, they were not a sign of damage being done but of healing from old scars. These tears began to feel cathartic to Jamal who eventually identified that he felt an almost constant tenseness and stress that was beginning to be loosened up in therapy. He later agreed to attending an 8-week mindfulness-based stress reduction course. On one of the weeks, Jamal's homework had been to notice feelings of discomfort in his day and to write down how they arose and what his response had been. This turned out to be something of an epiphany for Jamal. He reported, incredulously, that he had noticed he had very many uncomfortable feelings during his day, both the obvious ones he had known about, with feeling overwhelmed with patients, but also quite physical ones. For example, he said he had often needed to go to the toilet in the morning when he arrived at work but the surgery was busy and he usually immediately got caught up in tasks, often not managing to get to the toilet until the end of the working day! Feeling that he had to "hit the ground running" in this way, contributed to a build-up of tension through the day. After the session on the course, he had noticed the familiar physical discomfort of needing to go to the toilet one morning, but this time, he went. He said this put him back about 2 minutes with his patients, but it was fine, he felt comfortable and more able to focus on them, because he had tended to his own basic needs. A similar story unfolded about his lunch breaks. He had previously not taken a break as he was so busy, he hardly noticed his hunger and thirst. When we explored this, he noted that the culture in the surgery didn't help, it felt almost a badge of honour to be too busy to care for oneself and many other people didn't take lunchbreaks either. As well as challenging this idea of professionalism or being "up to the job", by sharing information about how hunger and thirst impact on our decision making, I set some homework of my own for Jamal. Now he had some experience of mindfulness, I encouraged him to practice a loving kindness meditation (a variety of these can be easily accessed online) each week and to challenge himself to hold kindness to himself and others in mind as he went through his day. When our session ended, it was this exercise and the epiphany about toilet breaks that Jamal reported as having the biggest impact on his life. He reported feeling much more resourceful when working with people in the surgery and tending to his own needs, even basic physiological ones, had seemed to re-energise him to help others. He also said that patients had asked specifically to see him because he "understood" them and they felt listened to. He found this very rewarding and, newly energised, began attending social engagements again. On one such occasion, he told his friends how much he had been struggling and how lonely he had been, despite not accepting their invitations to go out, for fear of being a burden. To Jamal's surprise, his friends were truly pleased that he had shared his feelings, assuring him they valued and loved him, however he showed up, and joking that next time he said he wasn't coming out, they weren't going to take no for an answer! A couple of them also shared that they often felt the same and Jamal was able to offer support.

4.4   Organisational Factors in Personal Spirituality and Self-Compassion

When discussing self-compassion and indeed, any form of self-care, it is important to remember that as an APN you do not exist in isolation. Seager and Bush (2017, p. 89) state that "human beings cannot simply create their own spiritual energy from a vacuum". The workplace environment and professional culture have a significant impact on the ability to nurture spirituality and practice compassionately. The burn-out that is indicative of low spiritual and compassion reserves, does not tend to happen suddenly. It is often a slow and corrosive process, heavily exacerbated by external factors, including unmanageable workloads, blame culture, poor support and leadership and other factors indicative of a non-learning organisation (Wright 2010).

It is important to note this because, if we only discuss personal spirituality and self-compassion in relation to our own qualities and competencies, we risk pathologising the individual, potentially bringing about feelings of shame and inadequacy and adding to the environment that limits their capacity in both areas.

In the same way good quality care requires the practice of compassion and spirituality, good nursing cannot be embedded in a spiritually depleted organisation (Seager and Bush 2017). Care cannot be spiritually competent unless the personal spirituality of practitioners is also continually supported and refreshed by the working environment. We must, therefore, create environments that engender a sense of belonging and safety for the people who work in them. Spirituality is not just an individual and relational practice, but a systemic and responsive one (Seager and Bush 2017) and the working environment must also be responsive.

In a learning organisation, there is an understanding of the systemic nature of the work. Values, practices and processes are in line with the cultural ethos and knowledge and competence are developed by responding to the experiences and ideas of staff and people who use the service (Syed 2015). Mistakes are seen as whole system phenomena that must be shared openly and honestly with the intention of learning. Granger (2020) suggested that non-learning cultures on the other hand are characterised by the use of shame. Often hierarchical in nature, people are discouraged from questioning practice, especially of senior members of staff. Reflective practice and creative thinking are suppressed in favour of adhering to target driven procedures (Senge 2006). These organisations can be characterised by their response to mistakes, where there is an emphasis on investigating in order to find an individual to publicly blame and punish rather than to understand what went wrong (Granger 2020). In his powerful book, Black Box Thinking, Matthew Syed identified that these cultures, actually contribute to an increase in mistakes as people dare not raise concerns, question others or admit their own vulnerabilities. To work in such an organisation is to keep a large part of yourself away from view. It is not a place where the flexibility required for self-compassion and personal spirituality can thrive and any vulnerabilities are a source of fear and shame which are used purposely as a threat. Blame and punishment are prioritised over the learning of lessons and improvements in practice and individuals are shamed if they raise concerns. Shame is a primal fear rooted in the fear of rejection from the group that in evolutionary terms could have been a life-threatening event, individuals are hard wired to avoid it at all costs (Sznycer et al. 2016). This means that mistakes are more likely to be hidden and lied about, or others blamed, than they are to be learned from (Syed 2015).

An individual in a fear culture will find themselves hypervigilant and defensive (Senge 2006). Granger (2020) recognises that individuals may betray their own values to be part of cliques for fear of rejection. She goes on to note, people impacted by a fear culture may find they don't take creative risks within strong professional boundaries, they will avoid stretching themselves, may not go for promotions rather than risk failure, and may miss other opportunities because they won't put themselves in development situations where they may face difficult feedback. Simultaneously, moved to a deficit mindset, they see other's gains as their loss. They may find themselves undermining or sabotaging others who they perceive as doing better than them (Granger 2020). In a physiological sense, in fear, humans literally become less able to be creative and flexible, teamwork and reflective practice are more difficult and individual IQ's can drop by up to 15 points. (Granger 2020). None of this bodes well for the health and success of the organisation concerned, the people they care for, or the individuals who work in the organisation.

The fear-based culture is the antithesis of a compassionate culture. A compassionate culture encourages a sense of belonging through shared values, and spiritually competent practice, mistakes are seen as systemic problems to be learned from and solved without shaming individuals. In a learning culture people are confident to respond flexibly and compassionately to others within the context of strong professional boundaries and good outcomes arising from this are shared and operationalised (Senge 2006). The quality of care given is dependent on the emotional state of the carer, which must be supported and nurtured in the working environment. Seager and Bush (2017) identify the ABC model of caring for the carer. In this, model, the relationship between carer (A) and recipient (B), are enriched by the spiritual and emotional needs of the carer (C) being factored into the caring process. The model outlines the three main characteristics of an organisation that provides a healthy environment in which staff can grow and learn. In a healthcare organisation like this, practitioners and other staff can be seen to model spiritually competent practice and self-compassion to peers and people they care for. These practices will be embedded in training, continuous professional development and reflective supervision and financial targets will not be prioritised over spiritually competent practice. This will be made possible by the development of assessment criteria for spiritually competent and compassionate practice based on qualitative research used to develop best practice guidelines. Crucially, in such an organisation, the values of the organisation are aligned with the values of the people working within it and this is enabled by more values-based training, supervision, mentoring and research.

When an APN cannot bring their whole self to work, their sense of hope, meaning and purpose is lost. When holistic care is reduced to financial and activity-based targets and only the technical aspects of the job are emphasised and stated, values around health improvement for patients are, in reality, overshadowed by the actual agenda of meeting targets. This can pose a sort of existential crisis for the APN. In a real way, when the APNs core values are not "seen" and validated in an organisational sense, the individual practitioner is not seen and this poses them an existential risk. "The greatest risk to psychological safety for all human beings is to be forgotten, lost from view and being "held in mind". This is arguably worse, even than having a negative identity in the minds of others" (Seager 2006, p. 276). Only when organisational values and targets are more aligned with holistic caring and health improvement, will nurses and other staff be able to address this existential crisis and this will only happen with more values-based research, training and mentoring (Seager and Bush 2017).

4.4.1 Illustrative Example, Maria

Maria was a fairly recently qualified Clinical Nurse Specialist (CNS) who had had a previous career in social work. Time spent working in a hospice had cemented her idea that she would transfer to nursing where she felt she was better placed to help people. She had undertaken her nursing training before training as a CNS in Cancer Care.

Maria was able to tell a strong and coherent story about her life. She had wanted to be a nurse as a child, but had chosen social work because she had not felt confident in her ability to study biology. Married with now grown-up children, Maria was comfortable and able to fund her degree in nursing. She had qualified with a distinction and had been working for 3 years in the role before training as a CNS. She noted though that she was increasingly unhappy. She expected herself to do everything perfectly, often not trying, rather than doing things that may face even the slightest negative feedback or being seen to make a mistake. She exhausted herself at work and home ensuring everything was done to the highest possible standard. She came to therapy describing severe anxiety and sleeplessness. She lived in fear of making mistakes at work and doubted her ability. She would take any feedback that was perceived as critical and ruminate about it for days. Increasingly, she felt less and less able to use her autonomy and lacked confidence to undertake even basic duties that she had previously done with very little thought.

Initially, we discussed Maria's tendency towards perfectionism and where she had learned this from, but it became evident that, prior to this job, she had been more tolerant of herself, seeing any errors or lack of understanding as learning experiences. Now, however, she responded with fear to any perceived lack of perfection in her work. She described this as being "real life" in nursing and was at pains to explain to me the responsibility of the job and how colleagues had been encouraged to leave or fired for even minor misdemeanours. The worst thing about this, said Maria, was her colleagues' unwillingness to come another's defence, even when everyone knew it wasn't just the fault of an individual nurse. Maria recalled her horror at colleagues making comments about "people that spent too much time with patients to avoid ward duties", comments she felt were aimed at her.

Nursing, she felt was not the path she should have taken, she thought she would be able to use the relational skills she had learned in the hospice and strengthen them with physical healthcare skills, but she realised now the job was more technical and less about people. Worse than that, she just felt she wasn't very good, that she didn't belong. She felt unable to change careers again as she would be seen as a failure but her anxiety about going into work was harming her to the point where she felt she may have a breakdown.

During our sessions, I used a narrative approach, accessing Maria's values through what, why, where, when questions (Beres 2014) `and Maria created new narratives with her responses. Before long, another narrative emerged. In this narrative, Maria described herself as having had the privilege of working for a spiritually competent organisation in which she had thrived and was inspired to revisit her childhood dream of becoming a nurse. Her concerns about her ability were outweighed by the meaning and purpose she found in this holistic care setting and she had achieved her dream. When she now found herself in an organisation that had many good features but lacked the spiritually competent, compassionate qualities, she was in a prime position to use her experience to influence the culture of this new organisation for the better. She had a choice, she said, she could shrink back and accept that her old workplace was unique and not replicable, or she could research how workplaces become spiritually competent learning organisations.

Over the following weeks and months, her research on this subject within the NHS in the United Kingdom meant Maria came in contact with key influencers in her organisation who shared her values. One of the senior CNS's was a researcher in the field of compassionate practice, well published, with a PhD and a respected practitioner. She told Maria that a number of people in her department had similar problems to Maria but didn't have experience of working in any other way. She approached Maria about mentoring other staff and this, eventually led to supervising and teaching students. Maria was able to go on leadership training and attended working groups concerned with compassionate practice. Following a promotion that she felt able to apply for, she began to do pieces of work and training on the subject of compassionate leadership, including training staff on reflective supervision and compassionate leadership. As her profile rose, Maria was approached by a number of people who shared her values and wanted to improve the culture of the organisation. Together, they were able to effect significant change, contributing to the organisation being recognised as a "Best Place to Work" in a special recognition award.

4.5 Conclusion

Health care is as much a relational as a technical practice. It requires an ability to identify with others, even in their pain and suffering and a willingness and ability to be in difficult emotional spaces, even when this brings up uncomfortable feelings in oneself.

Contrary to popular belief that nurses have to "develop a thick skin" and not be impacted by suffering (of self or others), caring requires the ability to be impacted by another and to experience empathetic concern, and for that concern to be obvious to the person being cared. "Seeing that one's suffering affects another is the very psychological and spiritual basis of change and transformation in suffering" (Seager and Bush 2017, p. 91).

If your spiritual reserves and self-compassion are not nurtured, maintained and supported, caring will come at an emotional cost to you, and the quality of care you give will be poorer. In the illustrative examples in this chapter, the APNs, people being cared for and organisation, all suffered.

There is much evidence of high profile failings in health and social care systems, globally, that have resulted in people being treated without dignity and compassion. These practice and organisational failures reflect the lack of attention given to compassionate and spiritually competent practice in health and social care research, training and procedures.

We cannot give to others to a greater extent than we can give to ourselves, APNs and other health and social care practitioners need to nurture their own personal spirituality and practice self-compassion if they are to be spiritually competent practitioners. As an APN you do not exist in isolation. You are unlikely to thrive if you are working in an environment and professional culture that prioritises financial and activity-based targets at the expense of compassionate, spiritually competent practice.

It is my hope and belief that as the research around compassionate and spiritually competent practice becomes operationalised, personal spirituality and self-compassion will be key aspects of practice and assessment requirements. It is through the embodiment of these qualities that professional culture will be influenced and you, the front runners, will become the researchers, teachers and mentors that will perpetuate a more holistic, compassionate, spiritually competent and effective healthcare system that future generations will enjoy.

References

Ali G, Wattis L, Snowden M (2015) Why are spiritual aspects of care so hard to address in nursing education? A literature review (1993–2025). Int J Multidiscipl Comparat Stud 2(1):7–31

Armstrong K (2011) Twelve steps to a compassionate life. Knopf Doubleday, New York

Beres L (2014) The narrative practitioner. Palgrave Macmillan, London

Brown B (2010) The Gifts of Imperfection: let go of who you think you're supposed to be and embrace who you are. Hazelden Publishing, Minnesota

Christian History Institute (2017) Christian History Institute. [online] Available at: https://www.christianhistoryinstitute.org/study/module/benedicts-rule/. Accessed 4 June 2017

Cosley BJ, McCoy SK, Saslow LR, Epell ES (2010) Is compassion for others stress buffering? Consequences of compassion and social support for physiological reactivity to stress. J Exp Soc Psychol 46:816–823

Department of Health (2012a) Compassion in practice. Nursing, midwifery and care staff: our vision and strategy. Department of Health

Department of Health (2012b) The NHS constitution for England. [online] Available at: https://www.gov.uk/government/publications/the-nhs-constitution-for-england. Accessed 19 Nov 2020

Epstein R, Franks P, Shields C, Meldrum S, Miller K, Campbell T, Fiscella K (2005) Patient-centered communication and diagnostic testing. Ann Fam Med 3(5):415–421

Fox M (2010) Compassion and peace. Available: https://philosophynow.org/issues/80/Compassion_and_Peace. Last accessed 18 Mar 2021

Gilbert P (2010) The compassionate mind. Constable & Robinson Ltd., London

Goetz JL, Keltner D, Simon-Thomas E (2010) Compassion: an evolutionary analysis and empirical review. Psychol Bull 136(3):351–374

Granger P (2020) Fear less: how to win at life without losing yourself. Vermilion, London

Hay D (1985) Suspicion of the spiritual: teaching religion in a world of secular experience. Br J Relig Educ 7(3):140–147

Jones J, Smith J, McSherry W (2017) Spiritually competent practice in healthcare: what is it and what does it look like? In: Wattis J, Curran S, Rogers M (eds) Spiritually competent practice in health care. CRC Press, Florida, pp 35–52

Kabat-Zinn J (2013) Full catastrophe living: using the wisdom of your body and mind to face stress, pain, and illness. Bantam Books, New York

Lazarus RS (1991) Emotion and adaptation. Oxford University Press, New York, p 289

McSherry W, Draper P (1997) The Spiritual Dimension: why the absences within nursing curricula. Nurse Educ Today 17:413–417

McSherry W, Smith J (2012) Spiritual care. In: McSherry W, McSherry R, Watson R (eds) Care in nursing: principles, values and skills. Oxford University Press, Oxford, pp 117–131

Mearns D, Cooper M (2017) Working at relational depth in counselling and psychotherapy, 2nd edn. Sage, London

Murthy VH (2020) Together: loneliness, health and what happens when we find connection. Profile Books Ltd, London

Najjar N, Davis LW, Beck-Coon K, Doebbeling CC (2009) Compassion fatigue: a review of the research to date and relevance to cancer-care providers. J Health Psychol 14:267–277

Narayanasamy A (2004) The puzzle of spirituality for nursing: a guide to practical assessment. Br J Nurs 13(19):1140–1144

Neff K (2003) Self-compassion: an alternative conceptualization of a healthy attitude toward oneself. Self Identity 2(2):85–101

Nicholas WS, Kerr J (2017) Practice educating social work students: supporting qualifying students on their placements. McGraw-Hill Education & Open University Press, London

Norcross J (ed) (2002) Psychotherapy relationships that work. Oxford University Press, New York, NY

Rogers C (1957) The characteristics of a helping relationship. Person Guid J 37(1):6–16

Rogers M (2016) Utilizing availability and vulnerability to operationalize spirituality. In: Beres L (ed) Practicing spirituality. Palgrave Macmillan, London

Rogers M, Wattis J (2020) Understanding the role of spirituality in person centered care. Nurs Stand 35(9):25–30

Seager M (2006) The Concept of 'Psychological Safety' – a psychoanalytically informed contribution towards safe, sound & supportive mental health services. Psychoanal Psychother 20(4):266–280

Seager M, Bush M (2017) Supporting the practitioner. In: Wattis J, Curran S, Rogers M (eds) Spiritually competent practice in health care. CRC Press, Florida, pp 87–97

Senge PM (2006) The fifth discipline: the art and practice of the learning organization (Revised and Updated Edition). Doubleday, New York

Slay G (2007) Lets get spiritual: the spiritual and religious aspects of Well-being are once again being recognised. Greg Slay discusses initiatives taken in West Sussex to include these neglected issues in mental health service assessments. Ment Health Pract 11(40):26–28

Strauss C, Lever Taylor B, Gu J, Kuyken W, Baer R, Jones F, Cavanagh K (2016) What is compassion and how can we measure it? A review of definitions and measures. Clin Psychol Rev 47:15–27

Swan L (2005) Engaging benedict: what the rule can teach us today. Ave Maria Press, Notre Dame, IN

Swinton J (2012) Healthcare spirituality: a question of knowledge. In: Cobb M, Puchalski C, Rumbold B (eds) Oxford textbook of spirituality in healthcare. Oxford University Press, Oxford

Syed M (2015) Black box thinking: the surprising truth about success. John Murray Press, London

Sznycer D, Tooby J, Cosmides L, Porat R, Shalvi S, Halperin E (2016) Shame and social devaluation. Proc Natl Acad Sci 113(10):2625–2630

Timmins F, Caldeira S (2017) Understanding spirituality and spiritual care in nursing. Nurs Stand 31(22):50–57

Upton KV (2018) An investigation into compassion fatigue and self-compassion in acute medical care hospital nurses: a mixed methods study. J Compass Health Care 5:7

Wattis J, Curran S, Rogers M (2017) What does spirituality mean for patients, practitioners and health care organisations? In: Wattis J, Curran S, Rogers M (eds) Spiritually competent practice in health care. CRC Press, Florida, pp 1–17

White M, Epston D (1990) Narrative means to therapeutic ends. Norton, New York

Wright SG (2010) Burnout – a spiritual crisis on the way home. Sacred Space

Zohar D, Marshall I (2004) Spiritual capital: wealth we can live by. Berrett-Koehler, San Francisco, CA

Introduction to Rogers' Availability and Vulnerability Framework for Operationalising Spirituality

5

Melanie Rogers

Abstract

This chapter introduces Rogers' Availability and Vulnerability framework which has been developed to help APNs operationalise spirituality. Spirituality is innately human and is influenced by the context we work in and how we emotionally engage with those in our care. Spirituality can be simply integrated into APN practice and operationalised through availability and vulnerability. Working in this way enables spirituality to be addressed on a practical level. Several examples from practice illustrate aspects of the framework.

Keywords

Spirituality · Availiablity · Vulnerability · Framework

5.1 Introduction

Chapters 6, 7, 8, 9, 10, 11, 12 and 13 present further APN case studies showing the integration of spirituality into practice in each of the World Health Organization global regions. They all follow the same format, starting with a brief overview of local APN practice for context. This is followed by a summary of how each country views and experiences spirituality in healthcare. The case studies illustrate how spirituality in APN practice relates to aspects of Rogers' (2016) Availability and Vulnerability framework. The premise of this framework is presented here to aid understanding and reflection.

M. Rogers (✉)
University of Huddersfield, Huddersfield, UK
e-mail: m.rogers@hud.ac.uk

Within Chap. 1 I identify those I work with as "patients" as this is the commonly used term in the area I work within, however I recognise that many areas utilise alternate terms. Sometimes the use of the word patient denotes a hierarchical relationship which is the opposite of what I suggest is the premise of holistic care. Therefore, please substitute the term as appropriate for your own area of practice and recognise that even though I use the term patient I am advocating a human-human relationship based on mutual respect based on acceptance and valuing one another.

Throughout my clinical practice as a nurse, Advanced Nurse Practitioner (ANP) and in my work as an APN educator I have often found that truly holistic care is hard to achieve owing to the many demands placed upon us. More "industrialised" styles of practice, with the need to reach targets, the lack of appropriate staffing and an emphasis on technical aspects of care provision, often leave some of the basic needs of patients' unmet (Wattis et al. 2017). Many of my patients talk to me about loss of hope, meaning and purpose as they face illness, stress and crises. This has been heightened dramatically with the Covid-19 pandemic where patients report feeling more isolated and unable to talk through their concerns due to social distancing, reduced general health care provision and support (Propper et al. 2020).

My doctoral studies focused on spirituality and whether the concepts of availability and vulnerability could be adapted to APN practice (Rogers 2016). In my own work over the last 30 years, I have often felt frustrated about not having the time to support patients holistically because of time pressures, targets and service demands. I have always been aware that patients are often in very vulnerable situations when they face illness and challenges, they need care from a clinician willing to connect with them and listen to their fears and anxieties. From the start of my career, I have worked hard to adapt my practice to have time to listen and to support patients holistically. I realised that patients often would ask me searching questions for example, Why me? What have I done to deserve this? How will I cope? I don't have the strength to get through this. I recognised that these questions and concerns were not just emotional but also existential in their meaning. At the same time, I also had my own questions about meaning and purpose and spent a lot of time studying, reflecting, talking to friends and colleagues, and considering what gave me hope, meaning and purpose. I took some time to go on a retreat to a Celtic Christian community in Northumberland. It was here that I was struck by the simplicity and radicalness of the principles of availability and vulnerability. In this community, relationship with God and others is mediated through availability and vulnerability (Northumbria Community 2020). Members of the Northumbria Community integrate availability and vulnerability through hospitality, care and concern for others, authentic relationships and being willing to reflect and change personally. I felt drawn to commit to living and working with these principles, not in a prescriptive way but as a guide to how I related to others. I considered whether these principles could be secularised and translated into clinical practice. This led to researching the concepts of availability and vulnerability with APNs, and more recently mental health clinicians (Rogers 2017, Rogers et al. 2019a, b, 2020, 2021). I describe the origins of the Availability and Vulnerability framework fully in Rogers (2016) and Rogers and Beres (2017).

Table 5.1 Rogers' Availability and Vulnerability framework for operationalising spirituality

Availability	
Availability to self	Self-reflection and self-awareness; this will help you to embrace spirituality by understanding your own meaning, purpose and direction in life
Availability to others	Welcome people into your care, be hospitable by offering your time, acceptance and understanding. This involves being truly "present" and listening attentively. It necessitates providing care and demonstrating concern through active participation in therapeutic relationships with patients
Availability to community	Develop your practice in response to the needs of the community and those in your care. The community may be your colleagues, organisation or the community as a whole
Vulnerability	
Vulnerability to self	Embrace the vulnerability of your role and the reality that you can never "know it all"
Vulnerability to others	Embrace accountability, engage in supervision and reflection, and accept constructive criticism
	Allow yourself to be vulnerable in your approach to practice. Acknowledging your mistakes and limitations. Be willing to share your uncertainty with patients to reveal your openness, honesty and transparency
Vulnerability to the community	Advocate for those in your care, question authority where necessary, keeping the interests of your patients at the Centre of care

(Rogers 2016, 2017, Rogers and Wattis 2020)

Spirituality is intrinsically linked to hope, meaning and purpose (Cook 2004; Wattis et al. 2017; Rogers and Wattis 2020). It is innately human and is influenced by context and emotional engagement and it can be operationalised through availability and vulnerability (Rogers 2016). Integrating availability and vulnerability into APN practice enables spirituality to be addressed on a very practical level. The concept of availability will be familiar as it is one of the premises of nursing; we offer time, care and presence to our patients. Yet, other aspects of availability may be new or more difficult to learn and apply, for example, being available to ourselves, or to the community as whole. Vulnerability is often viewed as weakness, something we should avoid. We may perceive vulnerability as being open to be hurt physically, personally or professionally. Of course, we need to protect ourselves from physical vulnerability but in the context of spirituality I am talking about us, as APNs, learning to be vulnerable in a way which enables connection with our patients and aids the provision of truly holistic care. Many of us will have been taught that maintaining an emotional distance from those we care for is an important aspect of professional boundaries. However, to fully connect to those in our care we need to be vulnerable enough to connect as a fellow human being (Thorup et al. 2012). My APN research, studies and reflection led to the development of a framework for operationalising spirituality for APNs (Table 5.1). Aspects of this framework are discussed here are illustrated through the following case studies in the following chapters.

Availability and vulnerability are not new concepts to nursing, they have been reported by notable nurse theorists especially those from the tradition of Caritas nursing. Caritas (Latin, Greek ἀγάπη, *agápē)* nursing aims to encourage the integration of care based on a holistic approach to nursing, where love and human-to-human connectedness is paramount (Martinsen 2006; Watson 2009; Thorup et al. 2012; Alvsvåg 2014; Lindström et al. 2014). The offer of love, charity, caring and compassion is the basis of Caritas in nursing. Within the concept of Caritas prescencing (being available) is paramount (Lindström et al. (2014). These concepts link to other concepts highlighted in health care, for example, compassionate engagement (NHS England 2021; Wattis et al. 2017), intelligent kindness (Ballat and Campling 2011), person-centred care (NHS England 2020). They also connect to the description of spiritually competent practice discussed in Chap. 2.

Love is not a prominent term in the nursing literature and may evoke conflicting thoughts and emotions for an APN. However, in the context of spirituality and healthcare the consideration of *agape* love, which is viewed as being *"unconditional"* based upon compassionate care for another, is fundamental to holistic care (Gordon et al. 2011; Clarke 2013). *Agape* is a Greek term (similar to the Hebrew *Chesed* meaning loving-kindness) denoting practical love, not something APNs should be fearful of, or run away from (Robinson et al. 2003; Gordon et al. 2011; Clarke 2013). It isn't *Eros* love which is romantic and sexual; *Agape* love is the basis of how we relate human-to-human (Clarke 2013).

Spirituality is entwined with love and relationship (Young and Koopsen 2011). Helming (2009) suggests that many APNs become nurses because of a vocational sense of love and care for others. APNs may feel called to compassion in alleviating human suffering which she terms *"spiritual work"* (Helming 2009). Stevens Barnum (2011) recognises that we have one *"medicine"* free to offer all our patients, which is *"love"*. I will never forget the first time I heard a nurse talk about love in terms of clinical practice. It was at a large medical conference where a Nordic nurse talked about what she believed is needed to revolutionise healthcare. The audience was a mix of medics and nurses and at the start of her presentation there was more than 200 people in the room. The audience appeared engaged as she talked about the demands of healthcare and research into the challenge's healthcare faces. She then moved on to discuss the need to fundamentally revise how we provide healthcare. She began to talk about how we needed to ensure love was at the centre of the care we provided. Once she started talking about love many of my medical colleagues got up and walked out of the session. For me, the presentation was incredibly powerful and insightful. She explained how throughout her career she had become a well-recognised nursing scholar, as well as advancing her clinical career. She had written widely on the application of nursing theories into practice. She talked of being careful about how she presented her work to ensure it fitted into the socio-political contexts of the time. However, she recognised that she had avoiding talking about the central tenet of her work because of how it would be received. This central tenet was "love" and for me it is a fundamental principle of spirituality and caritative caring. I wanted to highlight this point as I believe that compassionate love is fundamental to the way APNs should practice. It reminds us that we are fellow human beings who are navigating this life journey together and deserve care based upon love. Interestingly, I spoke to some of my medical colleagues over dinner and asked why they walked out of this session. Their answer was that there felt that there was no science to back this up and they felt that caring too much would make it harder for them to make clinical decisions about treatments and resources which may be limited. Christina Puchalski, a palliative care and internal medicine doctor and an international leader in spiritual care, has implemented major changes across medical education in the USA which challenges these views. Her work focuses on helping doctors recognise that compassion is an act of love which is at the heart of spiritual care, this has led to the "Call for Action" to develop healthcare systems that are based upon compassion and spirituality (Puchalski et al. 2014).

Working with compassion and spirituality means that our patients can be heard and respected in all aspects of their care (Treloar 2000; Ellis and Campbell 2004; Holmes et al. 2006; Hubbell et al. 2006; Helming 2009). Walker et al. (2007) suggests that APNs bring together the best of nursing and medicine to work holistically and provide the best possible care to their patients. I highlight the need for APNs to be careful not to embrace a biomedical model in their practice as this can often leave our patients feeling unheard and uncared for (Rogers 2016), a view echoed by other clinicians (Royal College of Psychiatry 2015). APNs need to focus on the bio-psycho-social- spiritual model to ensure patients remain the focus on their care (McCormack and McCance 2017; Sulmasy 2002).

5.2   Availability (Fig. 5.1)

Availability is defined as being free, present or ready (Merriam-Webster Dictionary 2020). Being available is key to APN practice and is taught early on in our training. The skills of being open and listening to patients to hear their story/concerns/presenting complaint often starts at the beginning of a consultation with an opening question, "how can I help?" (Neighbour 1987). We then listen as they identify their need/s or concern/s. APN education often focuses on being able to assess, diagnose and manage a wide range of presenting conditions. Maintaining a consultation approach which is holistic and not focused purely on the biomedical aspects is more likely to address the person's need/s and/or concern/s (Neighbour 1987). Rogers (2016) found that APNs recognise that working holistically, and not just addressing the presenting complaint, leads to a deeper relationship and a focus on person-centred care. Patients identify that they value the APN who is able to be fully present and willing to truly listen and empathise with them. Brown (2013) identifies key differences between empathy and sympathy pointing out that sympathy is about feeling for someone, whilst empathy is about true connection where you connect to the emotion someone is feeling. Creating a safe place for patients to talk about their concerns without judgement is viewed by APNs as an important aspect of APN's availability. In addition, practicing with kindness, compassion and empathy are all viewed as essential aspects of spirituality and holistic care. Rogers (2016) also found that to work in this way APNs needed to be self-aware, self-accepting and willing to engage in supervision as working in this way can lead to burn out. There is often a need for the flexing of professional boundaries in order to provide person-centred care, for example, sharing an aspect of our self to connect with those in our care as a fellow human rather than the historic hierarchy of the nurse-patient relationship which often places the nurse in a paternalistic position. Any sharing should be within our professional codes of conduct. An example could be sharing we have children which may reassure a mum who comes to see us worried about their child, or when recommending mindfulness to help reduce stress and anxiety by letting the patient know we found it helpful ourselves. These simple examples bring person-centred care to the fore and may help our patients see us as fellow humans. A key to sharing in this way is maintain the focus always being about the person in our care and utilised as a way of building therapeutic, never about making the consultation about ourselves.

Availability has several different aspects when thinking about the APN role: physical availability, emotional availability and vocational availability. All of them are important for enabling spirituality to be addressed and supported in clinical practice. Several authors link recognition of spirituality with holistic APN approaches where patients are welcomed, heard, valued and cared for (Treloar 2000; Hubbell et al. 2006; Helming 2009; Carron and Cumbie 2011).

5.2.1 Physical Availability

Physical availability is one of the basics of APN practice in that patients normally would have a face-to-face interaction with us during a consultation or interaction. However, physical availability is more than just being with our patient in a room. It involves choosing to be hospitable and welcoming, ensuring that we listen with empathy showing our patients that we value them as a person. Nouwen (1973) suggests that hospitality is part of perceiving that our work is as act of service to another which connects with the vocational nature of work as an APN. Nouwen (1973), p. 65) also states that "hospitality is a fundamental attitude towards our fellow human beings" and that it had the power to help professionals "retain their humanity" in their work. Although during this past year through the global pandemic of Covid-19 we may have changed our practice to remote ways of working we can still choose to be hospitable in our consultation approach.

Practicing physical availability through hospitality and welcome can help APNs bring spirituality into every consultation/interaction. How we welcome somebody in the first moment of contact is an opportunity for connection and is the start of whether a patient feels they can trust us to hear them and provide a safe place for them to share their deepest concerns. Rogers (2016) found that by framing a consultation simply as "*I am available and here for you*" can lead to a powerful interaction that has repercussions for the ongoing relationship between the APN and patient. The physical act of welcoming a person enables APNs to connect with many of the facets of spirituality including "*shared humanity*". Physically being with a patient and providing the context and space to understand what is happening for them is crucial to building relationship and integrating spirituality into care (Stevens Barnum 2011).

Availability, as described above, relates to what many nurses refer to as "presencing". Zerwekh (1997) suggests that presencing requires a deliberate stance of focused attention, connecting with another in awareness of our shared humanity. Sherwood (2000) suggests that presencing is an integral aspect of operationalising spirituality. Simply "being" with those in our care can help them to explore the many unanswerable questions about their illness and life. She continues by describing presencing as "one of the highest forms of human interaction", it does necessitate more than physical availability. Emotional availability is a key aspect of presencing.

5.2.2 Emotional Availability

Helming (2009) and Young and Koopsen (2011) identify that being available emotionally is important in spirituality as it helps to build relationship. This form of availability is a way APNs can facilitate trust and build rapport which may enable patients to share at a deeper level. Emotional availability appears to involve how we connect in a compassionate and empathic way, which offers hope (Rogers 2016). APNs report that being compassionate enables patients to feel safe enough to be honest and open about their presentation and concerns.

Emotional availability involves choice, intention, and potential risk, more so than physical availability which may be easier to implement. An APN can choose the level of connection with a patient though a choice to be emotionally available or not. An example from my own NP practice illustrates this.

Barry (name changed for confidentiality) was a 75-year-old man who presented to my practice in primary care. I welcomed him into my consultation room and introduced myself. I then asked the question I usually start with, "How can I help?" Barry began to explain that he had noticed that he was having diarrhoea with blood every day and felt exhausted. During a thorough assessment I discovered that he had also lost 14 kg in weight, was tired all the time and felt a little nauseous. He was managing to eat three meals a day but couldn't eat his normal intake. There was little to be found on examination apart from that he looked pale. During the assessment I talked to him about his concerns and how his symptoms were impacting him on a day-to-day level. He talked about being a carer to his wife with dementia and how he worried that should anything happen to him who would look after her. He also mentioned he didn't come any earlier as he liked to "put his head in the sand" about medical problems.

My provisional diagnosis was bowel cancer and I gently brought up this possibility. I explained that I needed to refer Barry urgently for investigations and that cancer was a possibility. Barry broke down in tears repeating that he couldn't have cancer as his wife needed him. We spent some time talking through his shock and anxieties. Barry stopped crying and asked me to talk to him about the investigations, possible treatment options and prognosis. It was here that I had a choice to be emotionally available and vulnerable with Barry or not. I could have easily told him the mechanics of the investigations and treatment, but I chose to be emotionally available. I told

Barry that my father had been diagnosed with Bowel Cancer 10 years ago having presented with very similar symptoms. I was able to share, briefly, his experiences of investigations and treatment. I was able to do this as this was not a current situation, I had personally worked through my own feelings of my father's cancer many years ago. I explained that his diagnosis may not be cancer but that being prepared for the possibility may help him manage the next few weeks of uncertainty.

Barry came back to see me 2 weeks later. He had undergone all the necessary investigations and had been told he had bowel cancer. We spoke for a long time about his feelings and his concerns. He was tearful throughout the consultation but towards the end he reached forward and took my hand. He looked me in the eyes and said it meant the world to him that I had shared my experiences with my father with him and that it had given him hope for the future.

This example of emotional availability (and vulnerability) had a positive impact; it was risky for me as a clinician as it moved away from a traditional historic approach to care involving emotional distancing. It illustrates shared humanity and a willingness to share an aspect of myself to support Barry and build trust. To practice in this way necessitated consideration and discernment. The focus must always be on the best interests or the patient and never the needs of the APN. I could share this experience with Barry because there was no emotional impact on me at this time. I chose to share the experience because of the distress and despair I witnessed when I told him that he could have cancer. It was a risk because it may not have been helpful. However, experience has taught me that a shared experience at the appropriate time can have significant positive impact for a patient.

Being able to make a choice of how and when we connect to our patients through emotional availability is important. APNs need to have excellent self-awareness skills and a willingness to have supervision to ensure working in this way is helpful to their patients. Rogers (2016) recognises that APNs are often able to be emotionally available and vulnerable when they are more self-aware and reflective about their practice. When APNs are exhausted, over-stretched or dealing with significant personal issues of their own, emotional availability becomes more limited. Rogers (2016) also found that APNs are able to recognise there are some consultations, depending on the patient and their own emotional wellbeing, where they might not be able to be emotional available. For example, one of Rogers research participants shared that returning to work after her mum had died she felt "empty" and unable to offer emotional availability until she had had time to grieve and heal. Another APN shared of a patient she felt was vulnerable, they were homeless and struggling with mental health problems and addiction. The patient always asked the APN questions about her own life, she could see that this patient was looking for a "friendship" which would be outside the professional relationship; the APN took care to still be available but limited what she shared to maintain a healthy boundary. Rogers (2016) found that APNs recognise that limiting their emotional availability may mean that the patient might be unable to share their deeper concerns. Recognising this and being able to discern when to utilise emotional availability reflects professional maturity; they were able to recognise that being emotionally available could have significant impact on them personally and professionally. Working intentionally, and using discernment, to provide emotional availability can increase hope, meaning and purpose for patients, and for APNs it connects to vocational availability.

5.2.3   Vocational Availability

Entering nursing for many of us is vocational or, as Young and Koopsen (2011) suggest, a "spiritual longing" to help heal others. Advanced practice nursing is an extension of this vocation where availability is paramount. Working autonomously and accepting the responsibility and accountability of our role can be viewed as an aspect of vocational availability (Rogers 2016). An extension of this vocation is the ability of the APN to provide holistic care which is beyond the bounds of traditional nursing practice whilst still embedded in nursing assumptions and philosophies.

Working in a way that encompasses vocational availability is often illustrated through the emotional sacrifices APNs choose to make in order to offer the best care possible. Encompassing emotional and physical availability within a vocational approach to care can have a significant positive impact on an APN connecting to their own sense of hope, meaning and purpose. Conversely it can also have the potential to lead to burn out. Professional boundaries are important to protect both patients and APNs and to ensure an ethical approach to care. There is a risk of being "*too available*" and as APNs we need to discern how much to give of ourselves, carefully flexing professional boundaries but not hiding behind professional "distance". O'Brien (2008) asserts that holistic care is the focus of vocation and that if nurses become too concerned with hiding behind the veil of professionalism spiritual care will be diminished. She suggests that there is a choice to provide service to patients which is mediated by agape love (O'Brien 2008).

Vocational availability involves the desire to help and support patients within professional boundaries. These boundaries may be moveable and at times the choice to be less physically and emotionally available could be intuitive and protective. Availability might depend on the signs being given by patients and the recognition that if we are moving away from a focus on the patient towards our own needs we need to pull back. According to Tacey (2004) self-awareness provides the necessary insights needed to maintain healthy boundaries and emotional health. Self-awareness is paramount to protect patients from dependency but also to prevent the APN giving too much of themselves leading to burnout. Knowing ourselves and being able to connect to our own spirituality appears to have a connection to how available an APN can be. King (2014) asserts that self-knowledge is needed to truly care compassionately (Fig. 5.1).

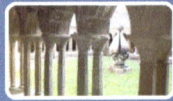
Be available to yourself in your inner life continuing as an APN to be self-reflective and self-accepting, embracing spirituality (broadly defined as understanding of one's meaning, purpose and direction in life) as key to your inner journey.

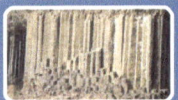
Welcome people into your care, be hospitable, offer time, acceptance and understanding whilst being truly present and listening attentively.

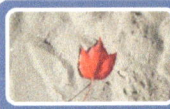
Offer care and concern to those in your care through active participation in therapeutiv relationships, creating a safe place for patients to tell their story as it is.

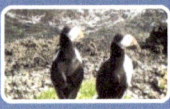
Being available and willing to develop your APN practice in response to the needs of those in your care and the community.

Fig. 5.1 Summarises availability (Rogers 2016)

5.3   **Vulnerability** (Fig. 5.2)

Vulnerability may be viewed as more contentious than availability as it is often more likely to be perceived as *"weakness"* or *"being hurt"*. The origins of vulnerability come from the Latin *"vulnerare"* to wound (Merriam-Webster Dictionary 2020). As APNs, many of us will have experienced vulnerability in this way possibly in terms of being physically put at risk by a patient but also in terms of our patients being vulnerable and at risk of being exploited or hurt. Physical vulnerability and patients' vulnerability need to be acknowledged when considering vulnerability, but are not specifically related to spirituality, though they could be. Professional and emotional vulnerability connect deeply to spirituality and are explored in this chapter, and further explored through the case studies in the following country chapters.

5.3.1   Physical Vulnerability

The impact of physical vulnerability often leaves profound anxiety. All of us working in healthcare settings will have experienced or seen events which have left them feeling physically vulnerable or at risk. Remarkably, although these events do occur, they often do not prevent us from still wanting to connect and support our patients, although they may make us more wary. The altruistic choice of still wanting to give of ourselves, despite the risks that may be faced, is laudable and connects with the vocational basis for nursing. Choosing to be present for patients will always involves an element of risk-taking. Maintaining boundaries and a safe environment are important. Contingency plans are needed when dealing with patients who may pose a physical risk.

5.3.2   Patient Vulnerability

Patients are vulnerable for many reasons when they consult an APN. They are vulnerable because they place their trust in us and share, often, very private information. They are vulnerable as they need to trust us to have the competencies and experiences to address their needs and they are vulnerable as they are often dealing with illness, stress and crises, which lower their resilience and ability to cope. APNs have to "*hold*" what patients share with them in confidence as patients don't always recognise that they are vulnerable through their sharing. We have a role in being an advocate for those in our care to ensure their best interests are paramount. Making the consultation a safe place is a necessary consideration for APNs and the acknowledgement of patients' vulnerability is important. Simply providing the gift of time, listening and being present in addition to creating a safe place enables a deeper connection to occur.

5.3.3   Professional Vulnerability

There are several aspects of professional vulnerability to consider within Rogers' (2016) framework. Firstly, the ability for the APN to recognise their own limitations and recognise they do not have all the answers. Sharing uncertainty with a patient is part of professional vulnerability and shows authenticity and courage. It opens an APN up to be challenged, but also creates an open and honest relationship where the power imbalance between APN and patient is reduced. This is not a sign of weakness, rather experience and maturity. As APNs we will never stop learning or know everything; we will always need to work collaboratively, to seek other opinions and keep updated with the constant changes in health care. Being able to recognise and have the capacity to manage professional vulnerability is part of our professional responsibility and self-awareness is needed. According to Tacey (2004), self-awareness provides the necessary insights needed to maintain healthy boundaries and emotional health. Reflection assists the process of self-awareness to develop understanding and meaning in practice (Sherwood 2000). Ballat and Campling (2011) assert that human connection demands self-awareness and take us to the heart of relationships where things can be messy, difficult, and painful. Being open to this and utilising supervision and self-reflection enhances relationship with those in our care.

Professional vulnerability is an important factor for APNs and includes how professional boundaries are maintained but also flexed appropriately. When integrating spirituality into care the issue of boundaries are significant. Rogers (2016) identified that some APNs have an unwritten moveable line in terms of boundaries which is contextual and relational where professional judgments are made in terms of flexing a boundary. This flexing of a boundary needs to be within the context of being self-aware and working within their professional code of conduct, whilst also responding to the needs of patients. There are clearly boundaries which are unethical to flex. However, boundaries relating to how APNs interact with their patients may be flexed positively in terms of professional vulnerability. This can lead to an increased depth of relationship with patients where there is a human-to-human connection that helps the patient move forward. Negative flexing of boundaries has the potential to lead to dependence from a patient and a sense that the APN had given too much. This may necessitate a pulling back to prevent burnout or a negative impact on the patient. Working through the relationship between spirituality and boundaries demands significant self-reflection and an opportunity to explore the context of boundaries. The tensions to consider within boundary flexing involve maintaining the balance of professional vulnerability between being too distant or too close and being too detached or being over-involved.

An additional consideration of professional vulnerability includes what is appropriate to share emotionally with a patient within professional boundaries. Williams (2001) suggests sharing our own life experiences with patients might be profoundly helpful for some patients, as it was for Barry. However, the choice of what to share needs to be made wisely with the patient's best interests at heart. Choosing to share something of ourselves could leave us feeling vulnerable and concerned about whether we have crossed a boundary, it could also be emotionally difficult. An example shared by an APN in my research was when she shared with a patient that she liked ceroc dancing as a way of relaxing, the patient asked some more questions about her dancing. Later that week the patient turned up to the APNs dance class and asked the APN if she would like to come to her house for dinner. The APN felt very uncomfortable, she had shared about dancing to try and help the patient recognise that finding a hobby may help her isolation. The APN declined dinner but the following week the patient came to see her and asked if she would like to go to another dance class together. The APN needed to clarify the boundaries which led to the patient becoming very upset and saying that she thought that the APN cared about her and was there for her. The patient left the consultation in tears and started to write to her regularly saying that she needed her and couldn't understand why they couldn't meet socially. The APN took this to supervision to work through how to maintain boundaries within this situation. However, it was clear that the patient was still struggling to understand the APNs perceived withdrawal and another clinician had to take over their care. I am sharing this example not to suggest not sharing but to illustrate that occasionally being available and vulnerable in this way can have a negative reaction. Alvsvåg (2014) suggests that giving of oneself should be offered with moral, practical and professional discernment. Professional/emotional distancing has historically been advocated in nursing however, it hinders deep connection. To truly offer holistic care and connect with those in our care emotional involvement is important. Professional/emotional distancing from patients is generally unhelpful as it is likely to reduce connection but in this example it was necessary.

Working as an APN is a privilege. We witness those in need and can offer our care, compassion, and empathy. Within this relationship a mutual vulnerability must be present partly due to the caring role but also shared humanity (Heaslip and Ryden 2013). As discussed earlier, boundaries may be flexed but utilising discernment can enable the APN to pull back if they feel this is unhelpful for the patient. Sherwood (2000) suggests that relationships between nurses and patients are reciprocal and that this is significant for patient healing and wellbeing. To fully connect with another there needed to be a willingness to connect with our shared humanity; this takes courage and a willingness to be emotionally vulnerable.

5.3.4   Emotional Vulnerability

Brown (2010) suggests that emotional vulnerability is about being willing to *"be seen"* authentically, to accept that it could be risky and uncertain but that it has powerful and significant impact on relationships. White (2006) recognises that spirituality has an emotional cost and if offering truly holistic care the practitioner must be prepared to realise this could be positive or negative. Rogers (2016) found that many of her participants were able to share experiences of when they had given of themselves emotionally to their patients. One participant identified that being open and using vulnerability consciously could help APNs *"reconnect with the core values of nursing and allow other aspects of our humanity to influence and guide us"*. For more detail about how this can occur Rogers and Beres (2017) wrote in depth about the experience of one APN, which illustrates a deep level of emotional vulnerability. One of the key agreements between APNs when discussing emotional vulnerability is that it should always involve choice and discernment. Young and Koopsen (2011) recognise that a deeply spiritual dimension can occur when a practitioner is willing to share something of their own life experience. I illustrated this with the experience of Barry when discussing availability, it was also an emotional vulnerable choice which could have been unhelpful for Barry and it could have resurfaced the distress I had experienced facing my dad's cancer. Nouwen (1972) states that it is impossible to help another person without becoming involved and willing to truly understand their situation. It can be risky, it can be painful, but it also reveals the depth of human connection and spirituality, which could help patients to find hope.

Despite emotional vulnerability being a way of relating authentically to a patient as a fellow human being it also demands choice and emotional energy. The desire to be real and human with those in our care can lead to excessive personal vulnerability, stress, and burnout. Burnout may be partially connected contextually with boundary issues, relationships and providing truly holistic care (White 2006). Giving too much of ourselves or being constantly available and present to patients can become draining and unsustainable. When choosing to be emotionally vulnerable burnout can be prevented by being self-aware about one's own limitations in addition to one's own needs and, of course engaging in supervision. Benner (1984) identifies that the ability to reflect on practice is key to being an expert practitioner. Finding supervision which has the balance of support and challenge is important, when successful it builds self-awareness and resilience, when not, it erodes confidence and self-belief (Reynolds and Mortimore 2021; Sharrock et al. 2013). APNs also often find informal support within the teams they work with. I found setting up a weekly coffee time with colleagues enabled us time to discuss difficult situations and learn from each other. The combination of supervision and informal support is necessary for safe and effective practice. Working in a way that is available and vulnerable necessitates being willing to be open and reflective about our practice, it leads to emotional and professional maturity and of course will benefit those in our care.

Brown (2010) wrote about vulnerability suggesting it was the birthplace of joy, love, and gratitude and that being vulnerable enables us to truly connect with another which is what human beings are hardwired to do. Her extensive research on vulnerability views it not as a weakness but as a courageous act. APNs continually show courage by turning up each day, being willing to be present and giving of themselves. Brown (2010) also suggests vulnerability without boundaries is not vulnerability. Vulnerability needs boundaries and to work in this way demands consideration of how much to give of yourself, how much you should share, how to connect deeply without losing the focus on the patient or burning out. Having boundaries connects with Rolheiser's (2004) view of not becoming a "*doormat*" by becoming so vulnerable and going to the extreme of letting every aspect of our lives "*hang out*". He suggests true vulnerability is held within the strength of being able to be present to another without the "*false props*" we often use to bolster our egos. Our need to be distant from our patient or not to share could be hidden behind a cloak of professional standards. Herrick and Mann (1998) write that being able to maintain boundaries but be fully present can lead to extraordinary freedom and connection with others and engender hope in them.

Availability and vulnerability enable APNs to operationalise spirituality. There is often overlap between the two concepts and how these are operationalised. Clinicians recognise that Rogers (2016) framework is a helpful way to operationalise spirituality with clinicians stating that it is "*absolutely essential to good practice*" (Rogers et al. 2021). Utilising availability and vulnerability links to truly holistic person-centred care. My hope is that you too will see how simple these concepts are to integrate into practice and how powerful they can be within a therapeutic relationship with those in our care (Fig. 5.2).

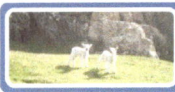 Embrace the vulnerability of the APN role and the reality that you will never 'know it all'

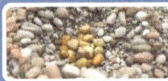 Embrace accountability: engaging in supervision, reflection and admission of mistakes. Be receptive to constructive criticism.

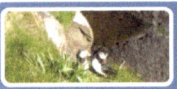 Be willing to share uncertainty with those in your care and be an advocate, if necessary questioning authority, being honest and truthful with the best interests of thosde in your care at heart.

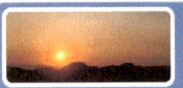 Be vulnerable and authentic in your approach to care.

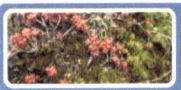 Be willing to be challenged and questioned without defensiveness

Fig. 5.2 Summarises vulnerability (Rogers 2016)

5.4 Conclusion

This chapter has introduced the concepts of availability and vulnerability as a way of operationalising spirituality. It has identified the benefits and challenges of integrating these into our practice. Fundamentally, it challenges us as APNs to be willing to work in a way which is truly holistic and person-centred. This demands our full intentional recognition of the spiritual dimension of practice which is evident in our *"human-to-human"* interactions with those in our care. Working in this way helps patients to find hope, meaning and purpose.

The following chapters illustrate global APN case studies which present stories of hope. They all include aspects of availability and vulnerability as the spiritual dimension is integrated into care. The case studies are from APNs working in a variety of settings.

References

Alvsvåg H (2014) Philosophy of caring. In: Alligood M (ed) Nursing theorists and their work, 8th edn. Elsevier, Missouri

Ballat J, Campling P (2011) Intelligent kindness: reforming the culture of healthcare. Royal College of Psychiatrists, London

Benner P (1984) From novice to expert. Addison-Wesley, Boston

Brown B (2010) The gifts of imperfection. Hazelden, Minnesota

Brown B (2013) Daring greatly: how the courage to be vulnerable transforms the way we live, love. Penguin, Parent and Lead

Carron R, Cumbie S (2011) Development of a conceptual nursing model for the implementation of spiritual care in adult primary healthcare settings by nurse practitioners. J Am Acad Nurse Pract 23:552–560

Clarke J (2013) Spiritual care in everyday nursing practice- a new approach. Palgrave, Hampshire

Cook C (2004) Addiction and spirituality. Addiction 99:531

Ellis M, Campbell J (2004) Patient's views about discussing spiritual issues with primary care physicians. South Med J 97(12):1158–1163

Gordon T, Kelly E, Mitchell D (2011) Spiritual care for health care practitioners- reflecting on clinical practice. Radcliffe, London

Heaslip V, Ryden J (2013) Understanding vulnerability. A nursing and healthcare approach. Wiley Blackwell, Chichester

Helming MA (2009) Integrating spirituality into nurse practitioner practice: the importance of finding the time. J Nurs Pract 5(8):598–598

Herrick V, Mann I (1998) Jesus wept: reflections on vulnerability in leadership. Darton, Longman & Todd, London

Holmes S, Rabow M, Dibble S (2006) Screening the soul: communication regarding spiritual concerns among primary care physicians and seriously ill patients approaching the end of life. Am J Hospice Palliative Med 23(1):25–33

Hubbell S, Woodard E, Barksdale-Brown D, Parker J (2006) Spiritual care practices of nurse practitioners in federally designated nonmetropolitan areas of North Carolina. J Am Acad Nurse Pract 18(8):379–385

King M (2014) The challenge of research into religion and spirituality. J Study Spiritual 4(2):106–120

Lindström U, Nyström L, Zetterlund J (2014) Theory of caritative caring. In Alligood M nursing theorists and their work, 8th edn. Elsevier, Missouri

Martinsen K (2006) Care and vulnerability. Akribe, Oslo

McCormack B, McCance T (2017) Person-centred practice in nursing and health care. John Wiley & Sons Ltd, Chichester

Merriam-Webster Dictionary (2020). www.merriam-webster.com. Accessed Nov 2020

Neighbour R (1987) The inner consultation. MTP, Lancaster

NHS England (2020) The comprehensive model of personalised care. https://www.england.nhs.uk/personalisedcare/comprehensive-model-of-personalised-care/. Accessed Online Feb 2021

NHS England (2021) Compassion in practice. http://england.nhs.uk/wp-content/uploads/2012/12/compassion-in-practice/pdf. Accessed Nov 2020

Northumbria Community (2020) Our rule of life. https://www.northumbriacommunity.org/who-we-are/our-rule-of-life/. Accessed Nov 2020

Nouwen H (1972) The wounded healer. Doubleday, New York

Nouwen H (1973) Reaching out. Fontana, London

O'Brien M (2008) Spirituality in nursing- standing on holy ground. Jones and Bartlett, Sudbury

Propper C, Stoye G, Zaranko B (2020) The wider impacts of coronavirus pandemic on the NHS. Institute of Fiscal Studies Briefing Note. April 2020

Puchalski CM, Vitillo R, Hull SK, Reller N (2014) Improving the spiritual dimension of whole person care: reaching national and international consensus. J Palliat Med 17(6):642–656. https://doi.org/10.1089/jpm.2014.9427

Reynolds J, Mortimore G (2021) Clinical supervision for advanced practitioners. Br J Nurs 30(7):422–424. https://doi.org/10.12968/bjon.2021.30.7.422

Robinson S, Kendrick K, Brown A (2003) Spirituality and the practice of health care. Palgrave Macmillan

Rogers M (2016) Spiritual dimensions of advanced nurse practitioner consultations in primary care through the Lens of availability and vulnerability. A Hermeneutic Enquiry. PhD, University of Huddersfield

Rogers M (2017) Utilising availability and vulnerability to operationalise spirituality. In: Practising spirituality. Palgrave Macmillan, London, p 145164

Rogers M, Beres L (2017) How two practitioners conceptualize spiritually competent practice. In: Wattis J, Curran S, Rogers M (eds) Spiritually competent practice in health care, pp 54–69. https://pure.hud.ac.uk/en/persons/melanie-rogers/publications/

Rogers M, Hargreaves J, Wattis J (2019a) Spiritual dimensions of nurse practitioner consultations in family practice. J Holist Nurs 38(1):8–18

Rogers M, Wattis J (2020) Understanding the role of spirituality in providing person-centred care. Nurs Stand 35(9):25–30. https://doi.org/10.7748/ns.2020.e11342

Rogers M, Wattis J, Khan W, Curran S (2019b) A questionnaire- based study of attitudes to spirituality in mental health practitioners and the relevance of the concept of spiritually competent practice. Int J Ment Health Nurs 28(5):1162–1172

Rogers M, Wattis J, Moser R, Borthwick R, Walters P, Rickford R (2021) Views of mental health practitioners on spirituality in clinical practice, with special reference to the concepts of spiritually competent practice, availability and vulnerability: a qualitative evaluation. J Study Spiritual 11(1):7–23. https://doi.org/10.10180/20440243.1857624

Rolheiser R (2004) The restless heart: finding our spiritual home in times of loneliness. Double Day, New York

Royal College of Psychiatry (2015) Spirituality and mental health. http://www.rcpsych.ac.uk/mentalhealthinformation/therapies/spiritualityandmentalhealth.aspx. Accessed Nov 2020

Sharrock S, Javen L, McDonald S (2013) Clinical supervision for transition to advanced practice. Perspect Psychiatr Care 49(2):118–125. https://doi.org/10.1111/ppc.12003

Sherwood G (2000) The powers of nurse-client encounters- interpreting spiritual themes. J Holist Nurs 18(2):159–175

Stevens Barnum B (2011) Spirituality in nursing: the challenges of complexity, 3rd edn. Springer Publishing, New York

Sulmasy DP (2002) A biopsychosocial-spiritual model for the care of patients at the end of life. The Gerontologist 42(suppl. 3):24–33

Tacey D (2004) The spirituality revolution: the emergence of contemporary spirituality. Brunner Routledge, Sussex

Thorup C, Rundqvist E, Roberts C, Delmar C (2012) Care as a matter of courage: vulnerability, suffering and ethical formation in nursing care. Scandinavian J Caring 26:427–435

Treloar L (2000) Integration of spirituality into health care practice by nurse practitioners. J Am Acad Nurse Pract 12(7):280–283

Walker R, Bindless L, Harrison F, Michael S, Firth J (2007) Combining the best of nursing and medical care- evaluation of the West Yorkshire nurse practitioner (primary care) development programme from 2001–2005. Yorkshire and Humber Strategic Health Authority, Leeds

Watson J (2009) Caring science and human caring theory: transforming personal and professional practices of nursing and health care. J Health Hum Serv Adm 31(4):466–482

Wattis J, Curran S, Rogers M (2017) Spiritually competent practice in health care. CRC Press, London

White G (2006) Talking about spirituality in health care practice- a resource for the multi professional health care team. Jessica Kingsley, London

Williams A (2001) The study of practicing nurses' perceptions and experiences of intimacy within the nurse-patient relationship. J Adv Nurs 35(2):188–196

Young C, Koopsen C (2011) Spirituality, health and healing- an integrated approach. Jones and Bartlett, Sudbury

Zerwekh JV (1997) The practice of Presencing. Semin Oncol Nurs 13(4):260–262

Global APN Case Studies in Spirituality-Stories of Hope from Africa

6

Christmal Dela Christmals

Abstract

This chapter presents spirituality in advanced practice nursing within the African context. Because the Advanced Practice Nurse (APN) role has only been recently formalised in a few countries in Africa, it is difficult to find a system-wide case study of the integration of spiritual aspects of care into APN consultation. As a result, the author explored individual patient encounters by APNs that involved issues of spirituality in some countries where APNs are formalised. Spirituality is part of everyday life of an African. Illness is often perceived as a form of suffering or punishment in a typical African society and is often attributed to a supernatural source. Africans are highly religious and associates spirituality with a deity (spirit). APN programmes are being established on the continent through the advocacy of various leaders and academics. It is essential that spirituality, as a component of holistic care, is built into curricula to ensure that future APNs are competent in spirituality and the provision of spiritual.

Keywords

Spirituality · Advanced practice nursing · Africa · Stories of hope

6.1 Introduction

In Chap. 1 of this book the authors describe spirituality and how it impacts Advanced Practice Nurses (APN). This chapter presents spirituality in advanced practice nursing within the African context.

C. D. Christmals (✉)
Centre for Health Professions Education, Faculty of Health Sciences, North-West University, Potchefstroom, South Africa
e-mail: christmal.christmals@nwu.ac.za

Contemporary authors (Hill et al. 2000; Hood et al. 1996; Rogers et al. 2020) have attempted the reconceptualisation of spirituality from its genesis (*spiritus, Latin origin*), which is intricately linked with a deity (spirit) (McGrath 1999; Rogers et al. 2020). They defined the concept, spirituality, as referring to "meaning, purpose, hope, and connectedness" which is mostly expressed theistically or secularly (Rogers et al. 2020). Spirituality is an essential aspect of healthcare, as forms of religion and spirituality have been established as a phenomenon capable of producing pathology and serving as an alternative treatment or coping mechanism as seen in the Amish (Hill et al. 2000; Hood et al. 1996).

Spirituality is an intangible base that underpins Africans' ontological perspectives which, in turn, drive actions and healthcare behaviour. Africans, before and after the introduction of western medicine, accessed healthcare provided by traditional healers, who shared the same cultural and spiritual beliefs as well as a common language with them (Dhamani et al. 2011; Mokgobi 2014). Western medicine is central in public healthcare in Africa, partly due to the increasing acceptance of its scientific nature and to the perceived abhorrence of traditional practices that are associated with traditional medicine practiced. Despite the strides made by western medicine in Africa, the achievement of holistic care, which encompasses spirituality and spiritual care, remains a dream. Evidence has shown that paying attention to spirituality in healthcare delivery helps the individual, family and community to cope with the disease process, especially in chronic and terminal illnesses (Dhamani et al. 2011; Olive 2004). It is recommended that patients, especially those receiving palliative care, be given access to faith healers; religious groups, leaders and services/rituals; counsellors; community support groups; complementary therapies and a quiet space in the units for personal reflections to promote spirituality (Selman et al. 2010).

6.2   The Role of the Advanced Practice Nurse in Africa

Advanced practice nursing is a fairly new concept in sub-Saharan Africa (SSA) (Christmals and Armstrong 2019b; Dlamini et al. 2018, 2020; Geyer and Christmals 2020). Several countries have instituted various APN programmes across Africa, with the support of, and in collaboration with, first world countries or institutions. According to Geyer and Christmals (2020), the development and implementation of these APN programmes encountered challenges, such as resistance from the medical profession, limited resources, regulatory inefficiencies, inability of nurses to influence national policy, and lack of context-specific benchmarks (Christmals and Armstrong 2019a; Geyer and Christmals 2020). Despite these challenges, there are positive examples from SSA regarding emerging APN roles (Christmals and Armstrong 2020; Geyer and Christmals 2020) drawing strength from the high proportion of rural population, acute shortage of medical practitioners and the inequitable distribution of health workforce in sub-Saharan Africa (Christmals et al. 2019; Dlamini et al. 2018, 2020; East et al. 2014). For example, the World Health Organisation (WHO) Regional Office for Africa (WHO/AFRO) noted that at least nine countries were already investing in APN roles. However, their requirement for appropriate remuneration, coupled with a lack of context-appropriate curricula frameworks for APN training, have limited the uptake in countries. Towards the resolution of some of these challenges, Christmals and Armstrong (2020) developed a curriculum framework to guide the development of context-specific APN curricula in SSA. Also, the Anglophone Africa Advanced Practice Nurse Coalition Project (AAAPNC) presented a proposal to the WHO/AFRO Health Systems Leadership to support the development of APN on the continent (International Council of Nurses 2020). These efforts are yielding results and may need to be intensified in advocating for APN in SSA (Christmals et al. 2019; Dlamini et al. 2018, 2020; East et al. 2014).

Even though nurses in many African countries have taken on APN roles, it is only a few countries, notably, Botswana (Family Nurse Practitioner), Ghana (Nurse Practitioner), Eswatini (Family Nurse Practitioner) and South Africa (Primary Care Nurse Specialist) that have formalised the roles for APN categories, and subsequently licensed them to practice (Christmals and Armstrong 2019a; Dlamini et al. 2020; Geyer and Christmals 2020). In some countries (for example, Seychelles, Namibia and Sierra Leone), the roles of APNs are formalised but lack local institutional capacity for training of APNs hence they rely on other countries for training. Advanced Practice Nurses serve in varying capacities in sub-Saharan Africa. In Botswana, the Family Nurse Practitioners (FNP) are licensed to provide Primary Health Care (PHC) services across hospitals, clinics, workplace, community and educational institutions—especially to the underserved rural communities where about 70% of the population dwells. In Ghana, Nurse Practitioners (NP) are trained and licensed to provide PHC services to rural and deprived communities (Christmals and Armstrong 2019a; Geyer and Christmals 2020). In the Kingdom of Eswatini, a FNP programme has been introduced to provide access to quality patient-centred care, especially for deprived rural communities (Dlamini et al. 2020). The programme was approved by the Eswatini Nursing Council which is expected to license the qualifying FNPs. The first cohort in this category graduated from the University of Eswatini in 2020.

In Eswatini the APN programme encountered some context-specific challenges. First, there were difficulties in transitioning students from the disease focused bachelor's curriculum to a family-centred health promotion APN programme. Second, it took a lot of effort to gather local texts for inclusion as these were not readily available. Third, students had difficulties completing their research projects and clinical practice hours simultaneously. Fourth, students who work in full-time jobs across the country preferred to do clinical placement at their workplace which created some challenges that needed to be resolved (Dlamini et al. 2020). Additionally, there were no masters level APNs in practice to serve as preceptors hence the need to use medical doctors who had little understanding of the FNP role but were willing to learn. There were PhD prepared academics, however they needed some clinical experience to teach in the APN programme. The programme was generally supported by all stakeholders though there were some policy challenges such as whether the FNP should report to nursing or medical leadership, improving the remuneration of the Registered Nurse post qualification as an FNP, availability of resources for the FNP and educating the health workforce and community on the role of the FNP (Dlamini et al. 2020).

6.3   How Spirituality in Health and Social Care is Viewed in Sub-Saharan Africa

Contrary to the views of many people, it is worth clarifying that, Africa is not a country but a continent of 54 countries, with thousands of cultures and languages (Woods 2019), Sub-Saharan Africa is the larger portion of Africa, mainly, to the south of the Sahara Desert. Despite the contemporary definition of spirituality, the African concept of spirituality is mainly, if not absolutely, seen through the lens of religion hence the necessity to briefly describe religion in Africa (Dhamani et al. 2011; The Harvard Gazette 2015). To affirm this view, Professor Jacob Olupona contends that: "African spirituality simply acknowledges that beliefs and practices touch on and inform every facet of human life, and therefore African religion cannot be separated from the everyday or mundane" (19, p. 2).

Before the encounter with the western colonialism, Africans have always had a monotheistic belief in the existence of a supreme being that occupied a supernatural realm, with sub-divinities and alienated spirits that were most often associated with traditional priests, witches and sorcerers (Paris 1993). Africans conceptualised life and nature as entities intricately interwoven with spirits (Lugo and Cooperman 2010; Tagwirei 2017; The Harvard Gazette 2015). Even though Christianity and Islam were in existence in sub-Saharan Africa, less than 25% of the population had embraced them by the year 1900 (Hill 2009).

Islam entered Africa through the trade between West and North Africa across the Sahara Desert, gradually converting people from African Traditional Religion through the influence of economic status, the message of Islam and the prestige of Arabic literacy. From 1900, the number of muslims in Africa south of the Sahara increased about 20-fold, to approximately 234 million in 2010. Currently, large portions of Senegal, The Gambia, Guinea, Burkina Faso, Niger, Mali, Nigeria and some east African countries are Muslim (Hill 2009).

Though Christianity was the dominant religion in Africa north of the Sahara desert in the second and third centuries, the population of Christians dwindled through wars and internal conflicts (Onyinah 2007). Christianity, however, came to sub-Saharan Africa through European missionaries (Onyinah 2007). Many attempts to proselytise traditional Africans to christianity from the fifteenth to the eighteenth centuries did not yield significant results, until missionaries from organisations such as the Basel Mission, Bremen Mission, London Missionary Society, Wesleyan Methodist Society, and various Catholic missions arrived in sub-Saharan Africa (Nkomazana and Setume 2016; Onyinah 2007). The number of Christians in Africa has grown about seventy folds that of the Muslims in Africa from 1900. Sub-Saharan Africa currently contains about 21% of the Christian population globally.

As of 2010, the population of Christians, Muslims and folk religions in sub-Saharan Africa were 62.9%, 30.2% and 3.3%, respectively. It is estimated that the

Christian population will drop to 58.5%, Muslim increase to 35.2% and folk religion decline to 3.2% by 2050 (Pew Research Center 2015). It is also observed that the practice of folk religion is dominant in rural communities where APN's are expected to expand access to quality healthcare. Providing care in a very complex religious environment demands that a APN is culturally competent, including having deep insights into the spirituality of the population served and the spiritual dimensions of healthcare.

In Africa, spiritual health needs are perceived through the expression of a patient and/or family about the need for spiritual care, or an expression of belief that witchcraft and devils are sources of disease or mortality (Dhamani et al. 2011). It is not uncommon for patients under treatment in health facilities to require the presence of their faith leaders, especially imams and pastors (priests) to pray with them during admission or treatment. Though there has been an enormous switch from traditional healthcare to western medicine, many Africans still seek care from traditional and spiritual healers. Recently, there has been a pressing call for the inclusion of indigenous knowledge systems and traditional medicine into the practice of healthcare in SSA, which some countries are piloting in selected health facilities. Also, advocates have often argued for the inclusion of indigenous knowledge systems into health professions education curricula (Dove 2010).

6.4   Integration of Spiritual Aspect of Care into APN Consultation/Interaction

It is difficult to find a system-wide case study of the integration of spiritual aspects of care into APN consultation, as the APN role has only been established recently in a few countries on the continent. As a result, the author explored individual patient encounters by APNs that involved issues of spirituality in some countries where APNs are formalised. These cases are presented from the perspective of the APNs.

6.4.1   Ghana

Conventionally, Ghanaians choose the type of care (western, herbal, psychological and spiritual) based on their family concept of causality of disease. Though the government has tried to inculcate herbal medicine and spiritual care into the western medicine (mainstream biomedical model of care), through the use of patrons, (religious leaders who are responsible for spiritual matters in clinical facilities), many Ghanaians still receive care from unregulated herbal and spiritual settings or persons. There remain concerns about the safety and scientific underpinnings of complementary medicine and indigenous knowledge systems that are included in Ghana's healthcare system (Aziato and Odai 2016). It is not uncommon for the causality of disease and disability to be associated with evil forces, especially terminal, disabling and chronic illnesses (Asare and Danquah 2017). As a result, it is very common for patients with terminal diseases to be referred to spiritualists, who are touted as the last source of hope (Opoku et al. 2018). It is, therefore, important that the APNs in Ghana pay critical attention to spirituality and spiritual care in their interaction with clients. To gain insights into what spirituality issues APNs in Ghana encounter, we contacted APNs to share their lived experiences of cases of spirituality in their practice.

6.4.1.1 The Experience of a Ghanaian APN with Mr. Abdul, a Patient with Advanced Hepatitis

Abdul (for anonymity) was a middle-aged married Muslim with three children. Abdul was a businessman in Kumasi, a city in the middle belt of Ghana, but hails from Bawku in the Upper East region of Ghana. He occasionally drank alcohol and smoked cigarettes.

Abdul reported to a health facility with swollen lower limbs, distended abdomen, and moderate jaundice. From physical assessment and further investigations, he was diagnosed with Hepatitis B. He presented advanced signs, such as hepatomegaly and anasarca with profound ascites. Abdul was admitted to hospital, near the community of residence where he was residing, for medical care.

The relatives, meanwhile, inquired of a soothsayer about why he was not being cured quickly. They were told by the soothsayer that Abdul had some misunderstanding with a friend, who cursed him by a river god. Upon hearing what the soothsayer said, the family decided to withdraw him from the hospital and send him to a known spiritual healer in his home community, whom they believed could overturn the curse. According to Abdul, although the spiritualist gave his best the condition was not improving, the spiritualist asked the family to take him back to the hospital.

I (the APN) tried to educate the family on the medical nature of the condition but realised later that they were more aligned with the soothsayer's verdict of the condition and only listened out of respect. They accepted Abdul's stay in the hospital for management. His condition improved and he was discharged on a weekly follow-up plan.

Abdul went back to the spiritualist, who gave him some herbal preparation he believed would rid the distended abdomen of its unwanted content. The preparation was later found to have a laxative effect, which resulted in excessive fluid and electrolyte loss. By the time the family rushed Abdul to the hospital, he was dead.

6.4.1.2 Putting Abdul's Case in Context: Perception of Spirituality in the Setting

There seems to be an unwritten law in the health system of Ghana that allows only Muslim and Christian spiritual leaders to attend to patients that request their services in the hospitals. This, however, makes it difficult for patients whose spirituality is not in alignment with these two religions to communicate their spiritual health needs. As a result, patients' relatives have to sneak spiritual items to such patients in the hospitals or request for discharge to visit their spiritualists. The APN stated that:

"sometimes we, the health workers, resist [prevent] patients from practising spirituality although there is no documented evidence that prevent them from doing so. I think if the family had understood us and done away with the superstition, the patient would have lived. Because there was a diagnosis of a curse by the soothsayer it left the patient at a crossroad of whether to accept healthcare or listen to the spiritualist. We were unable to convince him to see through his treatment at the hospital, hence his return to the spiritualist. Collaborative care with traditionalists is unrealisable because most of the spiritual care service providers are less educated, not registered and unrecognised, they are not able to come forth or disclose their preparations"—An APN from Ghana.

6.4.2 South Africa

Intricately linked with their past political struggles, South Africans could be described as people whose lives are enshrined in hope, meaning and purpose that cannot be separated from spirituality. The biomedical healthcare system has been very dominant, but the passing of the Traditional Health Practitioners Act (Act 22 of 2007) has enabled traditional healers to be recognised in the healthcare system (Ramgoon et al. 2011). Studies have shown that about 70% of South Africans seek various forms of care from traditional and spiritual healers (Ramgoon et al. 2011; Zuma et al. 2016). Primary Health Care Nurse Specialists (South African Nursing Council 2014) and other categories of APN must pay critical attention to spirituality and spiritual healthcare needs of their clients, especially in this context. The case study below represents such competence, as demonstrated by an APN who practises in an industrial PHC clinic.

6.4.2.1 The Experience of a South African APN in the Case of a 32-Year Old Lady B

Lady B was a 32-year-old unskilled worker with a waste management organisation in Johannesburg. She lived in one of the townships (a populated community of indigent South Africans, mostly near a city or a major town).

Lady B reported frequent seizures, so I (the APN) referred her for various examinations, including neurological assessment and a computerised tomography (CT) scan with a specialist. All the test results, including the CT scan, were negative of any physical aetiology of epilepsy.

In one of our consultation sessions, she indicated that she would like to consult a known "sangoma" (a traditional healer). I encouraged her to do so and report any findings and treatments prescribed for her to me before starting the treatment, just to be sure it is safe. She was told by the Sangoma that she is being punished by her ancestors for being a lesbian and that there is nothing medically wrong with her. Lady B believed what the Sangoma said and was ready to start treatment with her. She stopped the western medicines we prescribed for her. On her last follow-up session with me, she stated that she was getting better since the Sangoma had started treating her, citing reduced frequency of the seizures as proof.

6.4.2.2 Perception of Spirituality within the Context of Lady B Case

The APN stated that she believes that God can heal anything and hence did not have a problem with her patients if they believed in anything that helps them. She does educate them on the pros and cons of all the medicines and allows them to make their choices. She stated that

> "Knowing well that some of the spiritualists or traditional healers who present themselves as a source of hope and healing are charlatans, profiteering in the name of a supreme being and at the expense of the innocent patients desperately looking for help, I normally do ask my patients to take the spiritual treatment simultaneously with the orthodox medication knowing that they will receive medical healing from our orthodox medications while keeping their spirit in hope. This I do with caution, knowing that some of the traditional preparations may interact with the orthodox medications"—An APN from South Africa.

The South African context presents a complex environment with varying quality of healthcare and profound economic gaps and inequality on the basis of race and ethnicity (Rispel 2016), creating a tense political and racial atmosphere, requiring spirituality and spiritual care to cope with. The APN who provides care in the community must be aware of the particular spiritual needs of the patient, especially if they contract chronic diseases such as HIV/AIDS.

6.4.3 Kingdom of Eswatini

The state of despondency inflicted on many people and families in the Kingdom of Eswatini, by the levels of poverty and the heavy burden of HIV/AIDS-related complications and deaths, make spirituality and spiritual care an essential aspect of healthcare in the country (van Wyngaard 2013). Spiritual care has been integrated into the Essential Health Care Package (Magagula 2017) of the Kingdom, but only under palliative care. Though spirituality plays a role in healthcare for all conditions and levels of care, one cannot underestimate its role in caring for people living with incurable diseases (Selman et al. 2010). There are some organisations, such as Shiselweni Home-Based Care (SHBC), that provide holistic care, including spiritual healthcare to people living with HIV/AIDS in the poorer regions of the Kingdom (van Wyngaard 2013). The people of the Kingdom of Eswatini believe in ancestors as custodians of the life, culture and death. The belief in reward and punishment from ancestors for one's behaviour and adherence to cultural practices underpins the lifestyle of a traditional Eswatini, albeit Christianity has taken root in the Kingdom since its introduction in the 1840s by the Methodist church.

6.4.3.1 The Experience of an APN in Eswatini in the Case of Hlengiwe, a 50-Year Old with HIV and Tuberculosis

Hlengiwe (name changed for anonymity), a 50-year-old female, was referred from a health centre to a hospital, in the Kingdom of Eswatini, where I (the APN) currently work. She was a grade 8 leaver, unemployed and dependent on her husband who worked in the coal mines in South Africa. According to the referral notes, she reported to a health centre, where she was diagnosed with pulmonary tuberculosis (TB) secondary to HIV infection. She was also a known hypertensive. She was referred to our hospital because the health centre did not have a TB ward for admission. She went home for 2 months before coming to our hospital with the referral notes. She was bedridden with pressure ulcers on the knees and toes. She was on the TB treatment for 2 months, antiretroviral therapy (ART) for 8 years and antihypertensives for 9 years.

One day, while I was on Ward rounds, she said she wanted to talk to me. I made time during lunch to listen to her. She said she had a secret that had been haunting her for 30 years. She said three of her kids were not from her husband. She said she could remember the father and surname of only two of her three children. She wanted me to call her a pastor so that she could confess to him/her before disclosing the news to the elder son, who was a soldier. I arranged for the hospital Christian fellowship leader to see her. He spoke with her and prayed with her. She then sent for the son, who came with his sister to see their mother. The fellowship leader gave them space to have a private conversation. Because of the nature of the conversation we watched closely from a distance in case there was any physical aggression. They concluded their meeting and the son left. She told the fellowship leader that the son had forgiven her. The patient became critically ill and died 2 days after meeting with her son.

6.4.3.2 Perception of Spirituality within the Context
The APN interpreted this case as follows:

> "In Eswatini, most people believe in God and their ancestors. We hold the belief that no one dies peacefully if they have some secrets which need to be told. Even though the people are mostly Christians, they have traditional upbringings, which they continue to uphold. It is believed that if the mother did not tell the children about their true lineage, it would haunt the children and their generations because the ancestors who are supposed to watch over them will not recognise them"—An APN from Eswatini.

6.5   Discussion

This section discusses spirituality and spiritual care in SSA in light of Rogers' Availability and Vulnerability framework for Operationalising Spirituality (Rogers 2016; Rogers et al. 2020). It flows from case studies that contend that spirituality within the African context has not transcended the boundaries of religion and cultural practice to integrate the "secular" as defined by Cook (2004).

6.5.1   Availability

Being available to oneself, the patient and community are essential in recognising personal values and understanding the needs of the patient and community through asking and listening. The practitioner needs to create an atmosphere of trust and safety within which the patient or community can share their problems openly. The patient should be engaged in a way that portrays that the practitioner is physically, emotionally and professionally present to ensure the patient feels heard, respected and cared for (Rogers et al. 2020).

The cases from Ghana, South Africa and the Kingdom of Eswatini indicate that the APNs understood the patients' values and context of spirituality. It can also be deduced that their understanding of spirituality was limited to their traditional and mainly, religious context. The APN from South Africa, however, exhibited the application of a broader understanding of spirituality in saying that anything (to mean, not limited to religion or tradition) that helped the patient was important (Rogers et al. 2020).

Caring in the African context requires carers (usually family members) to be present, empathetic and share some connectedness with the patient (Paris 1993). APNs translate the African culture of caring and connectedness into the practice environment. The APNs were physically, emotionally and professionally present with the patients and their families. In all the cases presented above, the APNs took time to engage with, listen to and care for the patient in a safe atmosphere; this is the only reason why very personal issues and secrets held for many years by the patients were shared with the APN. The element of trust, however, seemed to be absent in the case of Abdul from Ghana as he and his family resorted to spiritualist without involving the practitioner.

6.5.2   Vulnerability

A typical issue of APN vulnerability among the cases presented is that from Eswatini, where the patient had communicable diseases that put the APN at risk. The APN was also at risk of community outburst and aggression from the children of the patient who were invited to listen to their mother. Had they not accepted the news in good faith, a form of aggression was likely, which could be directed towards anybody present representing the risk of physical vulnerability. That notwithstanding, the APN chose to be emotionally vulnerable in their interactions with the patient and provided holistic care to the patient. This was evident in the APN being willing to share the pain and suffering the patient verbalised by the secret that was being kept. The APN was able to show empathy and a non-judgmental approach in their care. All the patients in the case studies were suffering from incurable diseases, which made the practitioners vulnerable - lacking the power to change circumstances and choosing to connect with their patients. The Nurse Practitioner from Ghana acknowledged that the medical team were not sufficiently convincing in educating the patient and family about the aetiology of the disease, hence the family resorted to the spiritualist after the patient's discharge from hospital. The APN in South Africa referred the patient to specialist care, which indicated the recognition of professional vulnerability, and allowed the patient to consult the Sangoma on agreed terms.

The patients were very vulnerable as they were at a stage where they understood that any hope of getting back to living a normal life, without continuous dosages of chronic medications, was not possible. They relied on trust in the health professionals to guide and help them make meaningful decisions. In Ghana, the patient and family put their last hope in the spiritualist to reverse the curse that made the patient sick; this exposed the patient to any form of practice or medication that the spiritualist provided, finally leading to complications and ultimately death. The patients also shared personal information and deep secrets kept for many years with the practitioners. These secrets, if revealed to society, could lead to a social stigma that could smear the family for many generations. It is the duty of the practitioners to recognise such trust the patient have in them and be professional and ethical in dealing with patient information.

6.5.3 Ethical Considerations

Protection of personal information through strict adherence to ethical principles; autonomy, confidentiality, dignity and privacy, formed the foundation of the data and cases reported in this Chapter (Bos 2020). The participants in this study were fully informed and voluntarily agreed about the use of data in this book chapter. The author used pseudonyms to represent both the practitioners and the patients as agreed to ensure their rights, dignity, privacy is protected (Bos 2020; Staunton et al. 2021).

Regarding spiritual care, Sulmasy (2012) listed 'patient-centredness, holism, discretion, accompaniment, and tolerance' as key ethical principles that must be adhered to. In all the cases presented, the APNs adhered to all these principles, for example, in the case of South Africa, the practitioner tolerated the patient's discretion in seeking spiritual care and cooperated with her. She followed-up with the patient is protected from any form of scam or danger. Likewise, in the Kingdom of Eswatini, the practitioner invited the Christian fellowship leader upon the request of the patient. Due to the level of connectedness of oneself to the object of hope and sensitive nature spirituality, Advanced Practice Nurses must endeavour to adhere to the core ethical requirements when providing care for their clients, even if their believe system contradicts that of the practitioner.

6.6 Conclusion

Spirituality is part of everyday life of an African person. Illness is often perceived as a form of suffering or punishment in a typical African society and is often attributed to a supernatural source. Africans are highly religious and view spirituality as associated with a deity (spirit).

Advanced practice nursing is developing on the continent, with efforts from various leaders and academics across the continent. It is essential that spirituality, as a component of holistic care, is built into curricula to ensure that future APNs have a full understanding of spirituality and spiritual care and how Rogers' Availability and Vulnerability framework for Operationalising Spirituality could be fully implemented in their practice.

References

Asare M, Danquah SA (2017) The African belief system and the patient's choice of treatment from existing health models-the case of Ghana. Acta Psychopathol 3(4:49):1–4. https://doi.org/10.4172/2469-6676.100121

Aziato L, Odai PNA (2016) Exploring the safety and clinical use of herbal medicine in the contemporary Ghanaian context: a descriptive qualitative study. J Herbal Med 2016. https://doi.org/10.1016/j.hermed.2016.11.002

Bos J (2020) Confidentiality. In: Research ethics for students in the social sciences. Springer International Publishing, pp 149–173. https://doi.org/10.1007/978-3-030-48415-6_7

Christmals CD, Armstrong SJ (2019a) The essence, opportunities and threats to advanced practice nursing in sub-Saharan Africa: a scoping review. Heliyon 5(10). https://doi.org/10.1016/j.heliyon.2019.e02531

Christmals CD, Armstrong SJ (2019b) The essence , opportunities and threats to Advanced Practice Nursing in Sub-Saharan Africa: A scoping review. Heliyon 5:1–21. (e02531). https://doi.org/10.1016/j.heliyon.2019.e02531

Christmals CD, Armstrong SJ (2020) Curriculum framework for advanced practice nursing in sub-Saharan Africa: a multimethod study. BMJ Open 10(6):e035580. https://doi.org/10.1136/bmjopen-2019-035580

Christmals CD, Crous L, Armstrong SJ (2019) The development of concepts for a concept-based advanced practice nursing (child health nurse practitioner) curriculum for sub-Saharan Africa. Int J Caring Sci 12(3):1410–1422. www.internationaljournalofcaringsciences.org

Cook CCH (2004) Addiction and spirituality. Addiction 99(5):539–551. https://doi.org/10.1111/j.1360-0443.2004.00715.x

Dhamani KA, Paul P, Olson JK (2011) Tanzanian nurses understanding and practice of spiritual care. ISRN Nursing 2011:1–7. https://doi.org/10.5402/2011/534803

Dlamini CP, Kaplan L, Stuart-Shor E, Mathunjwa-Dlamini TR (2018) Report on the landscape assessment of readiness to introduce the family nurse practitioner role in Swaziland. http://seedglobalhealth.org/wp-content/uploads/2018/11/Landscape-Assessment-Report-Final.pdf

Dlamini CP, Khumalo T, Nkwanyana N, Mathunjwa-Dlamini TR, Macera L, Nsibandze BS, Kaplan L, Stuart-Shor EM (2020) Developing and implementing the family nurse practitioner role in Eswatini: implications for education, practice, and policy. Ann Glob Health 86(1):1–10. https://doi.org/10.5334/aogh.2813

Dove N (2010) A return to traditional health care practices. J Black Stud 40(5):823–834

East LA, Arudo J, Loefler M, Evans CM (2014) Exploring the potential for advanced nursing practice role development in Kenya: a qualitative study. BMC Nurs 13(1):33. https://doi.org/10.1186/s12912-014-0033-y

Geyer N, Christmals CD (2020) Advanced practice nursing in Africa. In: Hassmiller SB, Pulcini J (eds) Advanced practice nursing leadership: a Global perspective. Springer, pp 63–76. https://link.springer.com/chapter/10.1007/978-3-030-20550-8_6

Hill M (2009) The spread of Islam in West Africa: containment, mixing, and reform from the eighth to the twentieth century. http://www.metmuseum.org/toah/ht/08/sfw/ht08sfw.htm

Hill PC, Pargament KI, Hood RW, Mccullough ME, Swyers JP, Larson DB, Zinnbauer BJ (2000) Conceptualizing religion and spirituality: points of commonality, points of departure. J Theory Soc Behav 30(1):51–77. https://doi.org/10.1111/1468-5914.00119

Hood RWJ, Spilka B, Hunsberger B, Gorsuch R (1996) The psychology of religion: an empirical approach, 2nd edn. Guilford Press, New York. PsycNET

International Council of Nurses (2020) International Council of Nurses Guidelines on Advanced Practice Nursing 2020. https://www.icn.ch/system/files/documents/2020-04/ICN_APN_Report_EN_WEB.pdf

Lugo L, Cooperman A (2010). Tolerance and tension: Islam and Christianity in Sub-Saharan Africa. www.pewforum.orgi

Magagula SV (2017) A case study of the Swaziland Essential Health Care Package. https://equinetafrica.org/sites/default/files/uploads/documents/SwazilandEHBcasestudyrepfinal2017pv.pdf

McGrath AE (1999) Christian spirituality: an introduction, 2nd edn. Blackwell Publishers, New York

Mokgobi MG (2014) Understanding traditional African healing. Afr J Phys Health Educ Recreat Dance 20(Suppl 2):24–34. http://www.ncbi.nlm.nih.gov/pubmed/26594664

Nkomazana F, Setume S (2016) Missionary colonial mentality and the expansion of Christianity in Bechuanaland. J Study Relig 2(October 2015):29–55

Olive KE (2004) Religion and spirituality: important psychosocial variables frequently ignored in clinical research. South Med J 97(12):1152–1153. https://doi.org/10.1097/01.SMJ.0000146496.36652.54

Onyinah O (2007) African Christianity in the twenty-first century. Word World 27(3):305–314

Opoku JK, Manu E, Antwi EKE (2018) Spirituality and healing: perceptions and implications on the Akan of Ghana. Adv Soc Sci Res J 5(8):566–579. https://doi.org/10.14738/assrj.58.5042

Paris P (1993) The spirituality of African peoples. J Black Theol South Afr 7(2):114–124. https://disa.ukzn.ac.za/sites/default/files/pdf_files/BtNov93.1015.2296.007.002.Nov1993.6.pdf

Pew Research Center (2015) The future of world religions: population growth projections, 2010–2050. Pew Research Center. https://www.pewforum.org/2015/04/02/religious-projections-2010-2050/

Ramgoon S, Dalasile NQ, Paruk Z, Patel CJ (2011) An exploratory study of trainee and registered psychologists' perceptions about indigenous healing systems. S Afr J Psychol 41(1):90–100

Rispel L (2016) Analysing the progress and fault lines of health sector transformation in South Africa. South Afr Health Rev 2016(1):1–23

Rogers M (2016) Spiritual dimensions of advanced nurse practitioner consultations in primary care through the Lens of availability and vulnerability. A hermeneutic enquiry. University of Huddersfield. http://eprints.hud.ac.uk/id/eprint/28469/

Rogers M, Hargreaves J, Wattis J (2020) Spiritual dimensions of nurse practitioner consultations in family practice. J Holist Nurs 38(1):8–18. https://doi.org/10.1177/0898010119838952

Selman L, Harding R, Agupio G (2010) Spiritual care recommendations for people receiving palliative care in sub-Saharan Africa With special reference to South Africa and Uganda. http://www.apca.org.ug

South African Nursing Council. (2014). Competencies for primary care nurse specialist. https://www.sanc.co.za/pdf/Competencies/SANC Competencies-Primary Care Nurse Specialist.pdf

Staunton C, Adams R, Botes M, de Vries J, Labuschaigne M, Loots G, Mahomed S, Loideain NN, Olckers A, Pepper MS, Pope A, Ramsay M (2021) Enabling the use of health data for research: developing a POPIA code of conduct for research in South Africa. South African Journal of Bioethics and Law 14(1):33. https://doi.org/10.7196/SAJBL.2021.v14i1.740

Sulmasy DP (2012) Ethical principles for spiritual care. In: *Oxford textbook of spirituality in healthcare*. Oxford University Press, Oxford, pp 465–470. https://doi.org/10.1093/med/9780199571390.003.0062

Tagwirei C (2017) The "horror" of African spirituality. Res Afr Lit 48(2):22–36. https://doi.org/10.2979/reseafrilite.48.2.03

The Harvard Gazette (2015) The spirituality of Africa. The Harvard Gazette. https://news.harvard.edu/gazette/story/2015/10/the-spirituality-of-africa/

Woods J (2019) Africa is not a country and other things you need to know about the continent. Heifer International. https://www.heifer.org/blog/africa-is-not-a-country-and-other-things-you-need-to-know-about-the-continent.html

van Wyngaard A (2013) Addressing the spiritual needs of people infected with and affected by HIV and AIDS in Swaziland. J Soc Work End Life Palliat Care 9:226–240. https://doi.org/10.1080/15524256.2013.794064

Zuma T, Wight D, Rochat T, Moshabela M (2016) The role of traditional health practitioners in Rural KwaZulu-Natal, South Africa: generic or mode specific? BMC Complement Altern Med 16(1). https://doi.org/10.1186/s12906-016-1293-8

Global APN Case Studies in Spirituality-Stories of Hope from Israel

7

Caryn Scheinberg Andrews and Abby Kra-Friedman

Abstract

Israel is a country with deep religious roots. Many laws, major life events, and secular rituals are influenced by religion and religious values. Spiritual care in advanced practice nursing is about forming connection with patients at many levels of care in order to influence health. Rogers' Availability and Vulnerability framework offers a guide for culturally competent spiritual care for advanced practice nurses. In this chapter, we will describe the brief history of Advanced Practice Nurses (APN) in Israel and our experience integrating spiritual care into our own practice. Using two case studies we will show how Rogers' Framework guides our spiritual care practice in APN education and in-hospital midwifery care.

Keywords

Spirituality · Advanced practice nursing · Middle east

7.1   Introduction

This chapter provides a brief overview of the history of Advanced practice nursing in Israel and describes the current status of spiritual care in the health care culture. We describe two case studies that illustrate how two Advanced Practice Nurses

C. S. Andrews (✉)
Advanced Practice Nursing, MSN Program, Hebrew University School of Nursing at the Faculty of Medicine, Jerusalem, Israel

A. Kra-Friedman
Women's Health Nursing, BSN Program, Hebrew University School of Nursing at the Faculty of Medicine, Jerusalem, Israel

Duquesne University School of Nursing, Pittsburgh, PA, USA

integrate spirituality into APN education and patient care and conclude with a discussion of how to utilise Rogers' Availability and Vulnerability (A&V) framework to provide culturally competent spiritual care in our deeply religious country.

7.2   Advanced Practice Nursing in Israel

Israel's socialised medical system is considered to be among the most advanced in the world, and in 2020 was ranked number five on the Bloomberg Health Care Efficiency Index (Miller and Lu 2020). All Israeli citizens are entitled to access to a wide range of services at little to no cost as mandated by the National Health Insurance Law of 1995. It is estimated that nurses comprise 50% of the healthcare workforce and in Israel nurses provide basic services in Primary Care clinics at the four major national health maintenance organisations. Yet, despite a documented Primary Care Physician shortage, Advanced Practice Nurses (APN) are not widely accepted in the mainstream Israeli healthcare culture (Aaron and Andrews 2016).

In 2009, Israel introduced the first specialty APN role in palliative care (Collett et al. 2019). In 2013 four other specialties—diabetes, geriatrics, neonatal intensive care (NICU), and surgical intensive care (SICU)—were legalised for hospital-based APN practice. The Ministry of Health Division of Nursing named this level of nursing "Achot Mumchit", translated into English, "Expert Nurse". This translation has been responsible for many issues related to the role such as being considered an expert in nursing instead of advanced practice nursing with expanded roles and privileges (Aaron and Andrews 2016) and is possibly responsible for the conflict regarding the role in the healthcare system.

Up until 2013, the certification process required a post-basic certificate course, and the role was not associated with a master's degree. With the introduction of clear guidelines in 2013, APNs were required to have a master's degree, but not necessarily in nursing (Nohal Expert Nurse 2013). During this time, many were grandfathered into the role (due to years of experience on the job) and were allowed to be considered for the new role without actually obtaining the credentials now recognised as required for APN practice. The basic pillars of APN clinical education - physical assessment, pathophysiology, and pharmacology - had not previously been part of the education trajectory (Israel Ministry of Health 2020). While these nurses used the APN title, they lacked the required education and overall knowledge of the scope of practice for Nurse Practitioners (Aaron and Andrews 2016; Andrews & Kra-Friedman 2021).

Since 2018, a nursing master's is required to certify as an APN (Ministry of Health 2019). However, only one college (differentiated from university) in Israel offers a master's degree with an incorporated APN certificate course for both geriatrics and palliative care. Unfortunately, many graduates from these programmes have returned to their previous registered nurse positions on the wards because of lack of job opportunities in the healthcare system.

In 2020, the Henrietta Szold Hadassah Hebrew University School of Nursing at the Faculty of Medicine (where we both teach), received approval for their MA programme to be officially recognised as a Master's of Science in Nursing (MSN) degree in advanced clinical nursing. The curriculum follows ICN international guidelines for advanced practice nursing education (ICN 2020). It includes core courses of theory and clinical practice: advanced physical assessment, pathophysiology, pharmacology, and extensive articulation of the advanced practice role in Israel and in the world. A mandatory module on spiritual care in advanced practice has been incorporated into the curriculum for all master's students (Andrews 2020). In Israel midwives can access our MSc programme and are recognised as APNs, this is similar to the APN model in the United States of America. In 2016, two immigrant Family Nurse Practitioners (FNP) tried to tackle the implementation and integration of FNPs with an academic approach. After an extensive review of the literature and analysis of the APN role in more than 50 countries, they presented their findings to the Israel Health Policy Conference in Jerusalem (2016) and then subsequently published their findings. Aaron and Andrews (2016) recommended an expansion of new and existing APN roles to support the physician shortage. Despite their findings, the notion of integrating NPs in the healthcare culture in Israel has been very slow, and to date only the aforementioned subspecialties are allowed to practice (Collett et al. 2019).

In 2018, the Ministry of Health introduced a plan to integrate the Family Nurse Practitioner (FNP) into the community Primary Health Care system. The plan met the goals of the World Health Organization (WHO) for increasing primary care providers in the community to address population health needs outside of the hospital setting. This would be the first time that nurses were given this level of independence. After major opposition from the Israeli Medical Association, the plan was withdrawn for further evaluation (Siegel-Itzkovich 2018; Efrati 2018; Maslow 2018). In November, 2020 the Ministry of Health announced it would be moving forward with the "expert nurse in the community" (FNP) (personal correspondence, Goldberg 2020). However, the criteria for expanding the FNP role in the healthcare system is still not transparent.

Literature on NPs in Israel is scarce. In a 2018 study, researchers found a serious lack of familiarity with the role in community clinics. Community nurses working in the socialised medical system were wary of the scope of practice set out in the initial plan for FNP integration (Dickman et al. 2018). Still, there is progress. One Health Maintenance Organization initiated a programme to train FNPs in an international programme and integrate them into the Primary Health Care system. As of publication there are 11 FNPs working in community clinics (personal correspondence, Andrews, November 2, 2020) and several hundred APNs practicing in hospitals all over Israel (personal correspondence Gottesman, November 2, 2020).

Whether hospital-based or community practice, APNs in the community have been shown to bring added value to the Israeli healthcare system (Nissanholtz-Gannot and Shapiro 2020). Using the advanced training in pathophysiology, pharmacology and physical assessment, APNs provide holistic care and prove competency in addressing the physical, emotional, spiritual needs of patients and families (APRN Consensus Work Group 2008).

7.3   Israel's Religious Culture

While individual communities have their own belief and value systems and different frameworks for incorporating spirituality, Israel is a religion-based state. Legislature is driven by Jewish laws and values. State marriage, conversion, abortion and burial laws are all based on traditional Jewish law. The population is made up of Jewish (74%), Muslim (17.8%), Christian (2%), Druze (1.6%), and other groups such as Samaritanism, Baha'i and religiously unaffiliated (4%) (Israel Central Bureau of Statistics 2019). Most people polarise to one of these religions to find their religious connections. There is clear distinction by level of religiosity, as well. For example, even within the Jewish population, people group together according to the Ultra-Orthodox (very religious), Modern Orthodox, Traditional (moderate), Non-traditional, and Secular. It is interesting to note that among Jews, for example, despite the level of religiosity, most life cycle events related to birth, coming of age (12–13), marriage, and death are still celebrated in traditional ceremonies in line with traditional Jewish culture.

7.4   Spirituality in Israeli Health Care Culture

In Israel, the idea of spiritual care is just evolving (Bentur and Resnizky 2010). Jewish religious leaders called Rabbis are employed in hospitals and care centres to guide and support administration, staff, and patients to uphold Jewish law, not to provide spiritual care. Community Rabbis may come to visit the sick or administer spiritual care as part of their synagogue-based role, but patients unaffiliated with a specific synagogue or religious group are not exposed to this type of spiritual support.

Israeli society embraces the religious aspect of culture. The concept of a non-denominational spiritual perspective that embraces multi-culturalism does not really exist in healthcare. Spiritual care education in nursing is evolving. Up until very recently the idea of chaplaincy and non-religious spiritual care providers did not exist in Israeli hospitals. In response to a growing need for a "neutralistic" non-religious perspective in patient care an organisation called Life's Door-Tishkofet (2020) (Hebrew for "perspective") was formed through a very large grant to provide education to healthcare practitioners to function as spiritual caregivers (Bentur and Resnizky 2009). They call it "hope-based support". In addition, since 2004, one hospital in Jerusalem offers "in-Spirit Care" through its palliative care services, providing spiritual support to patients on their cancer journey. They staff a volunteer chaplaincy service trained specifically to address the spiritual care needs of patients, for what they call "spiritual care loneliness" (Shaare Tzedek 2020).

It is important to recognise that, specifically in Israel, spiritual care may be addressed by many healthcare professionals because of the religion-based culture. Bedside nurses are in a unique position to give spiritual care because of the avail-ability and vulnerability that Rogers and Wattis (2019) describes during a health crisis. Rogers' (2016) framework focuses specifically on the skills of the APN which demonstrate a holistic approach to primary care. Spiritual concerns during health crises in the community setting can be directly addressed by the APN. The focus on understanding the patient as a holistic being means APNs can offer spiritual care at a higher level than bedside nurses. Moreover, as advanced practice nursing evolves in Israel there is a question of how care provided by an APN care is different from nurses and other allied healthcare professionals. As nursing and APN educators we saw value in adding spiritual care competency to our APN master's programme.

7.5   Applying Rogers' Framework to Spiritual Care in Israel

Rogers' (2016) Availability and Vulnerability (A&V) framework for Operationalising Spirituality drew inspiration from a Christian community and was translated into a secular framework which mirrored Rogers' own personal and professional journey. It is with this in mind that we present an Israeli perspective of those aspects of spiritual care that are based on educating APNs in our Israeli APN programme from our personal and professional journeys. We have chosen to discuss the application of spiritual care from an APN midwifery perspective.

We began to incorporate Rogers' (2016) A&V framework into our spiritual care workshop for our MSN students in Jerusalem because we believe it offers APN students a theory-based higher-level nursing skill. It crosses cultural and religious lines and can be applied by and for all. Our 2018 study on spiritual care competency among our MSN/APN students showed that the ability to provide spiritual care did not change based on self-reported religion or level of religiosity (unpublished data, Andrews and Friedman, 2018). For us, we see the A&V framework as a way to develop a new universal neuturalistic perspective to spirituality that is not based on Judaism alone.

The following two case studies illustrate integrating spirituality into APN education and with a patient.

7.6   Case Study # 1: APN Spiritual Care Education

As an educator of APNs in Israel (Caryn), and a Family and Oncology Nurse Practitioner, my own advanced nursing practice is in my interaction with students, patients, and others. One of the first challenges in teaching Israeli APN students was the notion of "sharing oneself" with the patients. Israel is a paternalistic society that is based on a stoic-personality trait. Most Israelis have been in the army at age 18, right out of high school, they do not attend University until after the army when they choose their career training pathway. Introducing spiritual care was not easily accomplished since the faculty and students brought up with a stoical ideology did not really understand the purpose of learning about it. Over the years students evaluated the spirituality workshop positively and began to challenge their stoicism. Spiritual care is now an integral part of the programme for all APN nurses in our school of nursing whichever specialty they study (Andrews 2020).

I approached the notion of teaching spiritual care to the APN students in the oncology route of an APN program based in Israel, by introducing spiritual care competency and complementary care as part of the holistic oncology perspective. Though naive to the concepts posited by Rogers (2016), I recognised that spiritual care was often constructed as a personal journey nurses embark on with their patients. This is often seen as the "next level" of bonding, by forming relationships and partnerships with their patients exemplifying the concept of "advanced practice nursing".

This case focuses on the spirituality workshops we run for APN students. The aim is to share neutralistic strategies for providing spiritual care for APN students regardless of religion, with a new understanding of spiritual care as separate and distinct from religious support. We have evaluated these workshops and the APNs ability to assess spiritual care competencies with their patients. Our results showed that spiritual care competencies could be increased by providing spirituality workshops and engaging and enlightening the APN students through discussions about spirituality as part of their advanced practice nursing education (Unpublished data, Andrews and Friedman 2018).

Initially during the workshops, the first question that often arises from students is "what is spiritual care?" and "what does spirituality entail?" I reflect on my understanding of what spiritual care means, giving examples of aspects of spiritual care, which I have seen as helpful to my patients. I describe to my students that storytelling, music, and poetry can be used to initiate engagement and sharing of ideas. I describe looking for ways to stimulate the emotional connection (availability) and transcendence (vulnerability) that happens in a spiritual encounter (Rogers 2016). I then consciously utilise openness and honesty as a way of creating an atmosphere of "vulnerability and hospitality" by first opening myself, and then inviting the students into a more "open environment". The students often reflect on their own encounters in practice that they have previously never considered as spiritual. Many students reflect that it was just something they did because they cared. I often notice tears, laughter, nodding heads, and words of comfort as the students share their stories with each other. We continue the workshop discussing models of spirituality, specifically Rogers' (2016) framework. Presented with this framework APN students reflect that it has given them a new awareness that many of their acts of caring during their interventions with patients is based in the principles of spiritual care.

In one of the first workshops I held, a student who worked in the neonatal intensive care unit said "my patients don't have spiritual needs, they are premature babies!". This sparked a very heated discussion where the students began a reflective dialogue about the needs of the patient and her family. They asked: "what about the parents? How can you help the parents connect with these tiny vulnerable beings?", "How can you instill hope? Where are you with the parents when the baby doesn't make it?" "What about the siblings? The grandparents? How can we help them connect to this new family member?" I asked her if she ever talked to the babies. I asked her to picture herself caring for the infant and connecting prayer and hope to the care she was giving. Did she connect to that type of care? Could she picture herself practicing that way? I told her about my own experiences with chemotherapy nurses who gave chemo with a prayer for healing and hope. As the students reflected, they recognised that they often also worked in this way, otherwise they said "how else can we do this every day?". In the end, many students left crying, feeling more connected to themselves and each other. The stories and discussion, support and hugs lasted long after the class was over. Even 8 years later some come back to me and tell me how this has helped their own practices as APN's.

As a newcomer to the Israeli culture, I was surprised to learn that when I shared meaning from personal stories, that I viewed as "spiritual dimensions", it often evoked deep emotional responses in my students. At the beginning there was always a surprised hush when I shed a tear or two. In a culture that values stoicism, heroism, and paternalism it was challenging to break through this barrier of communication and engage the students to be more vulnerable with themselves and their patients. After the first few workshops I held, students asked for me to provide a day when they could share spiritual practices they were each drawn to such as yoga, aromatherapy, music therapy, and reflexology. Each student presented the scientific evidence of using this practice, and then each gave the class a group "experience". The classroom was darkened, chairs were pushed aside, candles were set around the room, and mats were laid out. We changed into comfortable clothes. After a couple of hours of the "experience" we sat on the floor and talked about connectivity and transcendence and how it affected our ability to give advanced practice oncology care. Each of us was drawn to a specific modality and described how this could be used in our APN practice. Taking the "classroom" out of the picture was a way for me to connect with the students and help them find their inner strength and connection. It created an open environment of hope. I still hear from these students from time to time. One has even begun to teach with me.

Being available as a teacher of spiritual care is challenging because there is always a question of where to draw the line. The students are hungry to know how to actually practice spiritual care. They ask: "how do you initiate a real spiritual encounter?" I discuss evaluation of the hospital room setting, how to develop a therapeutic relationship, where to sit, holding hands, praying with the patient or family, celebrating life, and directing the connection. By providing spiritual care to the group of APN students, I was able to increase their connection to providing hope, to embrace each other, and most of all to be able to carry this competency to their APN practice settings. As Rogers (2016) says "spirituality broadly defined as understanding one's meaning, purpose and direction in life is the key to our inner journey". I believe this can be facilitated by teachers. Most recently teaching spiritual care in a "zoom" setting has presented its own challenges, however, the students have still wanted to share their progress on their own spiritual journeys.

The idea of providing spiritual care for me comes from a place of giving care to others, working with my students we journey together toward the mutual goal of understanding each other and building up the belief within ourselves that we can provide spiritual care and make a significant difference to the patients in our care. Other faculty in our school have trouble identifying with this method of teaching which they view as "soft science" and experiential care. A senior level faculty member once asked to sit in my workshop. A true "Sabra" or Israeli born she stated before the workshop "I hope you don't get upset if I don't participate or cry". Needless to say she shared many beautiful stories as a nurse, nurse midwife, mother and wife, and she continues to attend the workshop year after year. She made me cry. She left the classroom crying. With the consistently excellent student evaluations and her support this spiritual care course is a mandatory course for APN education in our school.

7.7 Case Study #2: Advanced Practice Midwifery—Spiritual Care at a Stillbirth

Esther, a 19-year-old Hassidic, Ultra-Orthodox, Jewish woman arrived in labour and delivery (L&D) triage just before midnight in active labour with her husband, Shmuel, and her mother, Sarah (names changed for anonymity). It was her first pregnancy. She was experiencing regular contractions and was quickly connected to a foetal monitor. The midwife in triage was unable to find a heartbeat. The doctor was called to perform an ultrasound right away and the young couple was gently informed that their baby had died.

The contractions were coming every 3 min—there was shock, fear, tears, and great pain. The midwife asked Esther to rate her pain from 0–10 and through her wailing she screamed "PHYSICAL or EMOTIONAL??". Esther was 5 cm dilated and fully effaced upon vaginal exam. She was hysterically crying and asking for an epidural. The midwife called the Anaesthetist—Esther was whisked into L&D and handed over to my care as an APN Midwife. She was given an epidural right away—the physical pain was taken care of.

I (Abby) dimmed the lights so she could rest and I asked her how I could support her. I told her I was open to any, and all, of her questions—I would answer as truthfully and sincerely as I could. Watching me connect her to a foetal monitor she asked why she needed it if her baby was dead and I explained that we would continue to monitor her contraction pattern so we would know when it was time to deliver since she no longer felt contractions. She had so many questions and I told her I would answer what I could. We talked about what it would be like when the baby came out. She asked what it would look like and what we would do with it. I asked what she wanted to do with her baby. She said it was important to her that she get to hold her baby and say goodbye as she gave him back to God. She asked if we could arrange a Jewish burial and I told her our hospital was able to make arrangements with any local Chevra Kadisha (Jewish burial society). They would perform the burial rituals according to the letter of the law and would work with the family to arrange a burial plot if they wished.

Within half an hour, Esther was feeling pressure and had progressed to full dilation. Esther was stoic. She was quiet, reserved, and seemed to have turned into herself. I sat down next to her bed and asked her about the kinds of things she did to cope with difficult situations in other times in her life. She looked me in the eye and said quietly, "I pray." I told her that, as a midwife, every stillbirth I attend is painful and sad and that sometimes I find myself praying for strength and comfort. I asked her if she thought that praying alone or together with her family or me would help her get through the birth of her baby. She began to tear up and nodded her head. I asked her if she wanted me to remind her to pray when the baby was coming. She looked at me with what I experienced as a great sense of gratitude and said yes. I asked her if there was a specific prayer she would like to say and she named certain Psalms that are for times of mourning and great pain. I told her that when the baby was coming I would be honoured for us to pray together.

As we looked into each other's eyes, I instructed her to push with love and compassion. Their beautiful peaceful silent baby arrived in a dimly lit room. There was calm and serenity as we whispered the Psalms together. "The Lord is my shepherd; I shall not want...Yea, though I walk through the valley of the shadow of death, I will fear no evil: for thou art with me; thy rod and thy staff they comfort me...Surely goodness and mercy shall follow me all the days of my life and I will dwell in the house of the Lord forever."

The next day, I went to see Esther in the gynaecology ward where mothers are hospitalised after stillbirths. She was so happy to see me. She gave me a big hug and handed me a small plant she was planning on bringing me later in the day. There was a card which read: "My Dearest Abby, I could not have gotten through this birth without you. You opened yourself up for me and supported me and answered all my questions with compassion and a warm heart. You made every moment meaningful and special. Even in my great pain, I was able to find moments of serenity, closeness to my God, and comfort that I know came directly from Him. He gave you to me as a gift to help me get through the hardest time in my life. I will forever be grateful to Him for that and I will never forget you. With love and Gratitude, Esther".

As a Master's prepared APN, I was able to use my higher-level nursing skill to see my patient as a holistic being experiencing a crisis. I honed in on the spiritual needs of my patient and opened myself up to sharing my own spiritual space with her. While I am not Ultra-Orthodox, I am Jewish and practice at a different level of religiosity. My personal, clinical, and community availability helped me provide spiritual care and show my patient concern through active participation in the therapeutic relationship. I reflected on my own experience as a midwife during stillbirths and was truly "present" while listening attentively to my patient's description of her spiritual coping mechanisms. I exposed myself and my experience. I showed her that I did not know everything and that I would do the best I could to answer her questions. I reflected alongside my patient to find the safe space in which to express her connection to her God in a way that would bring her comfort during this unbelievably difficult time. In the end, Esther was able to express the way her spirituality was addressed to help her cope in crisis. For me this was a true example of providing spiritual care.

7.8 Discussion

As we reflected on these two cases from our own practice of spiritual care with patients and students, we began to see how Rogers' (2016) A&V framework is really a humanistic model for building connection (Rogers and Wattis 2019). Religion is significant, but it is also not the only way to find meaningful connection.

In Israel, religion has always been at the core of spirituality. Our history and multi-cultural society make it difficult to ignore. The concepts of A&V put religion aside and let people be people. We can all find connection and meaning through each other and as practitioners provide competent relationship-centred care. A&V leaves us open to connection on many levels and creates space for the other. Our experience as APNs has shown that application of the framework crosses all religions and creates a model for "neutralistic" spiritual care competency. It is possible that this care may need to be focused on a person's religious practice, but it is most importantly personal, holistic, and patient-specific.

We have identified many barriers in Israel to the notion of spiritual care. The APN role in Israel is in an evolutionary state. Mainstream APN education is still not at the Masters level in Israel as it is in many other countries. We are still trying to prove the added value of APNs in the nursing profession and healthcare system. Although the APN role is unique in that it is based on a multi-disciplinary perspective of nursing, medicine, psychology, and sociology there is still much resistance from all these disciplines (Nicoteri and Andrews 2004).

The workshop presented in the first case study is unique. We have found that seasoned and experienced APN's can teach the next generation about spirituality and spiritual care by sharing stories and connecting with them on a personal level. In this time of impersonal professional communication through emails, Zoom, Whatsapp, and "TEAMS", we must find a way to bridge the online horizon and support APNs in connecting to their patients by acknowledging spiritual needs. APNs need to be open and willing to respond to those in need. They provide holistic care by understanding the value of true connection. Our students can earn spiritual care competence by expanding their knowledge of spirituality and different worldviews. Additionally, APN students can be inspired to use this competence to become spiritual care providers by sharing hope and their own experiences from their APN education and practice.

Healing can be physical, emotional, or spiritual and by being available and vulnerable we can elevate our relationships with our patients as APNs. Rogers (2016) A&V framework discusses aspects of spirituality as being connected and holistic. When we open ourselves up to our patients at the individual, community, and care levels, we enter into a communal space where we can really know, respect, and connect with each other. We enter into a healing place. This is availability and vulnerability.

7.9   Ethical Considerations

The four principles of bio-ethics—autonomy, beneficence, nonmaleficence and justice—are key to providing spiritual care. Individuals must be allowed to self-govern and make their own decisions (Varkey 2021). The A&V framework calls for the reflective practice that is embedded in ethical decision-making. Use of this model ensures that providers are serving patients' needs and not their own.

Using the A&V framework, our case studies discuss the use of moral sensitivity (Wocial 2019), and identifying and bracketing of our own beliefs to support the patient and family on the journey they choose. By being explicit in our intentions, open to student and patient needs, and asking direct but sensitive questions, we aimed to do no harm, and create an environment for our students and patients to live their best life.

7.10   Summary

We are both committed to creating therapeutic relationships with patients by providing some form of spiritual care. Using a model like Rogers' (2016) A&V framework gives a structure to creating a higher connection between patient and provider. Using this approach helps encourage relationship-centred care acknowledging our patients as holistic human beings with their own worldview. Engaging students in learning spiritual care encourages creating relationships with patients by entering the sacred container and connecting to the other. It is in this safe, open, and non-judgemental space that we can take the spiritual care journey together. The APN responds to another person's needs and offers mutuality, reflection, reaction, and care. Availability and vulnerability reflect our purpose; to be there, to listen, and to love unconditionally. This is how we add another dimension to the APN care we provide.

References

Aaron EM, Andrews CS (2016) Integration of advanced practice providers into the Israeli health-care system. Isr J Health Policy Res 5:7. https://doi.org/10.1186/s13584-016-0065-8

Ami SB, Yaffe A (2015) Palliative care in Israel: The Nursing Perspective. J Palliat Care Med S5:009. https://doi.org/10.4172/2165-7386.1000S5009

Andrews CS, Friedman AK (2018) Evaluation of spiritual care competency following an advanced practice nursing program. International council of nursing rotterdam 2018

Andrews CS (2020) Spiritual care workshop for advanced practice nursing at Hadassah Hebrew University School of Nursing. November 2020

Andrews CS, Kra-Friedman A (2021) Development of the collaborative family nurse practitioner education using physician preceptors: A focused crtical ethnographic study. Education Today, accepted manuscript

APRN Consensus Workgroup (2008) Consensus model for APRN regualtion: licensure, accreditation, certification, and education. APRN Joint Dialogue Group Report July 7, 2008. https://www.ncsbn.org/Consensus_Model_for_APRN_Regulation_July_2008.pdf

Bentur N, Resnizky S (2009) Spiritual care in Israel: an evaluation of the programs funded by the UJA-Federation of New York. Myers JDC Brookdale. Catalog RR-526-09. https://brookdale.jdc.org.il/en/publication/spiritual-care-israel-evaluation-programs-funded-uja-federation-new-york/

Bentur N, Resnizky S (2010) Challenges and achievements in the development of spiritual-care training and implementation in Israel. Palliat Med 24(8):771–776. https://doi.org/10.1177/0269216310380490

Collett D, Feder S, Aaron E, Haron Y, Schulman-Green D (2019) Palliative care advanced practice nursing in Israel: bridging creation and implementation. Int Nurs Rev 67:136–144. https://doi.org/10.1111/inr.12555

Dickman C, Miller T, Muchow L, Ward-Smith P (2018) Israeli staff nurse knowledge and perception of the nurse practitioner role. Nurs Pract (12):42–48. https://doi.org/10.1097/01.NPR.0000547553.01883.ac. PMID: 30439774

Efrati E (2018) Israeli physicians protest plan to let nurse practitioners do doctors' tasks. Haaretz. https://www.haaretz.com/israel-news/israeli-physicians-protest-plan-to-let-nurse-practitioners-do-more-1.5809173

Goldberg S (2020) Chief nurse of Israel, personal correspondence to schools of nursing, November 5, 2020

International Council Of Nurses Guidelines On Advanced Practice Nursing (2020). https://www.icn.ch/system/files/documents/2020-4/ICN_APN%20Report_EN_WEB.pdf

Israel Central Bureau of Statistics (2019) Population by religion and population group. https://www.cbs.gov.il/en/subjects/Pages/Population-by-Religion-and-Population-Group.aspx

Israel Ministry of Health (2020) Application for Recognition as an Advanced Practice Nurse in Israel for Immigrant nurses. https://www.health.gov.il/English/Services/MedicalAndHealthProfessions/nursing/nursingExpertise/Pages/abroad.aspx

Life's Door (2020) Life's Door- Coping with illness and death. https://holisticunderstandingof-grief.com/portfolio-item/model-gallery/

Maslow J (2018) We should start adopting nurse practitioners instead of fighting against them. The Times of Israel. https://blogs.timesofisrael.com/we-should-start-adopting-nurse-practitioners-instead-of-fighting-against-them/

Miller LJ, Lu W (2020) Prognosis: Asia trounces U.S. in health-efficacy index amid pandemic. Bloomberg Index. https://www.bloomberg.com/news/articles/2020-12-18/asia-trounces-u-s-in-health-efficiency-index-amid-pandemic

Ministry of Health (2019) Circular of General Director. Update of expert nurse in the community. https://www.health.gov.il/hozer/MK07_2019.pdf

Nicoteri JAL, Andrews C (2004) The discovery of unique nurse practitioner theory in the literature: seeking evidence using and integrative review approach. J Am Acad Nurse Pract 15(11):494–500. https://doi.org/10.1111/j.1745-7599.2003.tb00338.x

Nissanholtz-Gannot R, Shapiro E (2020) Community nurses and chronic disease in Israel: professional dominance as a social justice issue. Nurs Inquiry. https://doi.org/10.1111/nin.12376

Nohal Expert Nurse (2013) http://www.health.gov.il/download/pages/11896709

Rogers M, Wattis J (2019) Understanding the role of spirituality in person centered care. Nurs Stand 35(9):25–30

Rogers M (2016) Utilising availability and vulnerability to operationalise spirituality. In: Practising spirituality. Palgrave Macmillan, London, p 145164. ISBN 9781137556844

Siegel-Itzkovich J (2018) Physicians, Israel medical association, clash on nurse practitioners. Jerusalem Post 19:32

Tzedek S (2020) Spiritual care services. https://www.szmc.org.il/eng/departments/oncology/units-and-clinics/beruach-spiritual-care-services/

Varkey B (2021) Principles of clinical ethics and their application to practice. Med Princ Pract 30(1):17–28. https://doi.org/10.1159/000509119

Wattis J, Curran S, Rogers M (eds) (2019) Spiritually competent practice in health care. CRC Press, Boca Raton. https://doi.org/10.1201/9781315188638

Wocial L (2019) Ethical decision making. In: Tracy MF, O'Grady ET (eds) Hamric and Hanson's advanced practice nursing; an integrative approach. Elsevier, St. Louis, pp 310–342

Global APN Case Study in Spirituality-Stories of Hope from United States of America

8

Beth DeKoninck and Jeremy P. Fyke

Abstract

This chapter will explore the formation of advanced practice nursing in the United States (U.S.) and will focus on the role of the Nurse Practitioner (NP). While there is a rich history that supports advanced nursing practice in the US, this chapter is only able to address the highlights. Similarly, the NP role has experienced many challenges through the years and, while many of those challenges still exist on some level, the ever-evolving world of healthcare continues to provide new opportunities and issues for the profession. The last half of this chapter will present an actual case study exploring the integration of the Adverse Childhood Events (ACE) questionnaire as an adjunct to spiritual care in the primary care setting.

Keywords

Advance practice nursing · Nurse Practitioner · Spirituality · ACE questionnaire

This chapter will explore the formation of advanced practice nursing in the United States (U.S.) and will focus on the role of the Nurse Practitioner (NP). While there is a rich history that supports advanced nursing practice in the US, this chapter is only able to address the highlights. Similarly, the NP role has

B. DeKoninck (✉)
Compassion Health Care, Yanceyville, NC, USA

J. P. Fyke
Belmont University, Nashville, TN, USA
e-mail: Jeremy.Fyke@Belmont.edu

© The Author(s), under exclusive license to Springer Nature Switzerland AG 2021
M. Rogers (ed.), *Spiritual Dimensions of Advanced Practice Nursing*,
Advanced Practice in Nursing, https://doi.org/10.1007/978-3-030-71464-2_8

experienced many challenges through the years and, while many of those challenges still exist on some level, the ever-evolving world of healthcare continues to provide new opportunities and issues for the profession. The last half of this chapter will present an actual case study exploring the integration of the Adverse Childhood Events (ACE) questionnaire as an adjunct to spiritual care in the primary care setting.

Advanced practice nursing began in the U.S. as early as the 1600s with the arrival of the first settlers. Midwifery consisted of lay healers who were the primary healthcare providers at the time and who had origins in Europe and Africa (Tracy and O'Grady 2019; Joel 2018). The nurse midwife profession became more formalised in the late nineteenth century, about the time nurse anesthetists began to emerge (Joel 2018). The growth of advanced practice continued into the early twentieth century with the advent of the Clinical Nurse Specialists (CNS), who devoted themselves to one area of interest in nursing. One of the oldest specialty areas for the CNS in the United States is the psychiatric nurse and, interestingly, the psychiatric CNS remains the most prevalent specialty in the CNS role today (Tracy and O'Grady 2019).

The forerunners of the Nurse Practitioner (NP) role were the public health nurses and the Frontier Nursing Service (FNS). Public health nurses were instrumental in the delivery of primary care for the poor immigrant population in the US in the late 1800s, with Lillian Wald leading the initiative through the formation of the Henry Street Settlement in Manhattan, New York. The Henry Street Settlement provided primary care for the poor of the area over a period of decades and many of their patients lived in overcrowded tenements with all of the public health concerns related to close living conditions and poor socioeconomic status, such as respiratory infections, asthma, injuries, diabetes, heart disease, mental health issues, etc. (Tracy and O'Grady 2019).

The FNS initially provided midwifery services to those in rural Kentucky and they were known for traveling circuits on horseback to care for their patients. These brave forerunners of Nurse Practitioners eventually provided primary care to families in these rural areas, most of whom had no access to any other form of healthcare. It is from this rich history that the Nurse Practitioner role was developed in 1965 by the first paediatric Nurse Practitioner, Loretta Ford, RN and her physician-colleague Henry Silver, MD (Joel 2018).

Ford and Silver developed an NP programme at the University of Colorado to prepare professional nurses who could fill the gap in healthcare providers which developed as a result of Medicare and Medicaid. These two forms of government-sponsored health insurance allowed for people who had suffered from lack of health insurance to enter the healthcare arena and obtain long-needed services. With the advent of formal preparation of NPs specializing in paediatric populations in lower socioeconomic areas, the profession branched out into primary care for adults across the lifespan (Tracy and O'Grady 2019). As often happens when established barriers are breached, controversy developed over the educational preparation, scope of practice, and prescribing rights of NPs—all of which continue to the present day, in one form another.

8.1   Current State of Advanced Practice in the United States

Today in the U.S., the Consensus Model recognizes four roles for the Advanced Practice Registered Nurse (APRN): Certified Registered Nurse Anaesthetist (CRNA), Certified Nurse Midwife (CNM), Certified Nurse Specialist (CNS), and Nurse Practitioner (NP). Each of the roles has a population focus and some roles have now moved past the population focus with an APRN specialty such as oncology, cardiology, nephrology, etc. (APRN Joint Dialogue 2008).

The CNS, CNM and NP may practice either in the primary care or acute care setting. CRNA's practice in the hospital setting as well as ambulatory surgery centers. Some APRN roles have specific ages of the population within their scope of practice. For example, paediatric NPs care for children ages birth through 21-years-old and family NPs are educated to care for ages across the lifespan (Tracy and O'Grady 2019).

There are more than 290,000 NPs licensed in the US and 69% of all NPs practice in primary care. Nurse Practitioners make up the greatest segment of APRNs and hold prescriptive privileges in all 50 states, however, the prescribing limitations vary by state (AANP 2020). Furthermore, the legal requirement for an NP to collaborate with a physician also varies by state, although the number of states allowing independent practice continues to rise.

8.2   Educational Preparation of NPs

Nurse Practitioners in the US must be registered nurses and hold a Bachelor's degree in nursing before acceptance to graduate programs. When the NP role was developed in the 1960s, educational preparation to move into advanced practice required only a certificate. As the educational preparation became more formalized, the master's degree was required in most states by the end of the 1990s (Tracy and O'Grady 2019). Today, the master's degree is still the required degree for entry to practice, but momentum continues to build for the Doctor of Nursing Practice (DNP) to become the terminal degree for NPs (Pulcini et al. 2019).

Several reasons exist for the DNP as the terminal degree including the rapid expansion of knowledge found in healthcare today, the quality of patient care and patient safety concerns. The complexity of patient care and healthcare systems also requires the highest level of scientific knowledge to ensure the best patient outcomes (Pulcini et al. 2019). In addition, the DNP aligns clinical practice with other health professions in the US that have moved to the doctorate as the terminal degree (e.g., Pharmacy, Psychology, Physical Therapy) (DNP Fact Sheet 2019).

At present, a national debate in the academic nursing arena continues regarding not whether the DNP should be the terminal degree for NPs, but when that requirement should be implemented. The Council of Accreditation for Nurse Anaesthesia Educational Programs (COA) required all CRNA educational programs to transition to the DNP effective January, 2022 and all CRNAs will need doctoral degrees by 2025 (Wood 2019).

While the National Organization of Nurse Practitioner Faculty (NONPF) has set 2025 as the most recent date for the DNP to become the terminal degree, accrediting and certifying bodies have not drawn the same line. As a result, many NP educational programs have added the DNP as an option for NP students, with the majority of schools offering both the master's and DNP. Still others continue to offer only the master's degree (Pulcini et al. 2019). Momentum is increasing as the number of DNP graduates continues to increase. The issue is complex and requires the unity of certifiers, accreditors and NONPF for a final determination on the matter.

8.3 Obstacles for Nurse Practitioners in the U.S.

The NP role has experienced many challenges since its inception 55 years ago, with the two greatest challenges being autonomous practice and prescribing privileges. Currently, 23 states and two U.S. territories enjoy full practice authority. Sixteen states and three territories have reduced practice and 12 states still have restricted practice (AANP 2020). While great progress has been made in the area of autonomous practice, there remains a significant amount of work ahead for the profession. Many NPs own their own practices and/or practice in rural areas and a requirement to maintain a collaborative agreement is an impediment as NPs endeavor to practice to the full scope of their education.

Prescriptive authority in the U.S. varies by state and is taken into consideration as the degree of practice authority is determined. While the majority of states allow NPs to prescribe schedule II-V drugs, there are still states that restrict NPs from prescribing certain schedules of drugs (AANP 2020). All NPs who work under restricted prescribing privileges find the work of caring for patients more difficult. Hence, the effort to obtain full practice authority in all states will continue as NPs provide a solution for an increasing need of primary care providers across the nation (Sheehan et al. 2020).

Other challenging practice issues for NPs are insurance reimbursement, the ability to sign death certificates, order physical therapy and order durable medical equipment. These important practice issues continue to be addressed by national and state professional organisations. The largest issue regarding the education of NPs is the transition from the Master's degree to the Doctor of Nursing Practice (DNP) as the entry level to practice. The DNP continues to gain traction as schools continue to transition their programs, but it remains a slow process without the regulatory requirement that certifiers and state boards of nursing could provide

8.4 Spirituality in U.S. Health Care

While spirituality and religion are similar, the two are often not distinguished by healthcare providers. Many healthcare providers in the U.S. focus on religion, perhaps because religion is easier to conceptualize and more comfortable to discuss. For example, if a healthcare provider were to be asked if they provide spiritual care for their patients, many would immediately think of the concepts such as faith community, church attendance, and denomination. A large majority of healthcare providers would not move past this connotation and, likely, would say they do not provide spiritual care for their patients. However, when specifically questioned, those same providers would be very likely to say that spirituality and spiritual care are important aspects of holistic care (DeKoninck et al. 2016).

In addition to other perceived barriers to spiritual care, NPs in the U.S. largely feel inadequately trained and unprepared to provide spiritual care. The majority report feeling uncomfortable with doing more than offering a pastoral referral or, possibly, offering to pray with the patient (DeKoninck et al. 2016; Helming 2009). In recent years, as the idea of holistic care has become more well-known and an expected method of care for NPs, the concept of spirituality and its positive effect on patient health outcomes has become better understood (Tanyi et al. 2009). While medical schools have moved to incorporate spirituality and spiritual care into their curriculum, most NP schools have not made that transition (Koenig et al. 2010; Helming 2009). However, even for medical schools with spiritual care content in their curriculums, there is great variation as to how much content is actually provided as well as the depth and impact of the content that is presented to medical students/physicians (Koenig et al. 2010).

Although many NPs would report that they do not provide spiritual care to their patients, it is more likely that in actuality they do provide aspects of spiritual care, but do not recognise it. Rogers and Wattis (2019) has operationalised the concepts of availability and vulnerability as aspects of spiritual care provided by NPs. Based on these concepts and the relationships that NPs develop with their patients, most NPs are performing spiritual care in some manner, even though they may not be aware of it.

8.5   Background for Case Study

I have been a Family Nurse Practitioner for 25 years and have worked in many settings, with most of my career spent in family practice. Spiritual care has become a very intentional part of my practice in the past 10 years. In hindsight, I always provided spiritual care on some level, but lacked actual awareness or intentionality in that aspect of patient care. Provision of spiritual care for patients is still a work in progress, with time being the greatest barrier. Time and lack of education are two main barriers NPs and physicians cite in providing spiritual care to their patients (Tanyi et al. 2009; Vincensi and Solberg 2017; DeKoninck et al. 2016). In the U.S., time pressures related to provider schedules are felt by all, especially in light of the aging of the population and a fee-for-service model.

Quite a few years ago a colleague introduced me to the Adverse Childhood Experiences (ACE) study, which was published in 1998. This landmark study opened my eyes to a new aspect of patient care which clearly demonstrated the importance of understanding "what had happened" to my patients as compared to "what was wrong" with them. While I might be treating them for hypertension, diabetes, depression or other chronic diseases, it was understanding the past trauma that many experienced as children which really provided a key to many of my patients' health issues.

The ACE questionnaire assesses for ten areas of trauma experienced before the age of 18. These questions ask specifically about physical, sexual and emotional abuse as well as neglect, and several other categories. An ACE score of four or higher is significant for increased risk of chronic disease, substance abuse, mental illness and suicide. The 10-item questionnaire is easy to administer and provides an indicator of potential physical/mental health risks of patients and allows for a trauma informed approach to care.

I implemented this questionnaire with all new patients hoping to understand past trauma as a factor of chronic conditions and in hopes of mitigating risk going forward. Unexpectedly, a more significant result emerged from the screening: it created a space for my patients to speak about the trauma they have experienced as children and, often, I am the first person they have told. Most of my patients are female and I have found them to be very honest on their ACE questionnaires with a large percentage reporting sexual, physical, and verbal abuse as children. Many of these women have suffered the consequences of sexual abuse: guilt, shame, posttraumatic stress disorder, poor relationships with men and the lack of ability to trust others—just to name a few. It is this questionnaire that opens the door for them to talk about their trauma, if they choose, and to be referred to counseling. This has also allowed me to practice from a trauma informed care approach and to practice spiritual care from a new perspective and on a new level.

8.6   Case Study

Leah is a 53- year-old white female who came to see me to establish care as a new patient. She moved from out of state 9 months ago and had not been seen by any healthcare provider since arriving in the state. She had run out of her blood pressure, depression, and anxiety medications, and needed a refill on her albuterol inhaler.

Leah did not remember when she had her last pap smear (cervical screening) and had never had a mammogram. She reported right foot pain, specifically in her heal, when she got out of bed first thing in the morning. She had a peroneal nerve injury from hip surgery in the same leg and was unable to wear her brace because of the heel pain. She had also developed hammertoes in the same foot with the sensation of continually being pricked by needles on the bottom of the right foot.

Leah began to cry and and said she had been off of her psychiatric medications for at least 9 months and was also diagnosed with bipolar disorder. She did not remember the names of her medications, but remembered sertraline and paroxetine did not help. She had a diagnosis of Post Traumatic Stress Disorder (PTSD) and had been unable to sleep for months because she ran out of her medication. When asked if she had ever taken trazodone, she remembered that was her medication for sleep and it did help.

At this point her ACE questionnaire revealed a score of four with positive responses in the areas of sexual and physical abuse. After explaining the ACE questionnaire to Leah and noting her positive response in this specific area, Leah began crying and said she was sexually abused from the time she was 8 years old until the age of 13. She was then raped at the age of 16. Leah went on to tell me that she had been married three times and her first husband was physically abusive and it had taken her 8 years to leave him. Leah continued to cry and said she couldn't trust anyone but her son and the friend she lived with because of all that had happened to her. She was hardly able to leave her home or even go to the grocery store because of her mistrust of people and triggers, such as certain smells, that caused her to have flashbacks and panic attacks. She denied any suicidal or homicidal ideation.

During this conversation with Leah, I was seated in front of her, I provided her tissue for her eyes and just listened. I affirmed to her that she did nothing wrong as a child and what happened to her was not her fault. I asked her what support she had regarding family or a faith community since she was not working and fairly new to the state. She replied that her son lived out of state, but they spoke by phone. She had no other support, but her friend who lived with her. She had no faith community and questioned if she even believed in God because "how could a man of God do this to me?" Leah then told me that her abuser had been her grandfather, who was a Pastor and well-respected man in the community. I told her how sorry I was that this had happened to her, especially by her grandfather.

Leah continued to cry and told me that she had "lost four people in the past five years"—her mother, father, aunt, and sister—mainly from cancer. She said that these things continued to happen to her and she did not understand why. At this point, I placed my hand on Leah's knee and told her I was available for her and we would work through these things together. I also let her know that I wanted to understand her triggers so that we could work to avoid those when she was in our office.

Her past medical history revealed no known drug allergies. She had Attention Deficit Hyperactivity Disorder in addition to the diagnoses already mentioned and right hip replacement in 2017. She was unemployed, did not smoke tobacco, or use alcohol. She did use marijuana and only had sex with females.

Leah's Review of Systems and Physical Examination were unremarkable except for a blood pressure of 161/92 and marked tenderness to palpation of the right heel, noted hammertoes of the second and third toes and inability to flex, extend, evert, or invert her right foot.

The plan for Leah consisted of X-ray of the right foot and referral to the sports medicine physician in our group. She was started on Lisinopril 10 mg daily for hypertension. Trazodone 50 mg was started for sleep disturbance. Cymbalta 60 mg daily was started for depression/anxiety and in hope that would decrease the paresthesia in her right foot. Her albuterol inhaler was refilled for prn use. Referral was made to our licensed counsellor and our Psychiatric Mental Health Nurse Practitioner (PMHNP). The counsellor would be able to see her within a few days, but the PMHNP would not be available until December. She would have fasting labs the next day consisting of a complete blood count, comprehensive metabolic profile, lipid panel, Thyroid Stimulating Hormone, vitamin D, and Vitamin B12. She was scheduled for a mammogram. Leah was schedule to return to my office to follow-up on her blood pressure, labs and medications in 2 weeks and we planned to continue to work through her mental and physical health issues. She needed a complete physical with a pap smear in the near future, but we planned for that once her anxiety improved and I better understood what her triggers were so that her pap smear could be as non-traumatic as possible. Leah had stopped crying at this time and, unfortunately, I had to move to the next patient.

8.7   Discussion

Leah came to establish care, address her heel pain, and to re-institute treatment for chronic conditions. However, as with many patients, the physical complaints brought her to the office, but it is the inner turmoil from her past trauma which continues to fuel the fires of her chronic diagnoses. While Leah has been on medication and received counseling in the past, she has been unable to move forward in her life because the ties of the past manifest in emotional, spiritual and physical pain.

As is the case for many NPs in the U.S., one of the greatest barriers I experience in providing spiritual care is time (DeKoninck et al. 2016; Tanyi et al. 2009; Vincensi and Solberg 2017; Helming 2009). I have 30 min appointments for new patients and Leah had significant physical complaints (hypertension and foot pain) that needed to be addressed combined with her emotional/mental health problems. Building rapport and trust with a patient is always important, but even more so with patients like Leah. There always exists in situations like this an inner stress for the NP: a patient who needs more time/attention than an appointment slot allows and the knowledge that other patients are waiting to be seen. This is a pivotal moment where a provider can exhibit spiritual hospitality, which builds trust/rapport, through presencing so that a patient feels cared about even though the visit must come to an end before all complaints can be fully addressed (Rogers and Beres 2017).

It is the "presence" of the NP that is most important in cases like the one portrayed above. The ability to fully focus on Leah, fully listen and empathise with her pain and her experiences; to provide compassion and kindness during the visit were my top priorities for this visit. Presencing, or being fully present with the patient, is practiced through listening in a non-judgmental manner, asking open-ended questions and the simple act of appropriate touch (Helming 2009; Rogers and Wattis 2019). These are practical but powerful forms of spiritual care which can break down walls between the patient and provider, especially during a first visit (Vincensi and Solberg 2017; Helming 2009; Rogers and Wattis 2019). Rogers' concept of availability to others through caring and welcome encapsulates the essence of the NP-patient relationship formed in this scenario (Wattis et al. 2017)

With an emotionally intense visit, the NP must be aware of their own spirituality in order to emotionally engage with the patient, while being acutely aware of maintaining professional boundaries. Rogers' concept of availability to ourselves explains this need for self-protection (Wattis et al. 2017). The image of a ship caught in a storm often comes to mind when my patients are in emotional/spiritual distress and have a life in disarray. As I sit with my patient and allow them to pull their ship in out of the storm for a brief respite, I am cognisant not to get into the ship with them. It is overstepping this boundary that can lead to ineffectiveness for the patient and burnout for the provider. Debriefing and self-reflection are also important with these intense visits in order to remain emotionally, spiritually and physically healthy (Wattis et al. 2017).

According to Rogers (Wattis et al. 2017), vulnerability encompasses a teachable spirit, willingness to be accountable, to advocate for patients and to be authentic in our patient/provider relationships. My first visit with Leah allowed me to practice availability in a much more obvious manner than vulnerability. I believe that my authenticity was felt by Leah, but I do not know that for certain. Because I have not had a similar life experience, I had a limited ability to make myself vulnerable with Leah although compassion and empathy were demonstrated during the visit. As I provide care for Leah over time, I am sure opportunities for me to embrace open, honest and transparent conversation will occur.

The greatest facilitator to spiritual care in this particular case was the ACE questionnaire and Leah's ability to feel comfortable enough with me to share her pain and history of trauma. Like a majority of NPs in the US, spiritual care training was lacking in all levels of my nursing education, but a desire for relationship with my patients naturally brought me into the arena of spirituality and spiritual care (DeKoninck et al. 2016; Tanyi et al. 2009; Vincensi and Solberg 2017; Helming 2009). Over many years, I have developed a comfort level for providing spiritual care in a variety of ways which are individualised and patient-specific through praying with patients, presencing, and making myself available and vulnerable.

8.8 Ethical Considerations

All healthcare workers must be guided by the ethical principles of beneficence, autonomy, nonmaleficence, and justice. However, this is especially important for APRNs, who maintain such intimate relationships with their patients and who can have great influence on patients and their families. Patient autonomy is imperative in the provider/patient relationship and this is exemplified with the use of the ACE questionnaire, as the patient always has the right to decline completing the screening. It is important that patients feel no sense of judgment in the provider/patient relationship. Of course, there is a difference between being truthful with our patient versus judging them or their behaviors. Truth is always important for a trusting relationship and it is the "art" of our practice that enables us to deliver truth in a compassionate, empathetic manner.

Spiritual care itself requires sensibility and responsibility by the practitioner so that the patient both understands and feels safe, respected and free to express themselves. The use of the ACE screening tool has often provided me with a great segue to many deep and personal conversations with patients, but care must be taken to ensure that no harm is done through re-traumatization, as an example of "do no harm." Fortunately, behavioral health specialists are available in my practice setting for patients, if they choose to be connected with licensed counselors.

8.9 Final Thoughts

In order to not just endure, but to maintain passion and thrive as an NP over many years, I have found it tremendously important to move past just addressing the physical complaints of patients. It is my desire to learn what happened to each patient and to understand what brought them to where they are in life. This sacred honor to glimpse into personal lives continues to fuel my passion for patient care after 25 years in practice as an NP. It is the notion that through availability and vulnerability I may be able to impact a patient enough to enable them to lead a more healthy and joyful life. While that may not happen for most, even one life impacted means success to me!

References

American Association of Colleges of Nursing (2019) DNP fact sheet. https://www.aacnnursing. org/News-Information/Fact-Sheets/DNP-Fact-Sheet

American Association of Nurse Practitioner (2020) State practice environment. https://www.aanp. org/advocacy/state/state-practice-environment

American Association of Nurse Practitioners (2020) NP fact sheet. https://www.aanp.org/about/all-about-nps/np-fact-sheet#:~:text=There%20are%20more%20than%20290%2C000,NPs)%20 licensed%20in%20the%20U.S

APRN Joint Dialogue Group (2008) Consensus model for APRN regulation: Licensure, accreditation, certification & education. https://www.google.com/search?q=aprn+joint+dialogue+grou p+report&rlz=1C1EJFC_enUS919US919&oq=aprn+joint+&aqs=chrome.0.0j69i57j0i22i30. 2557j0j7&sourceid=chrome&ie=UTF-8

DeKoninck B, Hawkins LA, Fyke JP, Neal T, Currier K (2016) Spiritual care practices of advanced practice nurses: a multinational study. J Nurse Pract 12(8):536–544

Helming MA (2009) Integrating spirituality into nurse practitioner practice: the importance of finding the time. J Nurse Pract 5(8):598–604

Joel LA (2018) Advanced practice nursing: essentials for role development. F. A. Davis Company, Philadelphia. Doi: 1098765432

Koenig HG, Hooten EG, Lindsay-Calkins E, Meador KG (2010) Spirituality in medical school curricula: findings from a national survey. Int J Psychiatry Med 40(4):391–398

Pulcini J, Hanson C, Johnson J (2019) National organization of nurse practitioner faculties: a 40-year history of preparing nurse practitioners for practice. J Am Assoc Nurse Pract 31(11):633–639

Rogers M, Beres L (2017) How two practitioners conceptualize spiritually competent practice. In: Wattis J, Curran S, Rogers M (eds) Spiritually competent practice in health care. CRC Press, New York, pp 53–68

Rogers M, Wattis J (2019) Understanding the role of spirituality in providing person-centered care. Nurs Stand. https://doi.org/10.7748/ns.2020.e11342

Sheehan A, Jones A, McNerlin C, Iseler J, Dove-Medows E (2020) How advanced practice registered nurse practice barriers impact health care access in Michigan. J Am Assoc Nurse Pract 00(00):1–7

Tanyi RA, McKenzie M, Chapek C (2009) How family practice physicians, nurse practitioners, and physician assistants incorporate spiritual care in practice. J Am Assoc Nurse Pract 21:690–697

Tracy MF, O'Grady ET (2019) Hamric and hanson's advanced practice nursing: an integrative approach, 6th edn. Elsevier

Vincensi BB, Solberg M (2017) Assessing the frequency nurse practitioners incorporate spiritual care into patient-centered care. J Nurse Pract 13(5):368–375

Wood D (2019) Raising the Bar in CRNA Education: What the 2025 deadline means. In: Staffcare. https://www.staffcare.com/physician-blogs/raising-the-bar-in-crna-education-what-the-2025-deadline-means/

Felitti VJ, Anda RF, Nordenberg D, Williamson DF, Spitz AM, Edwards V, Koss MP, Marks JS (1998) Relationship of childhood abuse and household dysfunction to many of the leading causes of death in adults. Am J Prev Med 14(4):245–258

Global APN Case Study in Spirituality: Stories of Hope from the Republic of Ireland

9

Kathleen Neenan and Jacqueline Whelan

Abstract

This chapter presents an overview of advanced practice nursing in Ireland followed by a discussion on how spirituality is viewed in healthcare. Using a case study, we explore the unique contribution of an Advanced Practice Nurse (APN) delivering spiritual care to an older person with dementia who was transferred from her nursing home to an acute care ward after a diagnosis of Covid pneumonia was made. Rogers' Availability and Vulnerability framework for Spiritually Competent Practice is used to illustrate how the person's distress was attended to by holding a safe space and supporting her to find hope and meaning during her illness. We outline the need for APNs to remain truthful to their own availability and vulnerability by highlighting the need to hold the interior and exterior, the visible and invisible, the human and divine, the known and unknown and the temporal and eternal together. There are times when we can truly offer our presence, deep listening, prayer, love, and compassion to another human being who is suffering. These are times that we can attend to the spiritual needs of those in our care. We chose this case study to illustrate spiritual care as there is a need for a greater focus on the spirituality of the older person, to better support and lead to enhanced inner peace.

Keywords

Spirituality · Spiritual care · Care · Compassion · Availability · Vulnerability mindfulness · Self- compassion

K. Neenan (✉) · J. Whelan
School of Nursing and Midwifery, University of Dublin Trinity College, Dublin 2, Ireland
e-mail: kaneenan@tcd.ie; whelanj1@tcd.ie

9.1   Advanced Practice Nursing in Ireland

Advanced practice nursing in Ireland is delineated as Advanced Nurse Practitioners (ANP) or Advanced Midwifery Practitioner (AMP) roles (Department of Health 2019). ANPs and AMPs are registered nurses/midwives, who pursue ongoing professional development and clinical supervision, to deliver care as independent, autonomous, and expert nurses and midwives (Department of Health 2019). Irish (Department of Health 2011) and United Kingdom (National Health Service 2015) reports suggest advanced and specialist roles reduce costs and improve efficiency by ensuring the best use of hospital consultant time, freeing up the time of other staff members, driving innovation and offering value for money. Over the last 40 years there has been significant developments in specialist and advance practice in Ireland; such developments have been spurred on by healthcare restructuring, increasing costs healthcare workforce supply and government policy (Wren et al. 2017).

The Nursing and Midwifery Board of Ireland (NMBI) is the national regulator who maintains ten register divisions of nurses and midwives within Ireland (Department of Health 2019). Preparation for nursing is a 4-year Bachelor of Science degree. Nurse roles in Ireland have undergone considerable change, the National Council for the Professional Development of Nursing and Midwifery (NCNM) set up in 1997 supported advance practise and specialists' posts (Department of Health 2016, O'Shea 2008). Since 2010, the National Nursing and Midwifery Board of Ireland (NMBI) hold statutory responsibilities for registration and accreditation of advanced roles (NMBI 2017). In keeping with international standards, Irish ANPs core competencies include autonomy in clinical practice, expert practice professional and clinical leadership, and research (Begley et al. 2010). ANP attributes are related to advanced clinical knowledge, autonomous decision-making, responsibility, and accountability for patient workload. These roles promote wellness, offer interventions, and advocate healthy lifestyles for patients in varied contexts in collaboration with other healthcare providers according to an agreed scope of practice (NMBI 2015c).

The NMBI's Advanced Practice Standards and Requirements recognise the level of knowledge, skill and expertise required of a registered ANP/APM; these roles are both regulated and title protected, endorsing care provision to patients and their families in diverse settings aligned to the values of compassion, care, and commitment (Department of Health 2016). These standards and requirements provide flexibility to higher educational institutions to be responsible and adaptable in providing evidence-based education programmes that equip nurses and midwives with the required competencies for registration. The essential criteria for advanced practice roles as set out by the NCNM and NMBI, are that the practice is carried out by autonomous, experienced practitioners who are competent, accountable, and responsible for their own practice (NMBI 2015a). There has been a major revision in the new model of training for ANPs with a 2-year timeframe from graduate level through to advanced practice, which is reflective of current international trends in this area. This model includes a process that allows the NMBI to recognise ongoing education training and supervision from initial registration of the nurse or midwife and recognising continuing achievements (Department of Health 2019). This permits the nurse or midwife to commence an advanced practice role whilst undertaking the formal education requirements.

The development of advanced practice in Ireland has been incremental since the first ANP post in 1997, with currently 445 ANP/AMP and 183 students in training to register. National policy aims to have 2% of the national nurse and midwifery workforce as ANP/ANMPs (Department of Health 2019). ANPs work across many areas including the acute medicine, ambulatory care, cardiology, epilepsy, haematology, heart efficiency, gastroenterology, care of older person, occupational health, rheumatology, stroke, urology, women's health, tissue viability, sexual health, respiratory, mental health, and more developing. The degree level of pre- registration education commenced in 2002 and further investment in nurse education has enabled opportunities for nurses and midwives to demonstrate the added benefit of enhancing their role further, e.g., nurse prescribing ionising radiation and improving services and patient care. Current national policy aims to maximise the nursing and midwifery response to current and emerging health service challenges. This policy provides a model to support the development from graduate to advanced practice that will assist in building a critical mass of nurses and midwives working at advanced practice level (Department of Health 2019). By creating a critical mass of advanced nurses and midwives, care delivery can be enhanced to meet health needs. Evidence suggests that creating a critical mass of nurses and midwives as specialist and advanced practitioners has benefits for service provision, such as improved timely access to services, hospital avoidance, reduced waiting lists early discharge and integration of services.

Sláinte care, the national 10-year plan to reform the health service, has outlined the pivotal role of specialist nurses and ANPs/AMP for to the development of services and delivery of quality health care (Government of Ireland 2019). ANPs and AMPs play an important role in care delivery across many areas and the value of these roles is acknowledged and adds to the quality of healthcare in Ireland (Government of Ireland Committee on the Future of Healthcare 2017). The vision in Sláinte care is being realised by ANPs. There are many areas of advanced practice that are currently underdeveloped and ANPs are now expanding and delivering the services and meeting patient care needs across all healthcare and community settings.

Advanced practice and case management are some of the nursing roles that are integral to the integration of services, creating end to end pathways for patients. Demonstrating impact is essential to service planning and development to ensure nurses and midwives are strategically placed to enhance patient and organisational outcomes (Nursing and Midwifery Board of Ireland 2017). It can be difficult to build a body of evidence to champion the role and to showcase outputs at national and international levels, however with support from educational and professional bodies and clinical sites Ireland is sustaining and building a critical mass of APNs.

9.2 Introduction to Spirituality in Healthcare in Ireland

Reverence for the ancient Celtic spirit and spirituality is unique in Irish culture. In the pre-Christian era, nursing constituted a noble act with a view to nourishing the soul of the ill through inclusion of prayer to Gods (Johnson et al. 2006). During Christian times, Celtic manuscripts tell us that nurses served as companions or spiritual guides called 'Anam Cara' (Irish for soul friend), with a view to creating connection and relational belonging towards the sick (Weathers 2019). Despite the disintegration of Catholicism by King Henry V111, following emancipation, historical accounts show how Catholic orders of nuns continued to expand an awareness of a transcendent reality integrating spirituality into nurses working lives (Fealy 2005, Meehan 2012). The subsequent adoption of a biomedical approach to care hindered patient connection until movement towards holistic patient-centred care approaches, that take full account of all dimensions of the person, was accepted (Mazzotta 2016). However, recent political, cultural, and socioeconomic changes in Irish society underpinned by materialism, population movements and significant church and religious orders scandals, have weakened our sense of identity and purpose, testing people's spirits (Flanagan and O'Sullivan 2019). Increases in secularisation does not necessarily imply a religious decline; rather it attempts to find common ground, as people continue to believe in metaphysical, transcendental phenomena and associated spiritual dimensions whilst exercising freedom and choice to adopt new forms (Flanagan and O'Sullivan 2019).

The World Health Organisation, the International Council of Nurses (ICN) and the Royal College of Nursing all acknowledge the importance of respecting and supporting a persons' spiritual beliefs, with the ICN proviso that Advanced Practice Nurse (APNs) work towards developing capacity and capability of meeting patients' unmet diverse needs by embedding spiritual care provision directly into practice (WHO 1984; ICN 2012; RCN 2011; ICN 2020). Contrary to such practice beliefs, a recent systematic review on the role of Advanced Practice Nurses (APNs) and Spiritual care (SC) revealed that spirituality is not a fundamental component of advanced practice (Younas 2017). Other evidence has illuminated that spiritual aspects are often conflated with psychological needs, leading to patients' spiritual needs rarely being considered or met (Chrash et al. 2011, Timmins et al. 2016a).

Research tells us that the definition, nature and meaning of spirituality across diverse contexts is constantly unfolding and changing (Streib and Hood 2016). Contemporary definitions of spirituality within healthcare clearly identify central aspects of spirituality, that are primarily concerned with seeking meaning, purpose, connectedness, transcendence and hope, which can be differentiated from religiosity whilst also inclusive of some religious aspects, (Pulchalski et al. 2014; Weathers et al. 2015; Timmins et al. 2016a) thus reaching a degree of consensus.

Census figures, with a population of 4.76 million, 1.15 million under 19 years, capture the extent of changes relating to religious beliefs; persons identifying as Catholic has decreased from 84.2% in 2011 to 78.3% in 2016, with a corresponding rise of persons indicating no religion from 5.9% to 9.8% to (468,400) with increases in Orthodox (37.5%), Hindu (34.1%), Muslim (29%), Apostolic and Pentecostal populations (CSO 2016). With a current ageing population of 604,000 over 65 years, expectations of annual rises of 20%, and those aged 85 years and above by 23%, it is accepted that the need for spiritual care provision will expand as chronic disease increases (CSO 2016). Such demographic changes capture the need for APNs to develop cultural competency to directly respond to the diverse complex health care needs (inclusive of cultural religious belief systems) of the population across the life span.

The 1998 Report on the Commission in Ireland (Government of Ireland 1998), and empirical evidence arising from Irelands' SCAPE Report, evaluating APN roles, found strong evidence relating to holistic assessment being undertaken as a core constituent of advanced and specialist practice (Begley et al. 2010). Whilst Irelands' Code of Professional Conduct and Ethics for the professions is premised on the principles of respect, dignity and core values of care, compassion, and commitment (NMBI 2014; DOH 2016); spirituality is nonetheless omitted from the Code. This may minimise practitioner's engagement with spiritual care provision and addressing patients' spiritual distress. Professional regulatory standards and requirements all direct practitioners to advocate for persons rights equally without discrimination, in the context of person-centred care and the nurse–patient relationship (NMBI 2015a, b, c, 2017). However, such core concepts need to be progressed further given evidence of bias towards developing biomedical focused ANP education programmes (Cronenwett et al. 2011). Carney (2014) evaluated 12 advanced practice programmes across the globe to ascertain best educational practices and core content; evidence identified the need to expand the scope of curricular content to include the adoption of a bio-psycho-social spiritual model. The NMBI scope of practice document makes succinct reference to spirituality as a nursing and midwifery function, role and responsibility aligned to holistic caring practice grounded '*in experiential evidence based on the understanding of the spiritual experiences of patients*' (NMBI 2015c pg. 8). Such guidance raises the question as to how spirituality as an educational imperative and a protective factor in health care, is addressed as an integral core component of ANP programme delivery.

In the ROI, a Palliative Care Competence Framework (HSE 2014) exists that focuses on 'awareness' and understanding of spirituality in the broad context of palliative care. However, development of generic spiritual care competencies at post-graduate level is overlooked which raises professional and ethical concerns as '*neglect of spirituality and a conflicted spirit can obstruct good practice and result in poor quality healthcare*'. (Wattis et al. 2017 pg. 14). National health and intercultural strategies, in conjunction with health standards, all espouse an integrated holistic care approach to respond to patients diverse needs to reduce care fragmentation as '*religious beliefs and practices impact significantly on patient's healthcare experience and recovery around key life events*' (HSE 2011; Health Information and Quality Authority 2012a, b; HSE 2019, p. 76). Analysis of policy documents reveals inconsistencies in national approaches to spiritual care and spiritual care provision, given that the focus is placed on generalised awareness and recognition, as distinct from concentrating on interpersonal, intrapersonal, assessment, planning, intervention and evaluative perspectives for ANPs to support patient's spiritual well-being compassionately and safely.

There is minimal research undertaken in the ROI that examines nurses' views of spirituality and spiritual care from advanced practitioner or specialised levels. Timmins (2013) undertook a self-reporting survey of general nurse's view and attitudes of spirituality based on the Nurses' Perception of Spiritual Care Inventory (SSCRS). Nurses expressed positive views of spirituality and were responsive to their role in spiritual care provision based on their personal knowledge that was not linked to religion, which has implications for how nurses are educated on the topic. Timmins et al. (2016b), using a tripartite methodological approach, also explored multi-faith and current approaches to, and facilities for, integrated spiritual care provision in Health Service Executive Voluntary hospital settings and long-term older care across 48 sites in the ROI. Results demonstrated that spiritual care was a component of hospital policy (73.5%, $n = 25$). Approximately 50% of respondents ascertained it was the responsibility of the team to hold overall responsibility for spiritual care, whilst chaplains (23.8% $n = 8$) and nurses (17.6% $n = 6$) viewed this as part of their role. There was strong agreement by nurses regarding the extent to which ten spiritual care activities for example, showing attentiveness, respect, spending time, providing support, reassurance, listening, and encouraging concerns were inclusive of the nurse's role. Some key recommendations included a single body mechanism with responsibility for chaplaincy in healthcare; education and training in spiritual care provision, caring for minority faiths and the role of the chaplain and nurses and consistent development of hospital policy spiritual care provision.

Spiritual competencies are necessary for nurses to embed spirituality into their practice. Whelan (2019, p. 170) refers to three core professional competencies found across the majority of competency framework models relevant for all nurses including the need '*to discern their individual worldview and beliefs of spirituality; the need to accommodate patients' diverse worldviews and experience and to enable relevant actions that fit with the patients frame of reference and needs'*. Supporting nurses to develop mindfulness, compassion, self-compassion knowledge, skills and practices are imperative to build sensitivity, empathy, resilience, thereby reducing stress and burnout (Neenan 2019). The following case study illustrates examples of these skills in practice.

9.3 APN Case Study

9.3.1 Introduction

As populations age globally, the number of frail older people in need of acute care service is increasing. Most overnight stays in acute hospital settings in Ireland are over 65-year-olds with 64% having multiple comorbidities (Health Service Executive 2020). Decline in physical health and cognition, is linked with becoming dependent on others (Rasmussen and Delmar 2014). The Covid-19 pandemic has led to significant global threats to public health, with approximately 77 million cases and over 1.7 m deaths to date (Clark et al. 2020). Older, frail medically compromised patients have poorer outcomes, with dementia being the most common pre-existing condition. Long-term residential and nursing care facilities have had high clusters of Covid-19, with many patients being transferred to acute hospitals for assessment and management (Kennelly et al. 2020).

A more person-centred and less disease focused approach to ANP practice, is important in acute care settings (Rogers and Wattis 2019). A holistic approach to my patients' clinical care combines the technical with the interpersonal whilst incorporating physical, mental, spiritual, and emotional needs of my patients. In my work with older people this acknowledges the person's dignity, culture, values, beliefs, and rights (Rogers and Wattis 2019). Spiritual care is important for all older people, especially those with chronic, acute illness and those with disabilities (Rogers et al. 2020). How nurses use their time when interacting and delivering care whilst paying attention to the spiritual dimensions of life, can be difficult to conceptualise and apply to practice (NMBI 2017). Rogers' (2016) Availability and Vulnerability framework can be embedded in APN practice to deliver holistic person-centred care, allowing meaning making of patients hopes and fears. I have chosen this case study as spirituality can be a source of strength for patients with dementia when ill and in times of progressive cognitive impairment (McSherry 2006).

9.3.2 My Patient

June is a 76-year-old lady with progressive dementia, she is ordinarily resident in a nursing home. June tested positive for COVID-19 and began experiencing severe coughing bouts with a marked deterioration in her health. She was transferred to hospital for her condition to be actively managed. She was alone, frail, agitated and disorientated, having been separated from her caregivers. Her immediate family are upset and fearful they may never see their Mum again as the hospital has stopped all family visits due to Covid transmission risks.

9.3.3 Integrating Availability and Vulnerability into June's Care

Integrating spirituality into holistic care starts with compassion and empathy in all human relationships which is particularly salient for dementia patients. Principles of availability in delivering spiritual care encourages APNs to reflect on and accept ourselves; thereby allowing us to embrace spirituality by understanding our own meaning purpose and direction in life (Rogers 2016). My (Kathleen) own spirituality integrates mindfulness which allows me to be available to my patients through presence, awareness and acceptance. Mindfulness helps me to build trust with others by living my life honestly and sincerely, cultivating respect and concern for others (Nhat Hanh 2006). It helps me to accept myself and helps me be motivated by loving kindness and compassion which I notice often brings calm to others. Kornfield (2002) describes loving kindness as having the ability to see the original innocence, dignity, and beauty of another human being. In all my interactions with June, I chose my words mindfully with loving kindness and welcomed and supported her on arrival to the ward. I carried out my initial assessment of June in a calm, non-rushed manner and facilitated opportunities for continual acceptance, understanding, and reassurance to ease her distress. The art of deep listening by someone who understands others anguish, despair, and fear allowed space for June to let go of her fear, misery, despair which appeared to bring her a level of peace.

The meaning of compassion is to suffer with, to feel the pain of the other person and to be motivated to relieve it (Nhat Hanh 2014). Gilbert (2017) suggests that compassion is a warm and loving emotion, that acknowledges others pain and suffering, it does not need to become one's own suffering and it can enable one to feel positive caring emotions. Six key attributes of compassion have been identified: motivation, sensitivity, sympathy, non-judgement, empathy, and distress tolerance (Neff 2011). By embodying Neff's compassion attributes whilst I delivered care to June, allowed both of us to connect at a deep level with no judgement.

Whilst caring for June I was aware of sensations and emotions within myself which called for me to show care and kindness to myself first. I recognised that I needed to ground myself to care for her (Nhat Hanh 1975). I tuned into my sensations and the feelings of sadness, loss and loneliness for June who had a potentially life-threatening diagnosis that isolated her from her family. I am aware that when I attend to myself, I can then offer patients in my care loving awareness. Being mindful in my work helps me to better support patients and demonstrate kindness, humanity, and interconnectedness to help them feel more at ease (Neff et al. 2007). Utilising loving awareness, I was able to connect deeply to June with compassion and understanding, whilst recognising my own humanity. Many who suffer find strength from the compassion of those who care for them, even finding personal meaning in facing suffering and death (Cadge and Catlin 2006).

In view of June's deteriorating medical status, I was continually reassessing her health status and care needs. I was cognisant of her dementia and needed to understand her level of cognition and how her dementia impacted her ability to ability to communicate. To ensure I understood June's needs, I was in contact with June's daughter daily by telephone, these conversations allowed us the space to discuss June's condition and her current care needs. It also allowed her family opportunities to ask questions, express their fears and anxieties, and remain involved in June's care. As her daughter and family could not physically be with June, I ensured they were invited to be part of the decision-making process throughout June's stay in hospital. Given June's isolation and loneliness issues, it was imperative to mitigate and protect June against further psychologic and social effects of Covid-19 especially the social distancing rules that hospitalisation posed for her and her family. I did this by promoting connection and representing all their interests whilst minimising harm. Whilst it was difficult for June to fully comprehend why her family could not visit connections were fostered and negotiated through increasing contact time by using digital technologies with an IPAD which served as an antidote in helping to reduce June's difficult psychological effects of been alone whilst also keeping family abreast of June's condition and care.

Spirituality can be a source of strength and connection when faced with the challenges of progressive cognitive impairment and new situations (Daly and Fahey-McCarthy 2014). It was clear that being out of her familiar environment and being unwell was causing her deep distress. Her daughter had told me how much June's faith meant to her and that her rosary beads and prayer were a source of comfort to her. The ethical principal of beneficence was demonstrated by sharing June's faith, I felt comfortable reciting prayers with her and quickly noticed that she visibly became less agitated. I felt comfortable doing this as her daughter and the nursing home staff had identified that this often-helped June when she was in distress. It is accepted that nurses in the ROI can share aspects of their faith as spirituality and religion are interconnected. Praying can give may patients solace, comfort and meaning, however, cognisance needs to be taken of the appropriateness of this practise and an awareness of the ethics of praying with patients if unsolicited.

Gauging her emotional state, I recognised June was expressing sadness born out of her existential concerns around death, she asked me several questions related to her faith and God. Having Covid and becoming unwell caused deep fear for June as she thought she may die. She told me that when she is unwell, she gains connection and comfort by praying to God and asked if she could see a priest. The importance of patient advocacy as a core aspect of APN practice is asserted through developing relationships and intentionally speaking up on behalf of a patient (Josse-Eklund et al. 2014, Rogers 2016), giving voice to what a patient has to say (Walent and Kayser-Jones 2008), safeguarding and protecting patients from harm (Xiaoyan and Jezewski 2007). I asked the hospital chaplain to visit June that day; both patient and chaplain were positioned to connect spiritually through praying together, thus providing June with a sense of meaning, purpose and a degree of control concerning her situation.

Compassion is the medicine we need as individuals and as a species to heal suffering (Kornfield 2002). I believe that my intentional practice of love and compassion practiced with wisdom and care ensured that I met all of June's needs and not just the physical care she needed for her pneumonia. This practice necessitates the development of a truly wise and caring heart which puts the patient at the centre of all we do as APNs. Caring for patients with dementia requires a special skill set that allowed me to enter June's world and support her with her needs. Embedding empathy in my care for June helped me to gain insight and patience which resulted in June been less agitated, calmer and more aware of her surroundings. Empathetic communication involved me being fully present and understanding June's feelings, emotions and experiences which were valid and important. I was able to be truly present in each moment by sitting down next to June, using good eye contact and offering physical touch like holding her hand or touching her back. Observing emotional clues and facial expression to detect anger, fear and sadness are all barometers of how June felt which allowed me to connect and be with June in a deep meaningful and caring manner.

Health care workers are under constant pressure to become more efficient and time spent with patients is at a premium. The principle of beneficence involves balancing the benefits of treatment against the risks and costs. It can be very difficult to spend time with patients when there are multiple pressing demands, this impacts on the ability to integrate spirituality into care (Puchalski 2012). As APNs we should focus on the whole person regardless of age and capacity in an ethically sensitive manner. Valuing our patients as fellow human beings and not treating them like machines that need fixing is paramount to spirituality. Spiritual competent clinicians often have to 'fight' the system for the welfare of their patients. The way services are managed and evaluated needs to maximise the potential for this kind of action and to provide essential connectedness to patient and their families (Wattis et al. 2017). In terms of June this necessitated me advocating for her return to the nursing home safely whilst ensuring the necessary precautions were taken i.e. isolation and use of full personal protective equipment when caring for Covid positive patients. Elements of fear whilst caring for Covid patients is a real factor as many health care workers have lost their lives (Goodman et al. 2020). This impacted me, as despite been vigilant with handwashing wearing personal protective equipment (PPE) and social distancing many healthcare staff had contracted Covid. Some staff were very unwell and unfortunately others died, this made me reflect on my own mortality.

Illness can be viewed as an existential threat, a shipwreck of sorts marked by uncertainty, frailty, isolation, dependence, loss of autonomy and loneliness which June experienced (Stein 2008, Daly et al. 2019). Vulnerability was of significant concern for June and me. June was vulnerable as she was alone, scared and confused about where she was and what was wrong with her. I was vulnerable because I was fearful of contracting Covid. Vulnerability is understood 'as susceptibility to physical, ethical or spiritual harm that includes illness and is accepted as a condition of authentic nursing practice' (Little et al. 2000, p. 495). However, Rogers (2016) challenges this definition of vulnerability by suggesting that vulnerability in terms of spirituality should be thought as a vehicle to how we connect deeply with patients in our care and connect to our own humanity.

The need to commit to a patient's welfare is regarded as a virtue ethics directed towards patient's needs, ascertaining what good care is, and what constitutes good action to inform the nurse–patient relationship. In preparation for meeting my patients, I always acknowledge my personal worldview, so that I can step out of my frame of reference to discern a patients' perspective and facilitate relevant actions that fit with their frame of reference and needs. Whilst aware of June's diagnosis, I was conscious of the serious threat that the Covid infection posed to her deteriorating condition which was juxtaposed with the fear and risk that the disease and possible transmission posed for me and my family. Whilst this fact constituted an ethical concern, nonetheless I recognised caring not as a dilemma but as an inherent life force borne out of professional obligation, concern, and commitment. To prioritise June's safety, minimise distress and to do good I chose to commit to being receptive to her plight which helped develop interpersonal relatedness and appeared to help June find a level of meaning in her plight.

Given June's dementia and being aware of how the presence of PPE impacted patients, I needed to be attentive to June's nonverbal and behavioural cues. Being sensitive to these cues helped me to act ethically and to get to know June as a person. I ensured that I could spend adequate time with her and be actively present with her. June recognised that I had time for her and valued her needs. My care was dictated by her pace which enabled us to build a trustful secure relationship by treating June as a fellow human being. I ensured that I minimised environmental stressors which allowed me to provide and coordinate essential, psychosocial, and emotional aspects of care, reduce her agitation, feelings of isolation, making her comfortable and feel safe (Ericsson et al. 2013). Authentic engagement and listening attentively to June's story led to new possibilities of knowing and learning which enabled me to optimise the care I provided for her (Falk-Rafael 2001). For Frankl, the spirit of the person with dementia never gets sick as the capacity for 'spiritual intelligence' remains (McFadden et al. 2000). June's dementia represented a burden for her due to impaired cognition, requiring assistance to undertake tasks, behavioural agitation and distress that often culminated in tears. Faith and prayer constituted important aspects of her family life, creating a sense of belonging, helping her to stay connected, acting as a coping resource in facing her loss of independence thus providing a source of hope.

Authenticity relates to practicing genuineness, having the capability to reflect, engaging in caring communication, being open and honest with oneself and others (Horton -Deutsch 2017). Attempting to hold what gives our patients hope, meaning and purpose can help them heal, it necessitates paying particular attention to responsibilities brought about by opening up and engaging in face-to-face interactions, which can risky and be difficult (Whelan 2018). Levinas (cited by Watson 2005) considers vulnerability as the cornerstone of ethics and reminds us that face-to-face encounters are an ethical imperative. When we as APNs encounter and look in the face of a patient we are caring for, we are holding the mystery of that person's life in our hands that imparts a responsibility in for taking care of June respectfully as a person and protecting her as a consequence (Whelan 2018). This ethical imperative empowered me to direct my energy and responsibilities towards driving care in response to June's holistic needs, acknowledging and reflecting what was mirrored and seen through our relational interactions and understandings of one another.

9.4   Conclusion

Care, compassion, and commitment are foundational to APN holistic practice. APNs need to consider and reflect upon authenticity and genuineness regarding how they practice, the way in which they practice, and the capacity to fully utilise their scope of practice. Recognising and incorporating spirituality, spiritual literacy and spiritual competent care provision within APN education and practice in fundamental to ensure that the fullest extent of holistic patient care is provided in an ethical sensitive way. Spiritual care is an integral component of the APN role. Rogers' (2016) Availability and Vulnerability framework for Spiritually Competent Practice provides a seminal lens to advancing accessibility, sensitivity, openness and commitment to person-centred holistic care provision within the context of advanced nursing practice, facilitating an active intelligent soul presence and comfort that takes account of both patients and practitioners vulnerabilities which is very much needed within healthcare. An APN's aim is to provide holistic care which should include presence, listening and engaging with each person in an ethical responsive way whilst recognising them as unique spiritual beings. Without such integration, APNs will not be positioned to respond to, be open to potential suffering or to advocate for and on behalf of spiritual aspects of patients, families, lives, or their colleagues.

References

Begley C, Murphy K, Higgins A, Elliott N, Lalor J, Sheerin F, Coyne I, Comiskey C, Normand C, Casey C, Dowling M, Devane D, Cooney A, Farrelly F, Brennan M, Meskell P, MacNeela P (2010) An evaluation of clinical nurse and midwife specialist and advanced nurse and midwife practitioner roles in Ireland (SCAPE). National Council for the Professional Development of Nursing and Midwifery in Ireland, Dublin

Cadge W, Catlin EA (2006) Making sense of suffering and death: how health care providers' construct meanings in a neonatal intensive care unit. J Relig Health 45:248–263. https://doi.org/10.1007/s10943-006-9012-2

Carney M (2014) International perspectives on advanced nurse and midwife practice regarding advanced practice criteria for posts and persons and requirements for regulation of advanced nurse/ midwife practice. Nursing and Midwifery Board of Ireland, Dublin

Central Statistics Office Census of Population (2016) Profile 8 Irish Travellers, Ethnicity and Religion. https://www.cso.ie/en/releasesandpublications/ep/p-cp8iter/p8iter/p8bgn/

Chrash M, Mulich B, Patton C (2011) The APN role in holistic assessment and integration of spiritual assessment for advance care planning. J Am Acad of Nurse Pract 23:530–536

Clark A, Jit M, Warren-Gash C, Guthrie B, Wang HH (2020) Global regional and national estimates of the population at increased risk of severe Covid −19 due to underlying health conditions in 2020: a modelling study. Lancet 8:1003–1017

Cronenwett L, Dracup K, Grey M, McCauley L, Meleis A, Salmon M (2011) The doctor of nursing practice: a national workforce perspective. Nurs Outlook 59(1):9–17

Daly L, Fahey-McCarthy E (2014) Attending to the spiritual in dementia care nursing. Br J Nurs 23:787–791

Daly L, McCarthy E, Timmins F (2019) The experience of spirituality from the perspective of people living with dementia; a systematic review and meta-synthesis. Dementia 18(2):448–470

Department of Health (2016) Position paper one values for nurses and midwives in Ireland. Chief Nursing Office, Dublin, p 2016

Department of Health (2019) A policy on the development of graduate to advanced nursing and midwifery practice. Stationery Office, Dublin, p 2019

Department of Health and Children (2011) Strategic framework for role expansion of nurses and midwives: promoting quality patient care. DOH, Dublin, p 2011

Ericsson I, Kiellstrom S, Hellstrom I (2013) Creating relationships with persons with moderate to severe dementia. Dementia 12(1):63–79

Falk-Rafael AR (2001) Empowerment as a process of evolving consciousness. Adv Nurs Sci 24(1):1–16

Fealy G (ed) (2005) Care to remember: nursing and midwifery in Ireland in the twentieth century. An Bord Altranais, Cork

Flanagan B, O'Sullivan M (2019) The Routledge international handbook of spirituality in society and the professions, 1st edn. Routledge International Press, Oxon

Gilbert P (2017) Compassion: concepts, research and applications. Routledge, London

Goodman J, de Prudhoe K, Williams C (2020) Uk Covid −19 public inquiry needed to learn lessons and save lives. Lancet 397:177–180. https://doi.org/10.1016/S0140-6736(20)32726-4

Government of Ireland (1998) Report of the commission on nursing. Government Publications, Dublin

Government of Ireland Committee on the Future of Healthcare (2017) Sláintecare report. Houses of the Oireachtas. Stationery Office, Dublin

Government of Ireland (2019) A Policy on the Development of Graduate to Advanced Nursing and Midwifery Practice Houses of the Oireachtas. Stationery Office, Dublin

Health Information and Quality Authority (2012a) A guide to the National Standards for safer better healthcare. HIQA, Dublin

Health Information and Quality Authority (2012b) A guide to the National Standards for safer better healthcare. HIQA, Dublin

Health Service Executive (2011) A question of faith: the relevance of faith and spirituality in health care. HSE, Dublin

HSE (2014) National Guideline for the Development of Advanced Nursing or Midwifery Practitioner Services

Health Service Executive (2019) Second National Intercultural Health Strategy 2018–2023. HSE, Dublin

Health Service Executive (2020) COVID-19 nursing homes expert panel examination of measures to 2021. Health Service Executive, Dublin

Horton -Deutsch S (2017) Thinking, acting, and leading through caring science literacy, in the caring science imperative: a Hallmark in nursing education. In: Lee SM, Palmeiri PA, Watson J (eds) Global advances in human caring literacy. Springer: Watson Caring Science Institute, New York, pp 59–70

International Council of Nurses (2012) ICN code of ethics for nurses. ICN, Geneva

International Council of Nurses (2020) Guidelines on advanced practice nursing. ICN, Geneva

Johnson RW, Tilghman JS, Davis-Dick LR, Hamilton- Faison B. (2006) A historical overview of spirituality in nursing. ABNF J 17:60

Josse-Eklund A et al (2014) Swedish nurses' perceptions of influencers on patient advocacy: a phenomenographic study. Nurs Ethics 21:673–683

Kennelly B, O'Callaghan M, Coughlan D, Cullinan J, Doherty E, Glynn L, Moloney E, Queally M (2020) The COVID-19 pandemic in Ireland: an overview of the health service and economic policy response. Health Policy Technol 9:19–429

Kornfield J (2002) Path with heart: the classic guide through the perils and promises of spiritual life. Rider, London

Little M, Paul K, Jordens CFC, Sayers EJ (2000) Vulnerability in the narratives of patients and their Carers: studies of colorectal Cancer. Health 4(4):495–510

Mazzotta CP (2016) Biomedical approaches to care and their influence on point of care nurses: a scoping review. J Nurs Educ Pract 6(8):93–101

McFadden SH, Ingram M, Baldauf C (2000) Actions, feelings and values: foundations in meaning and personhood. In: Kimble MA (ed) Dementia in Viktor Frankls contribution to spirituality and aging. The Haworth Pastoral Press, New York, pp 66–86

McSherry W (2006) Making sense of spirituality in nursing and health care practice an interactive approach, 2nd edn. Jessica Kingsley, London

Meehan CT (2012) Spirituality and spiritual care from a careful nursing perspective. J Nurs Manag 20:990–1001

National Health Service (2015) Non-Medical Prescribing: An economic evaluation. NHS Health Education: North West, Liverpool

Neenan K (2019) Being human: cultivating mindfulness and compassion for daily living. In: Timmins F, Caldeira S (eds) Spirituality in healthcare: perspectives for innovative practice. Springer, Cham, pp 211–225

Neff K (2011) Self-compassion the proven power of being kind to yourself. Harper Collins, New York

Neff KD, Rude SS, Kirkpatrick K (2007) An examination of self-compassion in relation to positive psychological functioning and personality traits. J Res Pers 41:908–916

Nhat Hanh T (1975) The miracle of mindfulness. Beacon press, New York

Nhat Hanh T (2006) Teachings on love. Beacon Press, New York

Nhat Hanh T (2014) The art of communication. Harper Collins: Beacon Press, New York

Nursing and Midwifery Board of Ireland (2014) Professional code of conduct and ethics for nurses and midwives. NMBI, Dublin

Nursing and Midwifery Board of Ireland (2015a) Post registration nursing and midwifery Programmes standards and requirements. NMBI, Dublin

Nursing and Midwifery Board of Ireland (2015b) Practice standards for midwives. NMBI, Dublin

Nursing and Midwifery Board of Ireland (2015c) Scope of nursing and midwifery practice framework. NMBI, Dublin

Nursing and Midwifery Board of Ireland (2017) Advanced practice (nursing) standards and requirements, vol 9(4). NMBI, Dublin

O'Shea Y (2008) Nursing and midwifery in Ireland: a strategy for professional development in a changing health service. Blackhall Publishing, Dublin

Puchalski CM (2012) Restorative medicine. In: Cobb M, Puchalski C, Rumbold B (eds) Oxford textbook of spirituality in healthcare. Oxford University Press, Oxford

Pulchalski CM et al (2014) Improving the spiritual dimension of whole person care; reaching national and international consensus. J Palliat Med 17:642–656

Rasmussen TS, Delmar C (2014) Dignity as an empirical lifeworld construction—in the field of surgery in Denmark. Int J Qual Stud Health Well Being 9. https://doi.org/10.3402/qhw.v9.24849

Rogers M (2016) Spiritual Dimensions of Advanced Nurse Practitioner Consultations in Primary Care through the Lens of Availability and Vulnerability. A Hermeneutic Enquiry. Doctoral thesis, University of Huddersfield

Rogers M, Hargreaves J, Wattis J (2020) Spiritual dimensions of nurse practitioner consultations in family practice. J Holist Nurs 38(1):8–18

Rogers M, Wattis J (2019) Understanding the role of spirituality in providing person-centred care. Nurs Stand 35(9):25–30. https://doi.org/10.7748/ns.2020.e11342

Stein M (2008) The lonely patient how we experience illness. Harper Perennial, New York

Streib H, Hood R (2016) (2016) semantics and psychology of spirituality. Springer, Dordrecht

The Royal College of Nursing (UK) (2011) RCN Spiritual Survey. RCN, London

Timmins F (2013) Nurses views of spirituality and spiritual care provision in the Republic of Ireland. J Stud Spiritual 3(2):121–137

Timmins F, Caldeira S, Murphy M, Pujol N, Sheaf G, Weathers E, Whelan J, Trinity College Dublin (2016b) An exploration of current in hospital spiritual care resources in the Republic of Ireland and review of international chaplaincy standards; a preliminary scoping exercise to inform practice development. HSE, Dublin

Timmins F, Murphy MA, Caldeira GE, King C, Brady V, Whelan J, O'Boyle C, Kelly J, Neill F et al (2016a) Developing agreed and accepted understandings of spirituality and spiritual care concepts among members of an innovative spirituality interest Group in the Republic of Ireland. Religions 7:30

Walent RJ, Kayser-Jones J (2008) Having a voice and being heard: nursing home residents and in-house advocacy. J Gerontol Nurs 34(11):34–42

Watson J (2005) Caring science as sacred science. F.A. Davis, Philadelphia

Wattis J, Curran S, Rogers M (2017) What Does Spirituality Mean for Patients, Practitioners and Health Care Organisations. In: Wattis J, Curran S, Rogers M (eds) Spiritually competent practice in health care. CRC Press, New York. 99-1141-7

Weathers E (2019) What is spirituality? In: Timmins F, Caldeira F (eds) Spirituality in healthcare: perspectives for innovative practice. Springer, Cham, pp 1–23

Weathers E, McCarthy G, Coffey A (2015) Concept analysis of spirituality: an evolutionary approach. Nurs Forum 51:79–96

Whelan J (2018) The Caring Science Imperative: A Hallmark in Nursing Education. In: Lee SM, Palmeiri PA, Watson J (eds) Global Advances in Human Caring Literacy. Springer: Watson Caring Science Institute, New York, pp 33–42

Whelan J (2019) Teaching and learning about spirituality in healthcare practice settings. In: Timmins F, Caldeira S (eds) Spirituality in healthcare: perspectives for innovative practice. Springer, Cham, pp 165–192

World Health Organization (1984) Regional Office for South-East Asia; spiritual aspects of health. WHO Regional Office for South-East Asia, New Delhi

Wren MA, Keegan C, Walshe B, Bergin A, Eigahn, J, Brick A, Brick A, Connolly S (2017) Projections of demand for healthcare in Ireland, 2015–2030: first report from the Hippocrates model ESRI series. https://doi.org/10.26504/rs67

Xiaoyan B, Jezewski MA (2007) Developing a mid-range theory of patient advocacy through concept analysis. J Adv Nurs 57(1):101–110

Younas A (2017) Spiritual care and the role of advanced practice nurses. Nurs Midwifery Stud 6(1):e40072

Global Case Study in Spirituality: Stories of Hope from Canada

10

Sheryl Reimer-Kirkham, Kimberley Lamarche, and Josette Roussel

Abstract

The integration of spirituality by Advanced Practice Nurses (APN) in Canada occurs in the context of a remarkably diverse citizenry. This diversity requires that the APN bring together self-awareness with literacy about spiritual practices, how religious diversity is respected and accommodated, and how spirituality can serve as a pathway to social inclusion and healing. In Canada, this includes responses to the 2015 Truth and Reconciliation Commission with its calls to address the impacts of colonization and intergenerational trauma on Indigenous communities. A case study is presented to demonstrate how the Availability and Vulnerability framework can be integrated into the Two-Eyed Seeing Framework to provide a lens to understand the importance of spirituality within APN practice.

Keywords

Indigenous health · Two-eyed seeing · Diversity · Spirituality · Advanced practice nursing

S. Reimer-Kirkham (✉)
Trinity Western University, Langley, BC, Canada
e-mail: Sheryl.Kirkham@twu.ca

K. Lamarche
Athabasca University, Athabasca, AB, Canada
e-mail: lamarche@athabascau.ca

J. Roussel
Montfort Hospital, Ottawa, ON, Canada

153

10.1   Introduction

The Advanced Practice Nurse (APN) role in Canada has been slow in being fully integrated into healthcare services. However, recently it has begun to expand as evidence has grown about improved health outcomes and the cost effectiveness of advanced practice nursing. Concurrently, spirituality in health has also had varying amounts of attention in Canada, with the nursing profession tending to subsume spirituality under the umbrella of culturally responsive care. In this chapter, we explore this interface between spirituality and the APN role in Canada. We write from our scholarship and expertise in spirituality (Reimer-Kirkham), advanced practice nursing (Lamarche), and health policy and nursing leadership (Roussel). We write as non-Indigenous scholars and allies to the cause of decolonisation, Indigenisation, and reconciliation in Canadian healthcare services and advanced nursing practice.

The Canadian Nurses Association's (CNA) (2010) position statement *Spirituality, Health and Nursing Practice* encourages nurses to

- practice therapeutic communication that can create an opening for discussions with individuals about their spiritual beliefs and values;
- take into account the unique spiritual beliefs and values of individuals, families and communities during decision-making, treatment and care, including the terminology used to describe such beliefs;
- demonstrate sensitivity to and respect for diversity in spiritual beliefs, support of spiritual preferences and attention to spiritual needs as nursing competencies; and,
- work collaboratively with other care providers to be attentive to the spiritual beliefs and values and the physical and psychosocial needs of individuals and families at all stages of life. (CNA 2010, p. 2).

In Canada, the British Columbia College of Nursing Professionals (2018) *Entry-level Competencies for Nurse Practitioners* includes one competency that relates to spirituality. In the competency category of client care, in the domain of assessment, competency #B2b states: "…Collect relevant information specific to the client's psychosocial, behavioral, cultural, ethnic, spiritual, developmental life stage, and social determinants of health" (British Columbia College of Nursing Professionals 2018, p. 8). With these professional guidelines, spirituality is understood as relevant to the APN role (Staples et al. 2020).

10.2   The APN Role in Canada

In Canada, advanced practice nursing refers to the integration of graduate nursing educational preparation with in-depth, specialised clinical nursing knowledge and expertise; this knowledge and skillset facilitate complex decision-making to meet the health needs of people (CNA 2019). Nurses in Canada are regulated at the provincial or territorial level (Almost 2021). There are two recognised APN roles: the Clinical

Nurse Specialist (CNS) and Nurse Practitioner (NP). CNSs spend more time on education, research, organisational leadership and professional development activities, with less time devoted to direct clinical care (Almost 2021). The NP, by contrast, is the only APN role with additional regulation and title protection beyond the registered nurse. NPs can autonomously make a diagnosis, order and interpret diagnostic tests, prescribe pharmaceuticals and treatments, and perform specific procedures within their legislated scope of practice (Almost 2021; CNA 2016a).

APNs deliver health services at the individual, family, community, and population health levels in a wide array of settings. They focus on clinical practice, whether through a direct relationship with people and/or through indirect activities such as care coordination and provide clinical expertise through consultation about the person's health with other healthcare providers. APNs are also involved in roles related to optimising the health system, education, research, and leadership (CNA 2019). Therefore, they have been instrumental to inform, influence and accelerate healthcare system level reform and policy (CNA 2019).

APN roles have been in place for more than five decades, but many reports highlight the lack of full integration of these roles (CNA 2019; Little and Reichert 2018; Martin-Misener and Bryant-Lukosius 2016). Legislative and system barriers are present and vary between Canadian jurisdictions. A significant barrier identified by Canadian researchers is the lack of integration and connection between health-care priorities and the lack of evidence about the benefits of APN roles to improve the health of Canadians, increase access to care, and reduce costs (Bryant-Lukosius and Wong 2018).

The history and role development of the CNS and NP came from different origins and health system needs. The CNS first emerged in the 1970s as patient care grew more complex. CNSs were focused on complex care and system issues that required improvements, which resulted in measurable positive outcomes for the people they served. The Canadian Nurses Association believes that the CNS role must be better understood, described and distinguished. Additional efforts are needed to deploy CNSs effectively, including the requirement of graduate education and the creation of structures to empower them if they are not to be separately regulated (Almost 2021). "A CNS is a registered nurse who holds a master's or doctoral degree in nursing and has expertise in a clinical nursing specialty" (CNA 2016b, p. 1). They provide support for quality practice and health system strengthening across the health-care continuum. The CNS role was introduced to respond to increased patient need, a demand for nursing specialisation and to support nursing practice at the point of care. However, even though the CNS has been part of the Canadian health-care system for many decades, they continue to face challenges.

The NP role originated in the work of nurses who, decades ago, provided care that was otherwise unavailable in rural and remote areas (CNA 2019). In 2019, there were 6159 NPs in Canada (CNA 2020), an 8.1% growth from 2018. NPs work in a variety of sectors, with the highest number (30%) working in community care. NPs gained formal recognition in the 1970s, when they were recommended by policy-makers as a way of providing healthcare to isolated populations (CNA 2019).

The Canadian Nurses Association's *Advanced Practice Nursing: A Pan-Canadian Framework* (2019) defines advanced practice nursing and describes how nurses in these roles build on clinical expertise in a specialty area by integrating research, education, leadership, consultation and collaboration within a health systems approach. APNs provide effective and efficient healthcare, delivered with a high degree of autonomy, to an identified population. They lead interprofessional and intra-professional teams and have extensive depth and breadth of knowledge. They draw on a wide range of strategies to meet the needs of clients and to improve accessibility, safety and quality of healthcare. APNs can initiate or participate in planning, coordinating, implementing and evaluating programmers to meet client needs, promote the health of communities, and support nursing practice. They can explain and apply the theoretical, empirical, ethical and experiential foundations of nursing practice. In direct-care activities, APNs demonstrate advanced expertise in assessment, judgment and decision-making; they integrate in-depth nursing knowledge, research and clinical expertise, as well as knowledge from other disciplines. Another characteristic of APNs is their expertise in research methods and ability to critically examine research for quality, relevance to practice and effect on healthcare and system outcomes. Finally, APNs in Canada use knowledge-mobilisation techniques to promote and implement research-informed practice. They provide consultation services to other health-care professionals and stakeholders whose services influence the determinants of health. APNs understand and apply improvement science to identify and lead quality improvement initiatives. They implement influential leadership and change management skills to initiate change to improve client, organisation and system outcomes, and they analyse and influence health policy and other policies.

10.3 Spirituality in Canadian Healthcare

Broadly speaking, in Canada spirituality and religion are seen as interconnected. Conceptualizations of spirituality and religion entail sacred referents (whether to do with a higher power, a theistic God, or that which is special or set apart in some way), beliefs (about the nature of reality, how to achieve wellbeing, and people's relationships to the metaphysical), values (signposts for what is considered moral comportment), meaning-making (giving purpose to life, including illness and suffering), and practices (rituals, relationships). In practice, religion is usually expressed through relatively formal social institutions and spirituality has been interpreted as more individual expressions of values and beliefs (Bramadat et al. 2013; Reimer-Kirkham et al. 2020).

Canada's spiritual landscape is characterised by a "new diversity" (Beaman 2017) of secularism and fading majoritarian religions; Indigenous[1] histories and

---

[1] In Canada, the term "Indigenous" is being used as the preferred collective noun for First Nations, Inuit, and Metis. "Indigenous" comes from the Latin word "indigena" which means "spring from the land; native". Indigenous Peoples recognizes that, rather than a single group of people, there are many separate and unique Nations. This terminology also aligns with the United Nations Declaration on the Rights of Indigenous Peoples. See: https://opentextbc.ca/indigenizationcurriculumdevelopers/front-matter/introduction-2/.

spiritualities; newcomers and diasporic religions; new spiritualities; and those who identify as "nones." This diversity requires the APN to be conversant with and responsive to a range of spiritual and religious identities. This diversity also means that definitions of spirituality and religion vary, depending on which client population an APN is working with, as well as on the APN's spiritual and/or religious identity. Although declining in numbers, about two-thirds of Canadians affiliate with Christianity to some degree (Statistics Canada 2011).[2] Within this sector, there is considerable diversity as to Catholicism and Protestantism, and subsets within these groups. There has been a steady decline in the numbers of affiliates and also the social influence of these religions on social life in Canada over the last decades. At the same time, increasing numbers of Canadians (24%) indicate "no religion" on census surveys (Statistics Canada 2011). Also referred to as "nones," this is a broad category that includes emergent spiritualities not tied to formal religions, as well as agnostics, atheists, and those who do not view themselves as spiritual. Emergent spiritualities relocate the sacred in a new individual and holistic manner, "away from hierarchical, regional, patriarchal, and institutional religion" (Sharma et al. 2012, p. 299). Many Canadians refer to themselves as spiritual but not religious.

Diasporic minority religions are on the rise in step with patterns of immigration to Canada. Immigration from Asia, the Middle East, and Africa has created ever-growing Buddhist, Hindu, Muslim, and Sikh communities, collectively representing 7.2% of Canada's population (Statistics Canada 2011). With our diverse Canadian citizenry, and the rising evidence of religion and spirituality as social determinants of health (Idler 2014), APNs' literacy about spirituality in healthcare must include consideration of the beliefs and practices of newcomer and diasporic religions. Indeed, the overlapping relationships between ethnicity, culture, and spirituality (likewise between religion and race) are such that the issue is less one of conflation (e.g., between culture and spirituality) and more so one of intersection. In this regard, Canadian healthcare services have received scrutiny as to the degree to which religious and spiritual diversity is accommodated (Taher 2021; Reimer-Kirkham and Cochrane 2016), and all the more so in the era of #BlackLivesMatter and emerging stories of racialised religions, including Islamophobia (Joshi 2006; Reimer-Kirkham 2019; Samari et al. 2018).

Also re-shaping the Canadian landscape is the young and growing Indigenous population and an overdue movement to acknowledge and reconcile the longstanding government history of land dispossession and colonial oppression, much of which was operationalized by the church through residential schools and Native Indian hospitals. More than 150,000 children were forcibly removed from their families over a period of 100 years (with the last school closing in 1996), with the goal of assimilating them into Euro-Christian Canadian ways. The Truth and Reconciliation Commission (TRC) (2015, p. 43) explains, "residential schools were part of a process that brought European states and Christian churches together in a complex and powerful manner." This legacy carries forward today in patterns of

---

[2] Statistics Canada collects religion-related census data every 10 years, next to be released with the 2021 census.

lower life expectancy, intergenerational trauma and social dislocation. The TRC's (2015) "94 Calls to Action" require the address of systemic racism that results in Indigenous peoples continuing to experience structural vulnerabilities (e.g., lack of access to culturally safe healthcare, lack of access to clean water, lack of access to food security, racism expressed by healthcare providers). There is a degree to which Canada's secularism that has placed spirituality in the realm of the personal and the private is disrupted by this coming-to-terms with our shared colonial past and present. Referred to as "indigenizing secularism" (Colorado 2020, p. 76/77), the move is to bring acknowledgment of this "immeasurable damage wrought by residential schools," together with appreciation for the resilience of Indigenous spiritualities with the view that "the sacred is embedded in all aspects of Indigenous life." As Canadian institutions—including higher education and healthcare—take up the TRC's (2015) Calls to Action in the spirit of decolonization, we see a way forward that can contribute to healthier relations and better health outcomes. APNs can play a vital role in addressing health inequities and cultural safety for Indigenous Peoples, as illustrated in the case study that follows.

A search in CINAHL with the intersecting search terms of advanced practice nursing, research, and spirituality/religion yielded few Canadian research studies. There is an emerging body of ANP literature on ethnocultural, refugee, and migrant populations (such as South East Asians in Canada) where religious affiliation and beliefs often function prominently in their health practices (Wright and Sweeney 2020). A further, but small ANP research literature where spirituality is integrated relates to Indigenous health (Prodan-Bhalla et al. 2017; Ziabakhsh et al. 2016).

10.4　Case Study

This case study will focus on spirituality related to the integration of the Indigenous Two-Eyed Seeing Framework within APN practice. Drawing on traditional Indigenous knowledges, Two-Eyed Seeing principles were developed by Mi'kmaq (a vibrant First Nation established as an Indigenous Band under Canada's *Indian Act* of 1876) First Nation elders Murdena and Albert Marshall to communicate bringing together the different world views of Indigenous knowledges with Western knowledges (Bartlett et al. 2012). Community members, healthcare workers, researchers, and research agencies such as the Canadian Institutes of Health Research have embraced these principles (Forbes et al. 2020). Two-Eyed Seeing principles allow healthcare workers to consider self-reflection and vulnerability while respectfully addressing the impacts of colonisation and intergenerational trauma. Two-Eyed Seeing helps clinicians recognise that a one eye focus on Western knowledge and medical practices is unhelpful when supporting those of Indigenous ancestry. There is a need to have one eye also open to Indigenous knowledge and experience to be holistic and person-centered.

This case study demonstrates how Rogers' (2016) Availability and Vulnerability framework can be integrated with the Two-Eyed Seeing Framework to further understand the importance of spirituality within APN practice. The clinical setting for this case is an interprofessional Primary Health Care clinic housed within a larger non-profit organization supporting people living with stigmatised illnesses such as Human Immunodeficiency Virus, Hepatitis C, mental health and substance use disorders. The inner city clinic supports those amongst the most vulnerable in society: homeless people; people in trouble with the law; women escaping domestic violence; sex trade workers; and people from the lesbian, gay, bisexual, transgender, queer and two-spirited (LGBTQ2) community. The team includes a primary healthcare Nurse Practitioner, family physicians, street- and clinic-based registered nurses, phlebotomists, a community based social worker, peer support workers, and safe needle exchange, overdose prevention and suicide prevention trainers.

The patient, Noel, identifies as a Mi'kmaq male who has experienced housing insecurity, ongoing intravenous drug use, and chronic Hepatitis C infection. He currently lives off the Indigenous reserve[3] and away from the cultural support of his family and elders (elders are esteemed leaders of Indigenous communities). His co-morbid medical and socio-economic needs combined with a shared colonial history of intergenerational trauma have contributed to a lack of trust in Western medicine and clinicians. Paramount to the effectiveness of any interventions is understanding intergenerational trauma not as an individual concept but rather as a convergence of multiple processes of historical trauma and extreme losses perpetrated by colonization and its aftermath (Nelson and Wilson 2017). Intergenerational trauma brings significant health effects such as addiction and mental health disorders, chronic diseases, and suicide (Marsh et al. 2020).

I, Kim, first met Noel when he was in what we term "crisis" from a Western perspective. Noel is a regular visitor to our clinic where I work as a NP. Although he lacks trust in the healthcare system, he attends our clinic mainly to receive prescription medication. I was aware of Noel's Indigenous background, and prioritised his immediate medical and social needs as I was concerned about the impact of his medical condition on his overall wellness. As a NP I use a harm reduction approach where I have been taught to meet patients "where they are," and incorporate wellness approaches in each encounter. In reality, this is difficult concept to incorporate when a patient is in crisis and we are concerned about their immediate safety or welfare. Our clinic is unique and routinely sees patients who are not cared for within the traditional healthcare system as they feel stigmatized by the system, and are often perceived as non-compliant and difficult to manage. As part of our clinic's strategy to overcome stigma, I have experience and training in supporting patients who are structurally vulnerable. Many of our patients tend not to seek healthcare because they fear being further discriminated against because of their lifestyle or medical history. Our Primary Health Care clinic aims to reduce these barriers by providing person-centered care through harm reduction services in a known

---

[3] Reserves are tracks of land set aside under Canada's *Indian Act* of 1876 and treaty agreements for the exclusive use of an Indian band. This colonial system of displacing Indigenous peoples to reserves was accompanied by the dispossession of traditional lands, changes to lifestyle, and crowded living conditions. The government then had access to the traditional Indigenous lands for settlement and development (Joseph 2018).

non-judgmental and caring environment. During this appointment with Noel I noticed that he was in a poor state of health. I recognised that I was rushing the appointment; as I struggled with workload pressures, I sensed I was not connecting with Noel.

Later that day I reflected on our consultation, realising I did not focus on "where *he* was." My consultation lacked the usual depth of relationship as I was focused on encouraging him to start a new Hepatitis C medication. I was extremely focused on what I interpreted as his urgent medical need and I neglected to engage in "mindfulness" which I often utilise in practice to see beyond the known, be present and to become vulnerable enough myself to consider his wellness and healing beyond a Western medical perspective. I struggled to experience a sense of authentic connection with Noel based on my measure of progress and was unsuccessful in meeting my Western goals which included initiation of treatment, supporting him to understand transmission principles, and getting him to accept harm reduction support such as safe needle exchange.

The next day I sought out guidance to help me support Noel the next time we were due to meet. I wanted to understand more about his spiritual and cultural traditions and understand his world view better. As it happened, the local community was having an organised group walk to raise awareness of the impact of overdose and to acknowledge and advocate for friends and family members who had lost their lives in this way. Many colleagues, patients and family members joined together in the open air after the walk to share stories and music about loved ones. I absorbed the stories, music, and family members' presence in order to learn and be present. It was during the sharing of a story about healthcare that I gained insight into the Two-Eyed Seeing Framework embedded into Mi'kmaq culture. The Two-Eyed Seeing Framework is about not becoming blinkered to one's own view but always considering the world view of the other. Again, I reflected on my own practice and specifically my consultation with Noel. I recognised that I had a very *one-eye* perspective on healing which was not helping Noel.

During this community day I had the opportunity to witness Mi'kmaq traditions used to restore health and balance. I witnessed the Mi'kmaq elders creating a safe space for sage cleansing. Sage cleansing (sometimes referred to as smudging) has been used traditionally to "cleanse" a person, group or place and remove unwanted spirits which may be causing harm. I was interested to see Noel and his girlfriend arrive for personal cleansing and engage whole heartedly in the process. I saw Noel leave the cleansing and observed an aura of peace and connectedness. I reflected that my consultation with Noel the day before caused him to be more agitated and certainly not connected with me as an NP. I wanted to learn to be more open within my work and consider how these practices may help some of my patients, and if integrated into my work could lead to a more robust form of caregiving. I realised that these practices were key to Noel's spirituality and offered something to him that I had not been able to provide during our consultation. I recognised that I needed to understand how my personal understanding of spirituality and beliefs could help, or through a different lens, hinder the more holistic approach to caregiving. I later spent time during group supervision with colleagues exploring this further and we considered as a clinic how we could support the spiritual practices of Indigenous patients and thereby recognise their world view better. I met with the Mi'kmaq elders over a few months and talked to them about their spiritual practices and how I could integrate the Two-Eyed Seeing Framework into my APN work. They taught me a great deal about different practices and suggested I consider integrating the sage cleansing into my work if appropriate.

At our next consultation, I explored with Noel what the experience of sage cleansing meant to him. I stepped away from my own agenda of starting a new medication and instead encouraged Noel to share about his personal story and his spiritual practices. I asked if he would like complete a sage cleanse during our time together. Noel looked at me and asked, "do you mean it?" He appeared delighted that I was willing to consider this as he told me never had a Western clinician ask him about his background and traditions. He said this would really help him to feel listened to and valued. He performed the sage cleansing in my office and told me that being able to incorporate his cultural practices in our consultation gave him a sense of peace. It enabled us to develop a deeper connection and created a safe space for Noel to be more open about his health and social care needs. This is something we are striving to curate as APNs but often do not achieve fully because we do not always listen to our patients' spiritual needs. Noel returned later that day with his girlfriend who had an appointment with me. She asked if she could also carry out sage cleansing, she told me Noel was so taken aback about the clinic being open to his cultural practices that she wanted to start working with us to deal with her own health and drug usage. She said she believed if we respected and were as open to her as we were to Noel she could partner with us to improve her overall wellness.

My consultations with Noel and his girlfriend on that day were instrumental to me adapting my practice to meet my patients' spiritual needs. I find that the Two-Eyed Seeing Framework has meant my practice is much more integrative. I saw how different my integration of Western approaches were when I made the decision to ask Noel about his Indigenous identity and what would help him. I have also found that Rogers' (2016) Availability and Vulnerability framework resonates with my own approach to spiritual care. Using the concepts of availability and vulnerability has provided a practical way for me to integrate spirituality into my consultations with patients, my colleagues and also the community as a whole. I now practice using these concepts as I work with marginalized, structurally vulnerable and Indigenous populations. I have learnt that by choosing to be available and vulnerable in my work, my patients feel valued and respected as individuals and fellow human-beings. My consultations have become much more collaborative and I am more open to exploring different practices with my patients. Of course, I am careful to maintain ethical boundaries and there are some practices which are not appropriate to integrate into a consultation. However, learning about sage cleansing enabled me to be willing to use it within the consultation as Noel led this practice rather than me, the practice led to a much deeper connection with Noel which ultimately enabled him to trust me enough to support him to make positive changes to improve his health.

Over the next 12 months, the therapeutic trusting relationship which typically defines APN practice transformed through integration of the Two-Eyed Seeing Framework. Fostering increased connection to Noel's Indigeneity made a significant difference to his health. He subsequently accepted and completed pharmaceutical treatment of Hepatitis C and has remained connected to our clinic. His experiences as a Mi'kmaq male, with his unique perspectives have additionally allowed him to participate in the care of other patients through peer support and shared spiritual practices. We have since had additional sage cleansing ceremonies in our clinic, and have welcomed drummers, elder teachings and other traditional Indigenous spiritual practices to our health community experiences. Being open to viewing care through two divergent perspectives allowed for long term improvement to care not only on an individual level for Neil and his girlfriend, but also contributed to the integration of critical elements from Western and Indigenous culture as standard practices within our clinic.

For this case, acknowledging the strength of Noel's personal spirituality and that of his community enabled it to be integrated within the Western harm reduction approach. It necessitated both Noel and myself being vulnerable and open to meeting each other human to human in the sacred space he welcomed during the sage cleansing that led to our connection deepening. Meeting people where they are at is a core harm reduction tenant, as well as core to holistic care. Harm reduction principles are tools, best delivered through increasing the connection of the patient to not only the APN but also to their own spirituality and community. Reflecting on those initial meetings, using the Two-Eyed Seeing Framework and being open to the role of spirituality, I came to understand that the patient did not perceive himself to be in need of my treatment in the way I viewed it. He wanted me to see him as a fellow human who would see him for who he is and support him to make positive choices. This fundamental understanding allowed me to appreciate that meeting patients where they are includes being open to their priorities in terms of spirituality and wellness. Indigenous wellness traditionally respects the balance between the spiritual, emotional, physical, and social aspects of individuals, regardless of their Western medical diagnosis.

Sharing elements of traditional Indigenous spirituality validated where Noel was and how he experiences spiritual wellbeing. To assist with reconnection to the spiritual practices important to him helped to rebalance the way he had felt compromised by his marginalised status in the community and his previous experiences. Understanding how spirituality fits within the dichotomy of Western medicine and Indigenous healing practices can guide APNs to become vulnerable in their own professional practice base, as well as empower patients who are structurally vulnerable to improve their perception of their health.

Through a lens of relational ethics (Bergum and Dossetor 2005), this case study illustrates the importance of self-awareness on the part of the APN, and how person-centered care relies on the ethical values of respect and dignity. Relational ethics also draw attention to the role of the social environment and colonial histories in contributing to equitable health outcomes.

10.5 Conclusion

This chapter has focused on the integration of spirituality into an APN consultation related to the presentation of a patient whose Indigenous identity has a significant impact on his spirituality, sense of self, and wellbeing. It has identified how the NP initially was unable to connect to the patient because of a one-eyed approach which did not integrate what was important to the patient, nor account for his social location and structural vulnerability. The Two-Eyed Seeing Framework and willingness of the APN to be available and vulnerable in her work and in her understanding of his spiritual needs led to a deep connection based on trust, respect and willingness to integrate two world views. This led to an improvement in the patient's health. This shift also changed service provision at the clinic to incorporate Indigenous practices and to thereby contribute to cultural safety, decolonisation, and reconciliation. In this way, we see how the relevance of spirituality for ANP practice plays out at the individual level in the patient-nurse encounter and at the organisational level of health services, all against the backdrop of historical, political, and social influences.

References

Almost J (2021) Regulated nursing in Canada: the landscape in 2021. Ottawa: Canadian Nurses Association. The publication is available at: https://www.cna-aiic.ca/en/nursing-practice/the-practice-of-nursing/regulated-nursing-in-canada. Accessed 09 Apr 2021

Bartlett C, Marshall M, Marshall A (2012) Two-eyed seeing and other lessons learned within a colearning journey of bringing together indigenous and mainstream knowledges and ways of knowing. J Environ Stud Sci 3:331–340

Beaman G (2017) Religious diversity in the public sphere: the Canadian case. Religions 8(12):259. https://doi.org/10.3390/rel8120259

Bergum V, Dossetor J (2005) Relational ethics: the full meaning of respect. University Publishing Group, Hagerstown

Bramadat P, Coward H, Stajduhar K (2013) Spirituality in hospice palliative care. SUNY Press, Albany

British Columbia College of Nursing Professionals (2018) Entry-level competencies for nurse practitioners in Canada. https://www.bccnp.ca/becoming_a_nurse/Documents/NP_entry_level_competencies.pdf. Accessed 27 Mar 2021

Bryant-Lukosius D, Wong S (2018) Global development of advanced practice nursing. In: Tracy MF, O'Grady T (eds) Advanced practice nursing: an integrative approach, 6th edn. Elsevier, St. Louis

Canadian Nurses Association (2010) Spirituality, health and nursing practice. https://www.cna-aiic.ca/~/media/cna/page-content/pdf-en/ps111_spirituality_2010_e.pdf?la=en. Accessed 27 Mar 2021

Canadian Nurses Association (2016a) The nurse practitioner position statement. https://www.cna-aiic.ca/-/media/cna/page-content/pdf-en/the-nurse-practitioner-position-statement_2016.pdf?la=en%26hash=B13B5142C8D02990439EF06736EA284126779BCC. Accessed 27 Mar 2021

Canadian Nurses Association (2016b) Position statement: The clinical nurse specialist. https://www.cna-aiic.ca/~/media/cna/page-content/pdf-en/clinical-nurse-specialist_position-statement.pdf?la=en. Accessed 27 Mar 2021

Canadian Nurses Association (2019) Advanced nursing practice: A pan-Canadian framework. https://www.cna-aiic.ca/-/media/cna/page-content/pdf-en/apn-a-pan-canadian-framework.pdf. Accessed 27 Mar 2021

Canadian Nurses Association (2020) Nursing statistics. https://www.cna-aiic.ca/en/nursing-practice/the-practice-of-nursing/health-human-resources/nursing-statistics. Accessed 24 Mar 2021

Colorado C (2020) Reconciliation and the secular. Social Compass 67(1):72–85. https://doi.org/10.1177/0037768619894510

Forbes A, Ritchie S, Walker J, Young N (2020) Applications of two-eyed seeing in primary research focused on indigenous health: a scoping review. Int J Qual Methods 19. https://doi.org/10.1177/1609406920929110

Idler EL (2014) Religion as a social determinant of public health. Oxford University Press, Oxford

Joseph B (2018) 21 things you may not know about the Indian act: helping Canadians make reconciliation with indigenous peoples a reality. Indigenous Relations Press, Port Coquitlam

Joshi KY (2006) The racialization of Hinduism, Islam, and Sikhism in the United States. Equity Excell Educ 39(3):211–226. https://doi.org/10.1080/10665680600790327

Little L, Reichert C (2018) Fulfilling nurse practitioners' untapped potential in Canada's health care system: Results from the CFNU Pan-Canadian nurse practitioner retention & recruitment study. Canadian Federation of Nurses Unions. https://nursesunions.ca/research/untapped-potential/ Accessed 27 Mar 2021

Marsh TN, Marsh DC, Najavits LM (2020) The impact of training indigenous facilitators for a two-eyed seeing research treatment intervention for intergenerational trauma and addiction. Int Indigenous Policy J 11(4):1–20. https://doi.org/10.18584/iipj.2020.11.4.8623

Martin-Misener R, Bryant-Lukosius D (2016) Guest editors' reflections on progress in the development of advanced practice nursing in Canada. Nurs Leadersh 29(3):6–13. https://doi.org/10.12927/cjnl.2016.24887

Nelson SE, Wilson K (2017) The mental health of indigenous peoples in Canada: a critical review of research. Soc Sci Med 176:93–112. https://doi.org/10.1016/j.socscimed.2017.01.021

Prodan-Bhalla N, Middagh D, Jinkerson-Brass S, Ziabakhsh S, Pederson A, King C (2017) Embracing our "otherness". J Holist Nurs 35(1):44–52. https://doi.org/10.1177/0898010116642085

Reimer-Kirkham S (2019) Complicating nursing's views on religion and politics in healthcare. In: Nursing philosophy. Published online 2 September. https://doi.org/10.1111/nup.12282

Reimer-Kirkham S, Cochrane M (2016) Resistant, reluctant or responsible? The negotiation of religious and cultural plurality in Canadian healthcare. In: Llewellyn D, Sharma S (eds) Religion, equality, and inequalities. Routledge, London, pp 65–76

Reimer-Kirkham S, Sharma S, Brown R, Calestani M et al (2020) Prayer as transgression? The social relations of prayer in healthcare. McGill-Queens University Press, Montreal

Rogers M (2016) Utilising availability and vulnerability to operationalise spirituality. In: Practising spirituality. Palgrave Macmillan, London, pp 145–164

Samari G, Alcalá HE, Sharif MZ (2018) Islamophobia, health, and public health: a systematic literature review. Am J Public Health 108(6):e1–e9. https://doi.org/10.2105/AJPH.2018.304402

Sharma S, Reimer-Kirkham S, Fowler M (2012) Emergent spiritualities and nursing ethics. In: Fowler M, Reimer-Kirkham S, Sawatzky R, Taylor-Johnson E (eds) Religion, religious ethics, and nursing. Springer, New York, pp 295–312

Staples E, Pilon R, Hannon R (2020) Canadian perspectives on advanced practice nursing, 2nd edn. Canadian Scholars Press, Toronto

Statistics Canada (2011) National Household Survey. https://www12.statcan.gc.ca/nhs-enm/2011/dp-pd/prof/index.cfm?Lang=E. Accessed 27 Mar 2021

Taher M (ed) (2021) Multifaith perspectives in spiritual and religions care: change, challenge and transformation. Canadian Multifaith Federation, Toronto

Truth and Reconciliation Commission of Canada (TRC) (2015) Honouring the truth, reconcil-
ing for the future: summary of the final report of the truth and reconciliation commission of
Canada. Truth and Reconciliation Commission of Canada, Winnipeg
Wright V, Sweeney S (2020) Refugee and migrant populations. In: Staples E, Pilon R, Hannon R
(eds) Canadian perspectives on advanced practice nursing. Canadian Scholars Press, Toronto,
pp 168–186
Ziabakhsh S, Pederson A, Prodan-Bhalla N, Middagh D, Jinkerson-Brass S (2016) Women-
centered and culturally responsive heart health promotion among indigenous women in
Canada. Health Promot Pract 17(6):814–826

Global Case Study in Spirituality: Stories of Hope from China

11

Junhong Zhu and Frances Kam Yuet Wong

Abstract

This chapter provides an overview of advanced practice nursing in China, followed by a discussion on how spirituality in healthcare is currently viewed. We conclude the chapter with an Advanced Practice Nurse case study which illustrates aspects of availability and vulnerability.

Keywords

Advanced Practice Nurse · China · Spiritual care

11.1 Advanced Nursing Practice in Mainland China

About half a century ago, China faced the 10-year Cultural Revolution that halted the country's progress in many facets, including healthcare and nursing. At the end of this significant event in 1975, the government gradually revived and picked up the development momentum (Wong et al. 2010). In 1983, China resumed higher education in nursing. During that period, the number of nurses was low, and nursing education was mainly at certificate or diploma level. After many years' efforts, nursing in China has dramatically advanced in terms of education and strength. Currently, there are over 4

J. Zhu (✉)
Nursing Studies, Medical School of Zhejiang University, Hangzhou, China
e-mail: Junhong_zhu@zju.edu.cn

F. K. Y. Wong
School of Nursing, Faculty of Health and Social Sciences, The Hong Kong Polytechnic University, Kowloon, Hong Kong
e-mail: frances.wong@polyu.edu.hk

© The Author(s), under exclusive license to Springer Nature Switzerland AG 2021
M. Rogers (ed.), *Spiritual Dimensions of Advanced Practice Nursing*,
Advanced Practice in Nursing, https://doi.org/10.1007/978-3-030-71464-2_11

million nurses (Wong 2018), 100 schools that provide master programmes and 27 schools offer doctorate programmes in nursing (Tang et al. 2020). The enhanced education level contributes to the development of Advanced Practice Nurses (APNs). Concurrently, service demands call for a higher nursing service to deal with complex client situations. Policies have a role in forming directives meeting societal needs. In the following paragraphs, we shall examine each of the three essential elements, service, education, and policy, that each contributes to the development of APNs in China.

11.1.1 Service Needs

The earliest national document that mentioned the need for developing APNs was in the 2005–2010 Chinese Nursing Career Development Plan (Ministry of Health of the People's Republic of China 2005). The subsequent Development Plan for 2011–2015 further provided details on the number and areas of specialty nurses' development required. The plans projected a total of 25,000 specialty nurses prepared in the areas of critical care, emergency, blood purification, oncology, and operation room nursing (Ministry of Health of the People's Republic of China 2012). The 2016–2020 National Nursing Career Development Plan (2016) repeated a need to educate a critical mass of clinical specialists to increase the nursing team's standards to meet multiple healthcare levels. In the same document, the identified service needs extending from hospital-based to community, highlighted the value of nurse specialists in managing clients with chronic illness, rehabilitation needs and long-term conditions, the elderly, and those requiring palliative care.

11.1.2 Education Development

The earliest specialty nursing training programmes were introduced in 2001 when the Chinese Nurses Association invited Hong Kong to deliver an Intensive Care nursing course in Beijing (Wong et al. 2010). Guangzhou Nanfang University worked with the Hong Kong counterparts to commence the first specialty postgraduate course in 2004, focusing on four specialty areas: intensive care, infection control, geriatrics, and diabetes care (Wong and Wong 2020). The Guangdong Ministry of Health then made a contractual agreement with the Hospital Authority of Hong Kong to prepare 614 Advanced Practice Nurses (APN) in 14 different specialties from 2007 to 2011 (Liao 2011). In the year of 2011, the Chinese Ministry of Education upgraded nursing to a first-level discipline. Postgraduate programmes in China have been mushrooming since then, currently there are 85 clinical master's programmes (Wong 2018) and over 100 programmes at the Master's and Doctorate level (Tang et al. 2020). Clinical master programmes aim to prepare nurses to practise at an advanced level, with the universities collaborating with the clinical sectors in curriculum design and clinical supervision (Wong 2018; Tang et al. 2020). In 2017, Beijing University launched a pioneer Nurse Practitioner programme. In alignment with the global development, the Nurse Practitioners will have prescription rights (Feng et al. 2020).

11.1.3 Policy Support

The policy support for APNs in Mainland China involves the overall national health policy and profession-specific directive. In October 2016, China's central government issued a "Healthy China 2030 Strategic Plan". The document facilitated the development of APNs since it calls for the implementation of health systems at provincial and municipal levels to provide accessible care to their people, conduct health education and healthy lifestyle modification at the population level, and disease management for specific target groups in the community. The strategic plan has a strong health focus that fits well with the nursing's nature of maintaining health, preventing illnesses, and controlling symptoms and complications among chronically ill clients. On the other hand, nurses need to go beyond the boundaries and take the initiative to assume greater professional responsibilities with enhanced professional autonomy. This extended and expanded nursing practice requires policy support to engage the nurses to practise to the optimal extent reflecting their education. In 2019, a nurse representative at the National Committee of the Chinese People's Political Consultative Conference submitted a proposal seeking legal support to empower nurses in extended practice, addressing needs, particularly in senior care. National Health Commission of the People's Republic of China (n.d.) response was positive, confirming the need to examine global professional and practice references to be applied in the domestic situation in establishing responsibilities, education requirements, the scope of service, and regulatory acts of APNs.

11.1.4 Conclusion

APNs are developing rapidly in China to meet service needs. The introduction of a clear clinical career pathway is needed to formally recognise the APNs and keep them in the service front so that these talented nurses will not be promoted away to management or education positions. The national groups develop a competencies framework, educational standards for theoretical and clinical training to prepare nurses to practise at the advanced level. Still lacking is a national certification system and regulation to protect the title of "APN". Regulatory measures to protect the safety of the APNs and the clients are required.

11.2 Spiritual Care in China

11.2.1 Spirituality and Spiritual Care as a Sensitive Topic in Mainland China

Education on spirituality, spiritual care and relevant ethical regulations are developing in Europe, North America, and most Asia-Pacific countries. Clinical staff are taught aspects of spiritual care roles and how to avoid unnecessary ethical conflicts (International Council of Nurses (ICN) 2005; Canada Nurses Association (CNA)

2010; Wright 2011; Jackson et al. 2016; American Nurse Association 2015; Fowler 2017; European Association for Palliative Care (EAPC) 2018). While APNs are integrating spiritual care in the countries mentioned above; mainland China still lacks formal curricula training in spiritual care for health professionals (Cao et al. 2020). In 2017, the Chinese National Health and Family Planning Commission first advocated providing "death education" (死亡教育) for patients according to hospice care practice guidelines. While nursing researchers interpret this advocacy as a state-level recognition and encouragement of spiritual care (Cao et al. 2020), the policy specifies neither "spirituality" (灵性) nor "spiritual care" (灵性关怀) in the Chinese language. Instead, it includes phrases such as "psychological support and humanistic care" (心理支持和人文关怀).

The terms "spirituality" and "spiritual care" are commonly conflated with "religions" in China. The Chinese government does not officially endorse religious practice and instead institutes Communism as its state ideology since the founding of People's Republic of China (PRC) in 1949. Education related to religions in higher education remains a sensitive matter which the state aims to discourage or even suppress. Although religious and spiritual care are distinct (Rogers and Wattis 2019), it is hard to raise these issues and challenge the need to introduce spiritual care into Chinese nursing curricula. Therefore it is of no surprise that the Chinese use "mind, soul, psychological or humanistic care" (心灵、精神、心理或人文关怀) to vaguely describe the psycho-social-spiritual dimensions of spiritual care without a clear conceptualisation of "spirituality" or "spiritual care".

11.2.2 Spiritual Care as an Anticipated Aspect of Holistic Care in China

By taking into account the language sensitivity of spirituality and spiritual care, we conducted a systematic review of spiritual care in China by searching the added alternative keywords to retrieve relevant literature published in Chinese from January 1, 2010 to September 30, 2020. The aim was to understand the historical development and current clinical status of spiritual care within the Chinese healthcare system. The study found that many Chinese nurses are aware of holistic care's four dimensions: physical, psychological, social, and spiritual (O'Brien 1982). Chinese health professionals have introduced spiritual care but this is mainly associated with palliative care (Zhu et al. 2020). The number of Chinese papers related to spirituality in healthcare has gradually increased from zero to 122 in the past ten years. Although most Chinese journals avoid publishing papers related to "spirituality" and "religions", different spiritual care styles in hospice care and palliative care are well represented in a number of clinical settings nationwide. The majority of studies were in the first pilot sites for hospice care reform since 2017, including Beijing, Shanghai, Guangdong, Zhejiang, Jiangsu, Henan, Hubei, and Hunan.

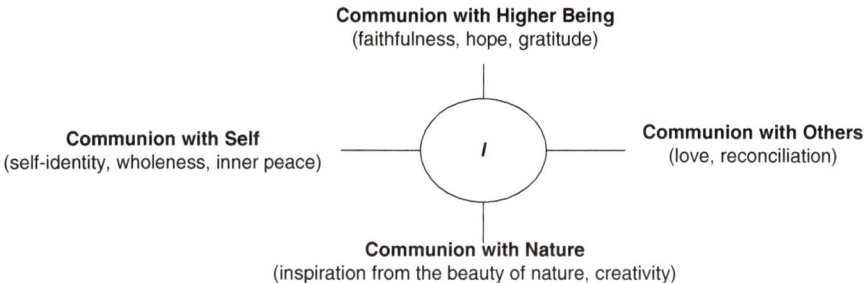

Communion with Higher Being
(faithfulness, hope, gratitude)

Communion with Self
(self-identity, wholeness, inner peace)

I

Communion with Others
(love, reconciliation)

Communion with Nature
(inspiration from the beauty of nature, creativity)

Fig. 11.1 The four dimensions of spirituality

Research and practice of spiritual care in mainland China is still in its infancy. However, spiritual care education has attracted attention in Hong Kong since the 1990s and Taiwan since the 1980s (Zhu et al. 2020). So far, under- and postgraduate nurse education in mainland China has not included spiritual care within their curricula.

Defining spirituality is difficult in mainland China. There are two main camps among those attempting to define spirituality: taking the West's definition or defining spirituality within the context of traditional Chinese culture, specifically, philosophic thought of Buddhism, Taoism, and Confucianism (Wei et al. 2018). However, there is little robust research evidence for understanding what are Chinese patients' actual spiritual care needs, except from a paper written by nursing researchers from Taiwan (Chao et al. 2002). Their hermeneutic study presents findings identifying essential aspects of spiritual care for terminally ill patients. They provide a theoretical framework of understanding spirituality through four constitutive patterns, including communion with self, others, nature, and higher being. The framework provides a meaningful definition of spirituality to humanity with practical value and applicability within Chinese culture (Chao et al. 2002, p. 242, Fig. 11.1).

It is noteworthy that nearly half of the Chinese studies in spiritual care were from Hunan Cancer Hospital. This facility serves as an outstanding example among the early spiritual care projects, and its achievements helped promote spiritual care locally and nationally. The hospital-based training is the only one consistently supported by the Association for Clinical Pastoral Education and Pastoral Counselling Education L (ACPE-PCE) in Hong Kong since 2007 (Xiao 2016). The Association had to sign a declaration that the education content would not be related to religions. The training could only be called "Mind Care" (心灵关怀). It provided spiritual care training leading to certificate in spiritual care after completion of the training which comprises of 4 units of 400 hours each. There are nearly 100 medical and nursing staff locally and nationwide who have completed units 1 and 2 of the training programmes at the Hunan Cancer Hospital (Xiao 2016). Units 3 and 4 of the training has been postponed due to the COVID-19 pandemic. Because of the signed declaration of 2007 development of nurses' practice of spiritual care is limited. To date only one nurse, who is also an APN, is able to work full time within the specialty of spiritual care (心灵关怀师) (See Case Study).

11.2.3 The Challenges Chinese Nurses Face in Practising Spiritual Care

To avoid the challenges "spirituality" or "spiritual care" may bring, Chinese authorities intend to address this aspect of care without any conflation to religion(s). This political edict has led to a great challenge for Chinese health professionals who may wish to embed spiritual care into practice. In China we are faced with an ethical dilemma. We can see the benefits of integrating spiritual care into practice but are challenged by the majority of nurses who have no knowledge or understanding of spiritual care and a lack of professional, organisational, and political support for nurses to address this (Zhu et al. 2021).

11.3 The Case Study in China

11.3.1 Introduction: My Role as a Nurse Consultant Supporting Nurses

Before introducing the case study I (Junhong Zhu) would like to share an aspect of my own work which I see as spiritual care. I am a registered nurse and nurse educator with 30 years' clinical experience in China. As a Nurse Consultant I actively provide consultation and support for nurses who feel burnt-out or vulnerable when they encounter personal or professional issues. I willingly devote time, share experiences, and provide advice and empathy with other nurses as a volunteer listener and advocate, in order to sustain their capability of caring with a positive attitude towards their nursing career. For me, this is an essential aspect of spiritual care.

Nurse consultants often fulfil many aspects of the APN role; however, this is not a recognised APN role across China. I believe the development of nurse consultant role will and should be recognised in China as an APN role. My work as a researcher has led my passion for supporting nurse colleagues. Several studies of nurses leaving nursing practice in China (Zhu et al. 2014, 2015, 2018; Zhu and Laschiger 2015), and the transition and retention of new graduate nurses in Canada (Laschinger et al. 2016) have revealed similar findings. Many nurses report that "*nurses take care of patients, but who will take care of us?*". We found that many nurses leave the profession or adopt a passive attitude towards nursing which directly impacts on their ability to take care of themselves, their family, their patients, and others in society (Zhu et al. 2015). These phenomena will negatively influence the safety and quality of healthcare and could be addressed through a recognition of the spiritual needs of nurses. Nurses who are well supported are more likely to provide compassionate care for patients. For me I see my role as a nurse consultant as someone who can support nurses with love and care from a person-centred approach by recognising and addressing their spiritual needs as well as their capability to provide spiritual care for patients.

I will briefly introduce the following case study a consultation shared with me by an APN before using Rogers' Availability and Vulnerability framework for operationalising spirituality (Rogers 2016). It reminds me how important it is to integrate spiritual care into APN.

11.3.2 Consultation with Ping, an APN as Spiritual Care Specialist in Oncology

Ping is a Chinese nursing specialist with a certificate in spiritual care working in the Hunan Provincial Cancer Hospital, the first Chinese hospital to initiate Mind Care (心灵关怀) training for health professionals since 2007, and later expanded the Mind Care training for more than 100 nurses in palliative care nationwide. Ping attended the training in spiritual care in 2007. I met Ping through my work as a researcher when she shared her experiences of providing spiritual care with me.

This case study illustrates how Ping views Mind Care and Spiritual Care. She introduces spiritual care in her daily practice as much as possible. However, Ping emphasises that for her spirituality (灵性) and religion (宗教) are separate constructs. Her main focus of work is on Mind Care which is widely accepted as it has a more scientific perspective. Hunan Cancer Hospital discourages patients to focus on religious superstitious beliefs. The focus of care offered is directed more towards offering psychological support and helping patients to manage the complex emotions experienced when dealing with a cancer diagnosis

Mind Care is defined by Hunan Cancer Hospital as giving psychological and spiritual support to terminally ill patients, or their family members as well, as clinical staff who face psychological or emotional difficulties (Liao 2021). The essence of Mind Care is the use of comprehensive psychological techniques to provide humanistic care for patients. It aims to promote communication between health professionals and patients, and to convey warmth, sincerity, respect, trust, and acceptance by focusing on a series of problems during cancer treatment. This is done through greeting, giving attention, listening, accompanying, sharing, and understanding patients from their viewpoints (Liao 2021).

Ping described her spiritual care practice in response to a 70-year-old man, Wang, in her care who had advanced bowel cancer. He was waiting for treatment when she first met him. On entering her patients' room, she found a frail elderly man who looked very sad and distressed. He had just been told that his prognosis was poor and that even with treatment he may not survive.

Ping noticed that there was appeared to be more than just the cancer diagnosis bothering her patient. Ping spent time with her patient over the following week and built up a trusting relationship. She hoped that he would begin to talk with her about his distress.

In China, the majority of people believe that emotions are considered as the major internal causes of disease. The practitioners in Traditional Chinese Medicine (TCM) believe that being overwhelmed by emotions causes imbalances in one's yin-yang energies. This imbalance, in turn, damages the internal organs and opens the door to disease. The seven emotions in TCM are joy (喜), anger (怒), anxiety (忧),

pensiveness (思), grief (悲), fear (恐), and fright (惊). Joy refers to a state of agitation or overexcitement; it is caused by the heart; anger covers a full range of associated emotions including resentment, irritability, and frustration; it is caused by the liver and gallbladder. Anxiety injures the lungs and the large intestine; pensiveness is considered to be the result of thinking too much, which directly affect the spleen and stomach; grief or sorrow causes disease of lung and colony; fear caused disease of kidney and bladder; fright primarily affects the heart and moves to the kidneys (Shen-nong Limited n.d.).

Ping understands that it is not easy for a Chinese older person to show their emotions in front of a nurse, but she said that she believed the key to relieving Wangs' distress was by understanding his emotional distress.

One morning, Wang opened up to her that he was plagued by insomnia due to the dreams he often had where he always saw the black and white image of people dying. She gently asked him if thought there was anything triggering these dreams. Her patient told her that his mother had died when he was only 11 years of age, closely followed by his father a year later. He was orphaned and this had a profound impact on his life. As he told her about his parents, he broke down and wept.

Ping felt compassion and empathy while listening to him and gently placed her hand on his arm to show that she cared and was present. In China touch is not common between patients and health professionals, but Ping felt this was the only way she could show her caring at that moment. She realised that prolonged grief and anxiety might have caused the patient to develop bowel cancer. She wanted to create a safe atmosphere for her patient to express his grief in a safe space.

Between sobs Wang went on to tell her that his first wife drowned shortly after their marriage in a freak accident. He did remarry but his second wife was severely depressed for many years and died 5 years ago. Upon hearing Wang's story Ping felt heartbroken: this man had gone through much trauma; he now faced cancer with very little family around to support him. At this point she felt unsure how to comfort him. She utilised skills she had learnt during her spiritual care training, she told him she was there to support him in any way she could and how saddened she was to hear about his losses over many years. She told him that in her experience grief of this magnitude could have a significant impact on one's life and asked him if he had ever talked about his grief. As a Chinese man he had been taught to be brave and independent. He told her that he had never talked about these things as he thought it was a weakness; but, now, as he faced cancer, he felt overwhelmed and was unsure as to how he could have dealt with his emotions.

They spent time talking about how he felt and Ping despite feeling unsure how to proceed was able to provide comfort by being with him and listening to his fears. It was clear there was much trauma in this Wang's life and she would not be able to address this herself. However, recognising that he was in distress, listening and being present was all he appeared to need at this point. After they had finished talking, his face brightened and he told her that although his dream showed all these people dying he actually felt some comfort as some of the people were family he had lost.

An important part of developing competencies in spiritual care as an APN is to have supervision and be aware of own's strength and weakness. Ping and I talked about this experience in supervision. She reflected to be how she felt helpless on hearing about all the losses Wang had experienced. She responded to him from a place of empathy and compassion but wondered if there was more she could have done. Ping asked me whether I knew of a better way to support her patient and offer him spiritual care. I told her that I admired her very much as she clearly cared deeply about her patient and his distress. I told her that I too would have felt very similar to her and that it was clear that she offered him what he needed at that time, she was there for him. We did talk through Chao's four dimensions of spiritual care (Fig. 11.1), as this can sometimes help patients connect to essential aspects of spirituality including self-awareness, relationships with others, and also relationship with the environment around them. It also addresses transcendence which may be particularly important in palliative care.

Chao's dimensions of spiritual care can be utilised to help patients gain a deep understanding of themselves and help them talk about their concerns and fears around death. It also can help nurses to understand the value of life, the meaning of life and death for the patient, and provide spiritual care accordingly. Ping was delighted to understand more about this approach and we spent time in supervision over the next few months exploring it together and recognising how to apply it to practice.

This case study reflects the essence of spirituality and of being human. Despite Ping feeling unsure how to comfort her patient she simply stayed present and expressed empathy and compassion for the deep grief her patient felt. There was no need to do anything more. Often nurses think spiritual care means "doing" something specific. This case shows that just "being" with her patient was all Ping needed to do.

11.4 Personal Reflection on the Availability and Vulnerability Framework as Applied to My Own Journey and Work as an APN

Working as an APN has been a powerful learning experience for me. It has enabled me to embrace spirituality by understanding my own meaning, purpose, and direction in my life and my nursing career.

Twelve years ago, I undertook my PhD in the United Kingdom. For many years I was troubled by seeing excellent nurses leaving the profession because of the poor moral experienced by many Chinese nurses (Zhu 2012). I had little awareness of spirituality and spiritual care in my personal and professional life mainly due to the Chinese ethos. Additionally, spirituality was never discussed in my nurse training or seen as a priority in healthcare. As with many growing up in China I was an atheist. However, during my time in the UK I became interested in the ideas from Christianity specifically the focus on unconditional love which mirrors my nursing philosophy. I was struck by Dr. Steve Tilley, my postgraduate directors' unceasing support and care for me as an international student. Over time I found out that he had a special interest in spirituality and we often discussed the concept and its application to nursing. For me, this also connected to my new found faith as a Christian but for many spirituality connects with meaning and purpose which is not informed by religion.

After my PhD I had the opportunity to work as a nurse educator in Canada where I had the opportunity to further research and learn about spirituality and the application of spiritual care. My vast experiences in China, the UK, and Canada have helped me developed my role as a nurse consultant with a special interest in spirituality and supporting nursing colleagues to find meaning and purpose again in nursing.

Understanding one's own spirituality is important as it informs our values and beliefs about patient care. For me unconditional love informs my approach to patient care. While from my Christian belief I maintain the necessary nursing boundaries of not proselytising to those in my care I recognise that having a faith helps me integrate spirituality into my work because of the values my faith has taught me. For others spirituality may informed by their work, their family, the environment for example. I found that as Rogers advocates availability for me is being accessible and serving others through relationship, compassion, and action, which is exactly what Ping offered in her approach to Wang (Rogers 2016).

As a researcher in human resources nurse management, I appreciate my colleagues who stay in nursing and continue to do a good job in resolving the problem of nursing shortage. The apppreciation has encouraged me to utilise my availability as a nurse consultant to support nurses who are burnt out or vulnerable. I trust that the consistent support to those in need will directly or indirectly influence their capability to take care of themselves, their family, and the society. During supervision and times of support I welcome them by offering time, I listen attentively and provide understanding and care through active participation in their problem-solving processes. I also feel passionately about supporting Chinese nurses who encounter ethical dilemmas and unfair treatment (Zhu 2020a, b; Zhu et al. 2020). For me I believe that supporting colleagues is also an important aspect of spiritual care.

In terms of vulnerability my work often encompasses this aspect of the Rogers' (2016) framework. I have chosen to speak out about some of the ethical issues that impact Chinese nurses, due to the current lack of spiritual care education in mainland China. Recently, I have tried suggest changes that could be made to nurse education reform by adding a curriculum on spiritual care. I have not convinced the education committee as of yet but will continue to promote spirituality as this is often the missing component in holistic care. As this moment, the Chinese government avoids talking about all matters related to religion. Although spiritual care is not confined to religion, it is hard to raise the voice to be heard. This is but one reason that makes the incorporation of spiritual care into nurse curriculum difficult. I think the best way to convince people about the importance of spiritual care is by providing solid research evidence and establishing formal training in spiritual care.

With Ping we were able to express our shared vulnerability as she shared how she felt about the patient who told her his story of grief. I felt we were able to learn from each other as we both began to see how spiritual care can be put into practice in China. This has led us both to work together in promoting spiritual care education for nurses in China. Understanding the concepts of vulnerability taught by Rogers (2016) allowed Ping and I to openly discuss concerns we have experienced by trying to raise the profile and implementation of spiritual care in China. We both agreed there is a need to learn more about spiritual care by providing a forum for nurses who are interested in promoting spiritual care to come together to research, discuss, and implement spiritual care into practice. We plan to develop collaborative research into spirituality, nurses' perceptions of spirituality and its implementation in practice. In China, we face multiple challenges as spirituality is still regarded as a sensitive topic which ought to be discouraged. In the view of the Chinese government, religious/non-religious belief can often become conflated with spirituality. Alignment to religion is not often apparent or seen among Chinese people.

However, all people, including those with no religious faith, have their own version of spirituality and personal beliefs that underpin how they understand life, health and illness, recovery and death. As nurses we need to be sensitive to these issues, respecting individuals' beliefs and offering care based upon the key principles of spirituality, kindness, compassion, and empathy.

As a nurse consultant who wishes to promote spiritual care in China, I must be open to further learning, cooperation, and advocacy. To encourage the integration of spiritual care into the nursing curriculum I have established a local, national and international professional social network through personal and professional activities. By comparing practical spiritual care and the relevant ethical principles in different countries, I have become more sensitive to the ethical dilemmas, which Chinese nurses have to face due to the insufficient knowledge of spiritual care (Zhu et al. 2021).

Spirituality is a universal phenomenon that extends beyond religious practices. I believe that we should try our best to do the right things as part of spiritual care for our patients and also our nursing colleagues whenever we have to face challenges. It helps nurses recognise their value, meaning, and purpose. Then they will be able to take care of their patients, themselves, their family, and the whole society, which will exert an optimistic impact on the safety and quality of healthcare in China.

Acknowledgments This case study is supported by Chinese Fundamental Research Funds for the Central Universities ((ZJU2021-12), and Authors also would like to express their gratitude to Dr Melanie Rogers, Dr Ching-Huey Chen, Dr Co-Shi Chao for their inspiration and support during the writing process. Authors declare no conflict interest.

References

American Nurse Association (2015) Code of ethics for nurses, with interpretive statements. American Nurse Association, Silver Spring

Canada Nurses Association (CNA) (2010) Spirituality, health and nursing practice-position statement. CNA, Jones & Bartlett Learning, LLC, Burlington

Cao YL, Kunaviktikul W, Petrini M (2020) A proposed conceptual framework of spiritual care competence for Chinese nurses. Nurs Health Sci 22(3):498–506

Chao CSC, Chen CH, Yen MF (2002) The essence of spirituality of terminally ill patients. J Nurs Res 10(4):237–244

European Association for Palliative Care (EAPC) (2018) 10th world research congress of the European Association for Palliative Care. Palliat Med 32(1_suppl):3–330

Feng S, Li X, Li L, Zhao Y et al (2020) Research progress and advices on nurse prescribing right in China. Chin Nurs Res 34(1):101–104. https://doi.org/10.12102/j.issn.1009-6493.2020.01.018

Fowler M (2017) Faith and ethics, covenant and code, the 2015 revision of the ANA Code of Ethics for nurses with interpretative statements. J Christ Nurs 34(4):216–224

International Council of Nurses (ICN) (2005) International Council of Nurses' code of nursing. ICN, Geneva

Jackson D, Doyle C, Capon H, Pringle E (2016) Spirituality, spiritual need, and spiritual care in aged care: what the literature says. J Relig Spiritual Aging. https://doi.org/10.1080/1552803 0.2016.1193097

Laschinger HK, Zhu JH, Read E (2016) New nurses' perceptions of professional practice behaviors on job satisfaction and career retention. J Nurs Manag 24(5):656–665

Liao XB (2011) Joint training program for specialized nurses in Guangdong Province in collaboration with Hong Kong. Chin J Nurs 46(12):1189–1190

Liao XB (2021) Hunan Cancer Hospital: healing the soul and protecting the safety of cancer patients. Available at https://m.voc.com.cn/wxhn/article/202102/202102031553044338.html

Ministry of Health of the People's Republic of China (2005) The Chinese nursing career development plan (2005-2010). Chin J Nurs 40(10):721–723

Ministry of Health of the People's Republic of China (2012) The Chinese nursing career development plan (2011-2015). Chin Nurs Manage 12(2):5–8

National Health Commission of the People's Republic of China (n.d.) Reply to the proposal a proposal on piloting the nurse practitioner system to help the development of senior care and other industries. In: 13th CPPCC meeting. Available from http://www.nhc.gov.cn/wjw/tia/202009/f8781cca71c443f6b09601dedfd124e0.shtml

National Nursing Career Development Plan (2016) Gazette of the national health and family planning commission of People's Republic of China. Int J Nurs Sci 11:24–30

O'Brien ME (1982) The need for spiritual integrity. In: Yura H, Walsh MB (eds) Human needs and the nursing process. Appleton & Lange, East Norwalk, CT

Rogers M (2016) Utilising availability and vulnerability to operationalise spirituality. In: Practising spirituality. Palgrave Macmillan, London, pp 145–164

Rogers M, Wattis J (2019) Understanding the role of spirituality in providing person-centred care. Nurs Stand. https://doi.org/10.7748/ns.2020.e11342

Shen-nong Limited (n.d.) What are seven emotions? Available at http://www.shen-nong.com/eng/principles/sevenemotions.html

Tang R, Lu Y, Jiang H, Jiang X, Zhou N, Li M, Shang S (2020) Nurse practitioners: a review of practice and prescription. Chin J Nurs 55(5):796–800

Wei D, Liu XY, Chen YY, Zhang M, Xu XH, Chen QQ (2018) Research progress on spiritual care at home and abroad. J Nurs Res 32(6):831–834

Wong FKY (2018) Development of advanced nursing practice in China: act local and think global. Int J Nurs Sci 5(2):101–104. https://doi.org/10.1016/j.ijnss.2018.03.003

Wong FKY, Wong AKC (2020) Advanced practice nursing in Hong Kong and Mainland China. In: Hassmiller S, Pulcini J (eds) Advanced practice nursing leadership: a global perspective. Advanced practice in nursing. Springer, Cham

Wong FK, Peng G, Kan EC, Li Y, Lau AT, Zhang L et al (2010) Description and evaluation of an initiative to develop advanced practice nurses in mainland China. Nurse Educ Today 30(4):344–349

Wright S (2011) The heart and soul of nursing. Nurs Stand 25(30):18–19

Xiao WX (2016) Hunan can hospital prescribes "mind care". China Hosp 2:72–74

Zhu JH (2020a) Ethical challenges faced by Chinese medical and nursing staff in coping with COVID-19. Caixin (in Chinese). http://opinion.caixin.com/2020-03-06/101524840.html

Zhu JH (2020b) Is it ethical to be a 'whistleblower' during COVID-19 pandemic? Ethical challenges confronted by health care workers in China. J Adv Nurs 2020:1873–1875

Zhu JH (2012) Towards an understanding of nurses leaving nursing practice in China: a qualitative exploration of nurses leaving nursing practice from recruitment to final exit. PhD Thesis, The University of Edinburgh, Edinburgh, UK.

Zhu JH, Laschinger HK (2015) Chinese nursing managers at crossroad: a nursing profession or professional nurses. Giving a presentation on May 1 2015 at the Iota Omicron Chapter, Sigma Theta Tau International 28th Annual Research and Leadership Conference, London, Ontario

Zhu JH, Rodgers S, Melia KM (2014) The impact of safety and quality of health care on Chinese nursing career decision making. J Nurs Manag 22(4):423–432

Zhu JH, Rodgers S, Melia KM (2015) A qualitative exploration of nurses leaving nursing practice in China. Nurs Open 2(1):3–13

Zhu JH, Rodgers S, Melia KM (2018) Understanding human resource wastage in the nursing shortage: lessons learned from Chinese nurses leaving nursing practice. Athens J Health 5(3):195–211

Zhu JH, Stone T, Petrini M (2020) The ethics of refusing to care for patients during the coronavirus pandemic: a Chinese perspective. Nurs Inq. https://doi.org/10.1111/nin.12380

Zhu JH, Wu HH, Zeng YC, Xiao J (2021) Discussions on spiritual care and ethical issues in China. Chin J Colorectal Dis 10(1):108–112

Global APN Case Study in Spirituality: Stories of Hope from Pakistan

12

Nasreen Lalani and Gulnar Ali

Abstract

Spirituality is central to health and healing in Muslim philosophy of care. Caregiving is considered sacred in Islam and therefore, families play an integral role at the end-of-life care in a Muslim context. Pakistan is a developing Muslim dominant country, where the concepts of spirituality and palliative care are slowly integrating in the healthcare education and practice. Similarly, Advanced Practice Nurse roles are gradually gaining importance in the Pakistani healthcare delivery system. Death and dying is a collective experience where patients, families, and caregivers, each goes through varying experiences of loss, grief, and suffering and requires meaningful care and support. These experiences bring a lot of spiritual concerns, uncertainties, and needs where both patients and families require compassionate care and support. Caring for dying patients and their families can be both challenging and rewarding for the advance practice nurses working in a palliative or hospice setting. Using Rogers' framework of availability and vulnerability and recognising that spirituality can enhance nurses' self-awareness, self-reflexivity, and self-compassion and assist them in providing meaningful care to their patients and families in palliative care and hospice settings in Pakistan is important.

Keywords

Suffering · Meaning-making · Palliative care · Muslim philosophy of care · Nursing in pakistan · Practice transformation

N. Lalani (✉)
Purdue University, West Lafayette, IN, USA
e-mail: lalanin@purdue.edu

G. Ali
University of Exeter, Exeter, UK
e-mail: g.ali@exeter.ac.uk

The following chapter will provide a brief context of the healthcare system in Pakistan along with the development of advanced practice nursing roles. It will then describe the role of spirituality and how it is viewed in the healthcare and social context of Pakistan generally and from nursing perspectives in Pakistan specifically. A case study will illustrate how spirituality was integrated into an interaction by an Advanced Practice Nurse (APN) in palliative care setting. Acknowledging the scope of availability and vulnerability model, this chapter will propose recommendations for establishing recognised advanced nursing care pathways in Pakistan.

12.1   Nursing Practice in Pakistan

Pakistan is a developing country where most people are Muslims. Pakistan has a population of 192 million people. Sixty-two percent of the Pakistani population live in rural areas and the remaining 38% live in urban areas (Organisation for Economic Cooperation and Development (OECD). OECD Health Statistics 2015). Sixty percent of the population live under the internationally defined poverty line of less than $2 per day (United States [US] currency). The healthcare system in Pakistan is gradually improving with new healthcare reforms including participation in Millennium Development Goal programme, initiating health programmes using Public Private Partnership in different urban and rural communities, reforming infrastructure, and improving human resource development (Kurji et al. 2016). Pakistan spent only 2.6% of its total budget on the healthcare of its population (World Health Organisation (WHO) 2016) compared to the 8.9% spent by Organisation for Economic Cooperation and Development (OECD) countries and 16.9% by the USA, excluding investments (Organisation for Economic Cooperation and Development (OECD). OECD Health Statistics 2015). Major barriers to an adequate and efficient healthcare system include poor governance, lack of access and availability of the resources, poor quality of health information management system, lack of regulatory and monitoring health planning and systems, and lack of human resource/trained worked force (Kurji et al. 2016). As a result, Pakistan is currently facing the double burden of communicable (38%) and non-communicable diseases (50%) (Naseem et al. 2016), high maternal and infant mortality rate, reduced life expectancy (65–67 years), and wide prevalence of malnutrition among women and children (World Health Organization (WHO) 2014).

Nursing in Pakistan is primarily a female dominant profession, with low image and status due to various religious, cultural and socio-political reasons (Parveen 2016). Lack of public awareness about the nursing profession is a huge factor that impacts negatively on the image and desirability of the nursing profession (Gul 2008). Furthermore, the low socio-economic status of nurses, unsafe work environment, lack of respect from doctors and the very nature of nurse's work create a dichotomy in society's attitude towards the nursing profession (Parveen 2016). There is an acute shortage of nursing workforce in Pakistan. The total nursing and midwifery workforce is 4.9 per 10,000 population, the precise number of nursing graduates is not known (Younas et al. 2019). The nurse-patient ratio is 1:50, the nurse-doctor ratio is 1:10. Pakistan Nursing Council (PNC) is an autonomous nursing regulatory body that works for the welfare of nurses and struggles to bring improvements in nursing education and practice. During the last decade, PNC has taken several initiatives to improve the standards and quality of nursing education and practice in Pakistan. PNC has gradually phased out the diploma in nursing and has mandated Bachelor of Science in Nursing (BSN) degree as the minimum educational requirement for a practising nurse. As per Pakistan Nursing Council (2017), there are approximately 166 recognised nursing institutions. Currently, there are four types of nursing programmes available in Pakistan including a one-year community health nursing programme for general nurses, community midwives, and health visitors; a one-year post basic diploma programme for nurses in specialised areas such as ward administration and teaching administration; a one-year licensed practical nursing programme; a four-year BSN, a 2-year Post Registered Nurse (RN) BSN (available only to those nurses who have done 3-year diploma in nursing in the past). Other than bachelor's in nursing, PNC also provides a two-year master's in nursing (MSN) programme (MSN) (Younas et al. 2019). One-year post diploma programmes are available post undergraduate training specifically design to prepare nurses for advanced practice. The curriculum for these programmes includes clinical practicum and preceptorship experiences in specialised clinical areas like medicine, surgery, cardiac, paediatric, and palliative care. These programmes also include education, research and management practicums to prepare nurses for faculty, researcher, and administrative roles. Younas et al. (2019) estimate that there are only 30 Master's and 9 PhD prepared nurses in Pakistan, most of whom working as educators/faculty in university and some work as administrators in hospital settings. A continuous struggle remains to retain the nurses in the profession, a high turnover of nurses exists due to low image of nurses, lower wages, lack of incentives, and managerial support, and unfavourable working conditions. Moreover, there are several barriers in terms of higher education, training and capacity building, and retention of nurses. According to Younas et al. (2019), barriers to higher education and training include lack of human and material resources. These barriers include shortage of Masters' and doctoral prepared nurse educators, lack of advanced teaching and learning spaces/facilities, limited research capacity and access to international literature, and minimal or no collaboration with international nursing regulatory bodies and institutions (Younas et al. 2019). Despite these shortcomings, APN roles are beginning to emerge in Pakistan with support from the PNC, several accredited universities, and the Higher Education Commission (HEC) of Pakistan. The emerging APN roles include case managers, Clinical Nurse Specialists (CNS) in medical, surgical, and palliative care areas, epidemiologists, public health nurses, infection control nurses, nurse managers, researchers, and educators. It is noteworthy that most of these nurses are Master's prepared, are a handful in numbers, with the majority serving in universities or bigger hospital settings mostly located in urban areas. There are no Nurse Practitioner programmes currently available in Pakistan. Struggles continue in meeting the millennium development goals and health indicators of the country (Younas et al. 2019).

Pakistan Nursing Curriculum is transforming gradually from a bio-medical model to bio-psycho-social-spiritual model of care. There is a limited focus in the nursing curriculum on psycho-social and spiritual aspects on care with patients and families in hospital and community settings. The concepts of spirituality and spiritual are rarely studied or given importance in the nursing or medical curricula in Pakistan (Lalani et al. 2019). Healthcare professionals do not receive any kind of specific training to spiritual care interventions or conversations with the family. Nonetheless, the cultural and religious beliefs and values do influence the caring values/practices of the healthcare professionals and impact the overall healthcare approach of the care facilities. Given specific care context, one would rarely find any kind of spiritual assessment or specific spiritual care interventions, policies/ protocols for the patient or family during their hospital stay. However, these areas may be slowly being addressed with higher education qualifications, emerging advanced nurse practice roles, increased awareness, and advocacy in policy and practice.

12.2 Spirituality in Healthcare and Healing from a Muslim Context

Muslim philosophy is the predominant cultural stance in Pakistan. However, the search for an ultimate reality or the divine can be pursued in various ways. Across all Muslim intellectual traditions, the concept of God is understood as an ultimate ideal and source of spirituality reflected in all aspect of human life (Esmail 1998). A major emphasis is placed on a personal search and self-awareness to recognise the spiritual aspects of religious life (Esmail 1998; Madelung and Mayer 2015). Religious experiences such as seeking wisdom, self-consciousness, and humility are multiple expressions of actualising the highest human potential (Walker et al. 2016). Rooted in a religious doctrine, the notion of intellect and knowledge is associated with the concept of revelation. Esmail (1992, 1995, 1998) analyses the meaning and articulation of the sacred in its social context and distinguishes theological doctrine from religious experiences. According to him, religion and spirituality provide a roadmap guiding human intellect, imagination, perception, conviction, emotion, and behaviour. In other words, religion and spirituality shape human life defining cultural values, language development, intellectual progress, social interactions, and symbolic interpretations in searching and encountering the sacred.

Within a health and healing context, religion and spiritualty are central to caring. Islam says all humans are spiritual beings and the spirit is immortal, care of the spirit and spiritual values are therefore essential for health and healing (Abudari et al. 2016). In Islamic literature, one of the attributes of God is *Shafi* meaning 'the one who heals or cures'. Quranic Verse 26:80 says: 'And when I am ill, it is He who cures me'. Prophet Muhammad (peace be upon him) is called as *Shaf* or *Shafeen*, which means Healer. Several Muslim scientists and philosophers have shown positive relationships between spirituality, health, and healing. Muhammad ibn Zakariya Razi, a Persian Muslim philosopher during the tenth century and famous Muslim physician and philosopher, Ibn-e-Sina, reflected on the significant role of spirituality in Islamic medicine and concepts of care (Johnson et al. 2016). Among Muslims, there is a concept of afterlife, adherence to religious values, beliefs, and practices transcends the soul with God, Almighty Allah, and enables an individual to attain the spiritual enlightenment (Hasnain and Rana 2010). Life is a blessing and therefore must always be cherished and protected, illness and suffering are inevitable parts of life and the moment of death is fixed by Allah. During illness, Muslims seek Allah's help and maintain a closer relationship with God. Religious and spiritual practices are sources of strength and coping during illness which promote healing (Lalani et al. 2018). Caregiving is viewed as sacred in Muslim families especially during illness and end of life. Altruistic values, selflessness, and service to others give meaning to the causes of suffering, and ways to achieve spiritual enlightenment (Lalani et al. 2019; Khan 2017). Care of a sick family member is a cultural and religious responsibility. The caregiving practices are highly influenced by religious and cultural values and beliefs. Caregiving is viewed as sacred and a source of spiritual enlightenment (Hasnain and Rana 2010). Muslims believe that God expects them to care for the weak, suffering, and outcasts of society, and that those who fulfill those expectations will receive special blessings and rewards in their afterlife (Khan 2012, 2017). However, with reference to nursing practice, a constant professional evolution is seen relating spirituality and religious experiences, acknowledging existential pain especially among patients and families at the end-of-life care. There is a dearth of literature around how spirituality, ethical values, and spiritual care needs are addressed especially among Muslim patients and families at the end of life (Lalani and Ali 2020).

Palliative and end of life (EOL) care bring multiple spiritual and existential concerns and are guided by cultural values, thoughts, and actions (Abudari et al. 2016). Spirituality is deeply rooted in Muslim culture and plays an integral role in healthcare attitudes and practices among people (Johnson et al. 2016). Family plays a significant role in palliative and EOL care decision making. Often a responsible family member or a male elder member of the family is a decision maker, and in some cases, families' preferences are valued over individual's wishes and rights (Ahmed et al. 2012). Talking about death and dying is often considered taboo and therefore families are not willing to openly communicate their needs and concerns as it is thought to bring bad luck, despair, and loss of hope (Barclay et al. 2007). Families often turn to prayers, religious rituals, and practices while caring for their family member with life-threatening illnesses. Palliative as well as hospice care is not well established in Pakistan and most terminally ill patients are kept in acute settings of hospital. Minimal psychological and spiritual support is provided to patients in these settings due to lack of staff, lack of palliative care training, unavailability of facilities and resources (Lalani et al. 2018). Like the Western model of Healthcare there are chaplains (*Imams, faith healers*) available to support the spiritual and pastoral care needs of a patient in Pakistan; however, those chaplains are not professionally recognised with relevant registered trainings in healthcare. Nonetheless, some hospice care settings do allow families to bring in religious scholars or *Imams* to visit the patients and perform healing rituals, as per the family beliefs and personal choice. Pakistani families often experience significant caregiving demands and pressures due to the lack of palliative care, poor socio-economic determinants of health, and socio-cultural expectations of caregiving. Keeping various cultural and religious values and beliefs, they often refrain to complain about their caregiving demands or sufferings (Khan 2012, 2017).

From the above description, it is evident that the notion of health and healing is deeply rooted in religious and cultural practices among the people in Pakistan, such philosophy of care is not very well integrated and practised in the health and healthcare delivery overall. Several barriers are reported in terms of adequate provision of spiritual care in the healthcare setting generally and palliative care setting specifically. These include non-integration of palliative care and spirituality concepts in the healthcare curriculum leading to lack of insight and training among the healthcare professionals. Other structural and organisational barriers include lack of focus on bio-psychosocial spiritual model of care, healthcare professionals finding lack of time and support in provision of spiritual care (Jawaid 2020). At the policy level, palliative and end-of-life care receives less attention and priority. Most healthcare funding and resources are directed towards other healthcare priorities such as maternal and child health and non-communicable diseases (Naseem et al. 2016). Patients and families struggling with their spiritual needs and care often visit the faith healers (saint, faith healer, or spiritualist), a common practice in Pakistan where they find more peace and comfort in comparison to the modern healthcare practitioners (Jawaid 2020; Qidwai 2003). Patients and families suffering from serious illnesses often visit places like *Mazars and ziarats* (shrines) to find cure and mental peace. They believe that faith healers or saints are closer to God, and that showing faith in them will please God (Jawaid 2020; Qidwai 2003).

Recent research studies in Pakistan demonstrate that spirituality is an integral aspect of care in religious societies like Pakistan and therefore, healthcare professionals need to understand the significance of spirituality and religion in care. A recent study conducted by Jawaid (2020) among patients and healthcare professionals in Pakistan reported that patients preferred physicians to discuss spirituality and spiritual aspects of care with them as spirituality helped them to cope with their condition better. The healthcare professionals in their study also supported similar views that spirituality plays an important part in a patient's illness and its prognosis; however, most reported several constraints such as lack of time and support, lack of training, lack of collegial support, and personal discomfort as major reasons for not discussing spirituality with their patients, whereas some believed it was a private matter. Similar findings have been reported in other Pakistani studies also. Ahmed et al. (2012) in their study about patients and physician perceptions on faith-based healing found that 93% of patients want their physician to express a prayer for them aloud and 88% accepted that physicians whom they think are religious would have a positive impact on their health. Similar other studies also found that religious and spiritual care values and faith healing practices including prayers helped in minimizing the psychological distress and suffering associated with their illness.

In the light of the above context, there is a possibility that drawing on faith and spirituality could play a significant and intentional role in supporting patients' and families' healthcare needs and wellbeing. Faith and spirituality can be major sources of coping and strength for families. The following case study will discuss spirituality and spiritual care at the end of life (EOL) from a family caregiving context in Pakistan. The case study will highlight the significance and role of APN including the barriers and facilitators providing spiritual care to family caregivers caring for their dying patients in a hospice setting of Pakistan.

12.3   APN and Spiritual Care: A Case Study from Pakistan

The following case study presents a 23-year-old female caregiver Sarah's story, caring for her father suffering from a terminal illness of cancer in a hospice setting of Karachi, Pakistan. I, Nasreen, worked with Sarah and her family in Pakistan as a CNS in palliative care. During this time, I was also collecting data for my doctoral research looking at the spiritual experiences of family caregivers while caring for their loved ones at the terminal stages of their illness in a hospice setting in Karachi, Pakistan. Most of my education and nursing experience is from Pakistan. I worked as a CNS and nurse educator for more than 25 years in medical-surgical and palliative areas in Pakistan before starting my PhD in Alberta, Canada. As a Muslim nurse from Pakistan with extensive experience, I have personally observed that the lack of palliative care and spiritual support given often causes family caregivers emotional, psychological, and spiritual distress. One would rarely find any kind of spiritual assessment or discussions of spirituality with the family during their hospital stay. As said earlier, the concepts of palliative care and spirituality are rarely studied or given importance in the nursing or medical curricula in Pakistan. Coming from a place where families are culturally and religiously held responsible to care for their sick family members (and must do so with limited facilities and resources), I was passionate to explore what provides meaning in daily family caregiving practices. I always had a strong desire to examine spirituality in the caregiving context of Pakistan.

Sarah was a young female caregiver caring for her father suffering from terminal stages of metastatic oral cancer for the last 5 years, currently admitted in the hospice setting. The hospice was 45 bed charitable cancer hospice setting in Karachi, Pakistan. Most patients admitted to the hospice were less educated, impoverished and had suffered from limited healthcare resources and other disparities. I still remember the hot summer day, when I met Sarah caring for her terminally ill father in the hospice setting. Sarah was wearing a full Hijab, only eyes were visible, sitting on the attendant's bench beside her father's bed. It was a male unit surrounded by four other male patient beds in the unit. Upon asking her history, she told me that her father was in the late stages of cancer, he had an oral neck resection surgery for the tumour which had been unsuccessful, he was now completely bed ridden. Her father was in a semi-conscious state, he couldn't talk and had a nasogastric tube in-situ for feeding. He needed a daily dressing of his surgical wound between his right cheek and neck area. When Sarah brought her father into the hospice, his wound was infected with maggots; however after regular daily dressings, it was now clean. While history taking, Sarah told me that over the last year they have been travelling to different cities on the bus to look for treatment and a cure for his father's cancer. They consulted multiple faith healers, tried alternative medicine and used spiritual healing practices, couldn't find cure for his cancer, the cancer is now metastasised in his body and now he is in hospice for palliative care. While her father was in the hospice, Sarah was residing at her relative's house and used to visit the hospice during the day only as women were not allowed to stay in the hospice during the night hours due to cultural reasons. Sarah was the eldest in the family and all the caregiving responsibilities were on her shoulder. When I heard Sarah's story, I could imagine that her suffering was not limited to her father's illness only but far more than that. Sarah was only 12 years old when her parents were separated. Sarah was left with her two younger siblings and her father. Being the elder in the family, she took the responsibility to take care of her younger siblings and the family. Sarah used to make bangles for a living to financially support the family. According to her, it was the immense love and affection for her father, her strong connectedness/bond with the family, and her faith in God that enabled her to transcend all the adversities in her life and made her a strong and resilient person. Sarah's staunch faith in God and unwavering love for the family provided her strength and courage to face all the suffering in her life and find meaning in her own journey as a caregiver. Sarah didn't want to leave a single stone unturned in the care of her father. Sarah expressed the love she felt for her father with these words:

> "If the sun does not rise a day, how would it be? If my father is not there, it would be like the sun not rising. It's his presence that gives me a lot of strength…. I have a kind of connection and closeness with him. So much so that if he moves his eyes (to ask for something), I get to know what he wants."

Providing care to Sarah and her father raised several questions around holistic and person-centered care aspects. First, I asked myself what are my own care values and philosophy? How should I ease her suffering? Am I better equipped to ease her suffering? What made her confide her sorrows and grief with me? How should I keep that trust? How should I help her in healing and finding meaning in all her sorrows and sufferings? All these were significant questions for me as an Advanced Practice Nurse in this caregiving situation.

My own care philosophy and values shaped by my own personal experiences along with the higher education and training in nursing played a critical role in understanding and internalising the care needs and preferences of Sarah as a caregiver and her father as a patient. Being part of Sarah's culture and religion enabled me to resonate with her caregiving needs and concerns, while my education and clinical experience enabled me to adopt a person-centered approach. Using a person-centered approach, I was able to offer Sarah, personalised care with an empathetic attitude, dignity, and compassion. Such an approach also helped me to recognise her spiritual care needs and concerns, to build a strong trusting relationship and to help her endure and transcend the suffering in the dying process. Sarah stated:

"Last night, I reached home late at night. Due to cold weather, my cousins didn't allow me to shower and I couldn't pray. I felt so restless and couldn't sleep the whole night. I felt like crying and got mad at my cousins…. If I miss my prayers, I feel strange and sinking. I feel like something is missing. Until I pray, I remain restless. My biggest strength comes from Allah. The days when I do not pray, I experience strange feelings, anxiety, and sadness. When I say my prayers, I refresh and reenergise myself."

The above statement indicates that for Sarah, prayers and religious practices were important spiritual attributes that provided her peace and strength in her spiritual suffering. For many people in theistic traditions, prayers are integral ways for liberating oneself, and transcending grief and worries, and finding peace and comfort in higher being or God. Being aware of her faith practices, I planned to arrange a religious counsellor for her, however, I couldn't find one in the hospice setting. I looked for alternatives and found a quiet place in the hospice setting where she could sit, offer her prayers and provided her with some holy books for recitation to help her find comfort and peace in spiritual distress. I also connected her with other family caregivers in the hospice setting who were suffering from the similar situations. Such strategies helped her to ventilate her feelings and make new connections to help her in healing.

Spiritual care interventions are complex especially when you are unaware of your own caring values and are working under limited resources. Despite being a hospice nurse for several years, I sometimes feel limited and vulnerable to my own fears and emotions and at risk of moral and spiritual distress. I am happy that I could provide some support to Sarah in her suffering and was able to build a special bond with her to help her in her grieving process. At the same time, I realised that I also needed lot of support and self-care on an ongoing basis. Often after leaving the workplace, I found myself in the shadows of her suffering and was unable to detach myself completely from her story. I felt her trauma, pain, and grief as it was mine and found myself unable to concentrate, that often prevented me from my personal self and family care. These experiences had both positive and negative impacts on my personal and professional lives. On one hand, I was also feeling despair and was unable to concentrate on my personal and family life. On the other hand, I found myself full of gratitude and forgiving towards others. I started journaling all these events, shared my pain with my close family members and friends. With continuous self-reflections, I was able to find some relief in my despair and continue working as a compassionate nurse in the similar setting. This was a journey of personal and self- transformation resulting in a self-empowerment, strength, and growth.

12.4   Discussion

The above case study indicates that dying is a collective experience, where patients, caregivers, and healthcare providers each goes through varying experiences of loss, grief, and suffering. Such experiences often generate the need for a search of meaning and connectedness. In times of suffering, spiritual issues become the central concern and therefore, should be the focus of care (Narayanasamy 2007).

Recognising and responding to the spiritual needs and concerns of patients and families in a hospice setting is a compound and multifaceted task that requires specialised skills and aptitude (McSherry and Jamieson 2011). Showing presence, compassion, listening attitude and respecting values and practices are important aspects in the provision of spiritual care (Lalani et al. 2018, 2019). According to Rogers' (2016) framework of Availability and Vulnerability (A&V), the notion of being aware of the needs and values of patients and families, being authentic in care, and showing presence and empathy in the care provision has been referred to as 'Availability'. In the above case study, we can infer that the APN was able to respond to her spiritual values and beliefs using self-awareness, knowledge, and understanding of faith, and utilising the principles of person-centered care. Understanding the cultural and religious values were essential aspects of spirituality and spiritual care (Jawaid 2020). Religion and spirituality provide foundations for making sense of existence and serve as a protective factor in times of loss and grief (Lalani 2020). From a Pakistani cultural context, the majority patients and families are Muslims who view health and healing in connection to several religious principles and values (Jawaid 2020; Lalani et al. 2019). Studies conducted in Pakistan showed most healthcare attitudes, decisions, and practices at EOL are influenced by religious and spiritual values and beliefs. Such values and beliefs help people to endure suffering and enable them to cope with loss and grief (Jawaid 2020; Lalani et al. 2019; Ahmed et al. 2012; Khan et al. 2012). Faith healing practices such as prayers and other religious rites and rituals are reported to minimize psychological distress (Jawaid 2020), prayers improve healing, and could curtail the duration of disease (Qidwai et al. 2009). Provision of spiritual care provides valuable support for patients and families by offering hope, self-efficacy, comfort, peace and strength and hence improves the quality of life of patients and families at the EOL (Lalani et al. 2019; Gijsberts et al. 2019).

Rogers (2016) Framework of A&V also emphasises that spirituality should be embedded in our routine acts of caring. Our small daily acts of kindness and of love (Sinclair et al. 2006), witnessing patient's suffering, careful listening, creating a healing environment, and inviting reflections can promote supportive care with authenticity and compassion (Deal 2011). Adequate spiritual assessment and communication are significant tools to offer adequate spiritual care to patients and their families (Buck and McMillan 2008; Ross and Austin 2015). Lalani et al. (2019) in her study reported that nurses' positive attitude, good communication, active listening, and humour instilled strength, hope, and courage in them. Similar findings have been reported in other studies (Kim et al. 2014; Sinclair et al. 2012). Furthermore, provision of adequate spiritual care to patients and families helps them to transcend their known and unknown fears and anxieties during end-of-life care, foster resilience, and spiritual transformation (Bhatnagar et al. 2017; Delgado-Guay et al. 2013; Lalani et al. 2019; Paiva et al. 2015).

The case study presented directs us to the fact that working as an APN in palliative or EOL care settings is emotionally challenging and may expose nurses to their own vulnerabilities and finitude (Tornøe et al. 2015). Self-reflection, self-acceptance, self-care, and supervision are therefore vital for building trusting relationships especially working in a palliative care nursing. A consistent reflection on one's journey brings the authentic self, increased compassion, and self-acceptance (Rogers 2016; Ali and Lalani 2020). Rogers (2016) stresses that a nurse should be willing to share uncertainty with patients and act in a way that is open, honest, and transparent. While working as an APN in the palliative care setting, I faced a lot of vulnerabilities such as not being resourceful and having difficulty meeting the spiritual care needs of Sarah in the case study. Nonetheless, embracing those vulnerabilities such as working with limitations while consistently demonstrating accountability and advocating allowed me in the provision of holistic care approach. In other words, embracing spirituality may enhance the availability and at the same time reduces the vulnerability by allowing openness, making us aware of our own inner selves, and eventually providing meaning and purpose to our caring actions and attitudes. Such principles direct our nursing care.

12.5   Way Forward: Transforming Nursing Practice and APN Roles in Pakistan

The above case study illustrates the significance of spirituality as well as APNs role in recognising cultural and spiritual beliefs in addressing the spiritual needs and provision of holistic person-centered care within the nursing and health context of Pakistan. Nursing care philosophies need to recognise the role of self-awareness, vulnerability, and reflexivity to apply the whole person care concepts (Rogers 2016; Wattis et al. 2019; Ali and Lalani 2020). It is vital to establish the concepts of spirituality and spiritual care in care-giving attitudes which could further be developed through nursing education and practice in the Pakistan Nursing curriculum. The need to incorporate spirituality and spiritual concepts in the nursing programmes at all levels would make a significant impact in nursing and for patient care. A strong relationship exists among spirituality, culture, and religion and is evident in the Muslim health and care philosophies (Lalani et al. 2019; Lalani and Ali 2020). APN programmes should include concepts of spirituality and palliative care concepts in the given cultural and religious context. This will enhance the scope and practice of APNs and will enable them to develop and apply innovative spiritual care models in their own care contexts. An authentic and transformative learning approach should be adopted to integrate spiritual care in clinical practice settings (Ali and Lalani 2020). Ali et al. (2018) encourages focusing on vocational aspect of nursing to encourage transformative learning approaches in clinical care and education, occurring at three levels: knowledge sharing (epistemological), being and becoming (ontological) and performance (skills and action) (Snowden and Ali 2017). Martinsen (2006, 2011) also suggests developing a perceiving eye in order to recognise and respond to a patient and family's spiritual need. Intuitive learning and transformative practices will allow embracing the concept of availability and vulnerability. By acknowledging personal fears, limitations, and knowledge deficiencies, APNs can be facilitated to develop an authentic self that could then be sensitive and available to understand spiritual care needs of others (Rogers 2016). Continuous funding and training support for nursing are needed in the areas of family caregiving and spirituality. Embracing spirituality and spiritual care in APN education and practice will improve the standards of care specifically and health generally and will enhance quality of life of patients and families at the end of life.

12.6   Conclusion

Spirituality provides an ethical foundation in making healthcare choices and decisions in Muslim traditions. Given the diverse cultural and social context of Pakistan, understanding spirituality and spiritual values of majority of Muslim population towards health, illness, and dying is paramount. Religious and spiritual values guide the ways in defining how Muslim patients and families define their health seeking attitudes and behaviors (Lalani and Ali 2020). Lack of spiritual care competency among nurses could lead to role ambiguity and anxiety as well as mistrust and lack of holistic patient/family-centered care (Ali 2017). Self-awareness education, and practice is therefore essential in acknowledging religious and spiritual needs of people near death and dying. Introducing advanced nursing care pathways focusing on professional authenticity, transformative leadership, and embracing spirituality in health education, policy and practice should be important considerations in the provision of holistic care in a wider Muslim context of Pakistan.

References

Abudari G, Hasim H, Genetec G (2016) Caring for terminally ill Muslim patients: lived experiences of non-Muslim nurses. Palliat Support Care 14(6):599–611

Ahmed W, Choudhry AM, Alam AY, Kaisar F (2012) Muslim patients' perceptions of faith-based healing and religious inclination of treating physicians. Pak Heart J 40(3-4):249

Ali G (2017) Multiple case studies exploring integration of spirituality in undergraduate nursing education in England. Doctoral thesis submitted to the University of Huddersfield. http://eprints.hud.ac.uk/id/eprint/34129/

Ali G, Lalani N (2020) Approaching spiritual and existential care needs in health education: applying SOPHIE (self-exploration through ontological, phenomenological, and humanistic, ideological, and existential expressions), as practice methodology. Religion 11(9):451

Ali G, Snowden M, Wattis J, Roger M (2018) Spirituality in nursing education: knowledge and practice gaps. Int J Multidiscip Comparat Stud 5(1-3):27–49

Barclay JS, Blackhall LJ, Tulsky JA (2007) Communication strategies and cultural issues in the delivery of bad news. J Palliat Med 10(4):958–977

Bhatnagar S, Gielen J, Satija A, Singh SP, Noble S, Chaturvedi SK (2017) Signs of spiritual distress and its implications for practice in Indian Palliative Care. Indian J Palliat Care 23(3):306

Buck HG, McMillan SC (2008) The unmet spiritual needs of caregivers of patients with advanced cancer. J Hosp Palliat Nurs 10(2):91–99

Deal B (2011) Finding meaning in suffering. Holist Nurs Pract 25(4):205–210

Delgado-Guay MO, Parsons HA, Hui D, De la Cruz MG, Thorney S, Bruera E (2013) Spirituality, religiosity, and spiritual pain among caregivers of patients with advanced cancer. Am J Hosp Palliat Care 30(5):455–461

Esmail A (1992) The Institute of Ismaili studies: the intellectual issues of the decade. The Ismaili 1:1–8

Esmail A (1995) Islam and modernity: intellectual horizons. In: The Muslim almanac: the reference work on history, faith and culture, and peoples of Islam. Gale Research, Detroit, pp 453–457

Esmail A (1998) The poetics of religious experience: the Islamic context. IB Tauris, London

Gijsberts MJH, Liefbroer AI, Otten R, Olsman E (2019) Spiritual care in palliative care: a systematic review of the recent European literature. Med Sci 7(2):25

Gul R (2008) The Image of Nursing from Nurses' and Non-Nurses' Perspective in Pakistan. The Silent Voice 1(2):4–17

Hasnain R, Rana S (2010) Unveiling Muslim voices: aging parents with disabilities and their adult children and family caregivers in the United States. Top Geriatr Rehabil 26(1):46–61

Jawaid H (2020) Assessing perception of patients and physicians regarding spirituality in Karachi, Pakistan: a pilot study. Perm J 24:214. https://doi.org/10.7812/TPP/19.214

Johnson J, Hayden T, True J, Simkin D, Colbert L, Thompson B, Martin L (2016) The impact of faith beliefs on perceptions of end-of-life care and decision making among African American church members. J Palliat Med 19(2):143–148

Khan RI (2012) End of life care in Pakistan: Some ethical issues. J College Phys Surg Pak 22(12):745–746

Khan RI (2017) Palliative care in Pakistan. Indian J Med Ethics 2(1):37–43

Khan ZH, Watson PJ, Chen Z, Iftikhar A, Jabeen R (2012) Pakistani religious coping and the experience and behaviour of Ramadan. Ment Health Relig Cult 15(4):435–446

Kim SS, Hayward RD, Reed PG (2014) Self-transcendence, spiritual perspective, and sense of purpose in family caregiving relationships: a mediated model of depression symptoms in Korean older adults. Aging Ment Health 18(7):905–913

Kurji Z, Premani ZS, Mithani Y (2016) Analysis of the health care system of Pakistan: lessons learnt and way forward. J Ayub Med Coll Abbottabad 28(3):601–604

Lalani N (2020) Meanings and interpretations of spirituality in nursing and health. Religion 11(9):428

Lalani N, Ali G (2020) Methodological and ethical challenges while conducting qualitative research on spirituality and end of life in a Muslim context: a guide to novice researchers. Int J Palliat Nurs 26(7):362–370. https://doi.org/10.12968/ijpn.2020.26.7.362

Lalani N, Duggleby W, Olson J (2018) Spirituality and family caregiving: an integrative literature review. Int J Palliat Nurs 24(1):112–124

Lalani N, Duggleby W, Olson J (2019) Rise above: experiences of spirituality among family caregivers caring for their dying family member in a hospice setting in Pakistan. J Hosp Palliat Nurs. https://doi.org/10.1097/NJH.0000000000000584

Madelung W, Mayer T (2015) Avicenna's allegory on the soul. IB Tauris, London

Martinsen K (2006) Care and vulnerability. Akribe, Oslo

Martinsen E (2011) Care for nurses only? Medicine and the perceiving eye. Health Care Anal 19(1):15–27

McSherry W, Jamieson S (2011) An online survey of nurses' perceptions of spirituality and spiritual care. J Clin Nurs 20(11-12):1757–1767

Narayanasamy A (2007) Palliative care and spirituality. Indian J Palliat Care 13(2):32

Naseem S, Khattak UK, Ghazanfar H, Irfan A (2016) Prevalence of non-communicable diseases and their risk factors at a semi-urban community, Pakistan. Pan Afr Med J 23:151. https://doi.org/10.11604/pamj.2016.23.151.8974

Organization for Economic Cooperation and Development (OECD). OECD Health Statistics. (2015). Health Policies and data. Retrieved from http://www.oecd.org/els/health-systems/health-data.htm

Paiva B, Carvalho A, Lucchetti G, Barroso E, Paiva C (2015) Oh, yeah, I'm getting closer to God: spirituality and religiousness of family caregivers of cancer patients undergoing palliative care. Support Care Cancer 23(8):2383–2238

Pakistan Nursing Council. (2017). List of PNC recognized institutions for diploma program, degree program and post basic diploma program. Retrieved from https://www.pnc.org.pk/PNC_Recognized_Institutes.htm

Parveen S (2016) Acute shortage of nursing professional in pakistan. Int J Nurs 2:1–6

Qidwai W (2003) Use of services of spiritual healers among patients presenting to family physicians at a teaching hospital in Karachi, Pakistan. Pak J Med Sci 19(1):52

Qidwai W, Tabassum R, Hanif R, Khan FH (2009) Belief in prayers and its role in healing among family practice patients visiting a teaching hospital in Karachi, Pakistan. Pak J Med Sci 25(2):182–189

Rogers M (2016) Utilising availability and vulnerability to operationalise spirituality. In: Practising spirituality. Palgrave Macmillan, London, pp 145–164

Ross L, Austin J (2015) Spiritual needs and spiritual support preferences of people with end-stage heart failure and their careers: implications for nurse managers. J Nurs Manag 23(1):87–95

Sinclair S, Raffin S, Pereira J, Guebert N (2006) Collective soul: the spirituality of an interdisciplinary palliative care team. Palliat Support Care 4(1):13–24

Sinclair S, Bouchal S, Chochinov H, Hagen N, McClement S (2012) Spiritual care: how to do it. BMJ Support Palliat Care 2(4):319–327

Snowden M, Ali G (2017) How can spirituality be integrated in undergraduate and postgraduate education? In: Spiritually competent practice in health care. CRC Press Taylor and Francis Group, London

Tornøe KA, Danbolt LJ, Kvigne K, Sørlie V (2015) The challenge of consolation: Nurses' experiences with spiritual and existential care for the dying-A phenomenological hermeneutical study. BMC Nurs 14(1):62. https://doi.org/10.1186/s12912-015-0114-6

Walker P, Simonowitz D, Poonawala I, Callataÿ G (2016) Sciences of the soul and intellect (part I): an Arabic critical edition and English translation of epistles. OUP/Institute of Ismaili Studies, Oxford, pp 32–36

Wattis J, Rogers M, Ali G, Curran S (2019) Bringing spirituality and wisdom into practice. In: Practice wisdom: values and interpretations. Brill-Sense Publishers, Rotterdam

World Health Organization (WHO) (2014) Cancer mortality profiles: Pakistan. Retrieved from http://www.who.int/cancer/country-profiles/pak_en.pdf?ua=1

World Health Organization (WHO) (2016) Pakistan: country profile. Retrieved from http://www.who.int/countries/pak/en/

Younas A, Rasheed SP, Sommer J (2019) Current situation and challenges concerning nursing education in Pakistan. Nurs Educ Pract 41:10238. https://doi.org/10.1016/j.nepr.2019.102638

Global APN Case Studies in Spirituality: Stories of Hope from the United Kingdom

13

Melanie Rogers, Joanne Pike, and Angela Windle

Abstract

Spirituality is not routinely integrated into healthcare practice in the United Kingdom (UK). Many practitioners, when asked, are confused about the definition of spirituality and routinely conflate it with religion. However, when you talk to practitioners about holistic care, they will often use terminology which connects to spirituality, for example person-centred care and compassionate care. This chapter firstly discusses the Advanced Practice Nurse role in the UK before exploring how spirituality in healthcare is understood. Two case studies are then presented to illustrate spirituality being integrated into practice by Advanced Nurse Practitioners in a primary care and hospital setting.

Keywords

United kingdom · Advanced Nurse Practitioner · Spirituality · Availability · Vulnerability

13.1   Introduction

In the United Kingdom (UK) there are four countries: England, Scotland, Wales and Northern Ireland, each with a devolved government responsible for developing health policy. Each country has developed advanced practice roles in response to

M. Rogers (✉) · A. Windle
University of Huddersfield, Huddersfield, UK
e-mail: m.rogers@hud.ac.uk; a.f.windle@hud.ac.uk

J. Pike
Wrexham Glyndwr University, Wrexham, UK
e-mail: j.pike@glyndwr.ac.uk

their own specific needs. The term Advanced Practice Nurse (APN) is not used in the UK; however, the term Advanced Nurse Practitioner (ANP) is common, as is the term Advanced Clinical Practitioner (ACP). Both ANPs and ACPs attain the same competencies. ACPs however, are allied healthcare practitioners, for example paramedics, occupational therapists, physiotherapists and pharmacists. ANPs and ACPs in the UK have in the past been educated to diploma and degree level but now are usually educated at master's level with a full master's degree recommended to practice. The UK also has Clinical Nurse Specialists (CNS), some of which meet the criteria of advanced practice, while others are qualified to work as specialist nurses.

ANP, ACP and CNS roles are not regulated and historically do not have legal protection of their titles. This has led to significant issues across the UK including variation of education, titles, and role confusion. The Royal College of Nursing (RCN), the largest nursing union and professional body in the UK, has tried to address issues of education and practice and has produced extensive guidance for ANP education and practice. In addition, they have set up a voluntary register of credentialed ANPs. The Nursing and Midwifery Council (NMC), who regulate nurses in the UK, have historically insisted that ANPs do not need individual regulation as they should work within their code of professional conduct. For many years, nurses, educators and policymakers have lobbied the NMC to reconsider this position and in 2010, a report by the Prime Minister's Commission on the future of nursing and midwifery stated that the NMC should be responsible for the regulation of ANPs (Sell 2010). Finally, in 2021 the NMC is considering ANP regulation as part of a major review of its regulation process.

In recent years, Health Education England (HEE) who support the delivery of healthcare through education, training and workforce development have developed a multi-professional advanced clinical practice framework. This has been a driving force towards setting standards for advanced practice in England (Health Education England 2017) and has led to plans to establish a Centre for Advanced Practice which will provide governance for education and practice (Council of Deans of Health 2018). Scotland has three Academies of Advanced Practice which maintain a database of all advanced practitioners working there. The plan in England is to have a single Centre which will accredit university courses meeting the national standards for advanced practice. The Centre will also keep a database of all advanced practitioners in England.

England is the largest of the four countries in the United Kingdom and has chosen to follow Wales' lead (National Leadership and Innovation Agency for Healthcare (NLIAH) 2010) in developing a Multi-Professional Framework for Advanced Practice (Health Education England 2017). Both country frameworks clearly identify their vision for ensuring advanced practice is possible for all health professionals, not just nursing. Northern Ireland published their Advanced Nursing Practice Framework in 2016 (Department of Health, Social Services and Public Safety (DHSSPSNI) 2016), followed by releasing the Advanced Allied Health Professional Practice Framework in June 2019 (Department of Health 2019), signalling its commitment to advanced practice in all health professions. There has been much debate about this, but the idea of developing a workforce which enables professionals to advance their scope of practice and extend the boundaries of their profession is welcome (Rogers and Gloster 2020). Only Scotland has limited advanced practice to nurses only at this time.

Advanced practice in the UK is viewed as a level of practice rather than a specific role. In all four countries, four pillars of advanced practice have been widely accepted as the foundation for all education and practice. The pillars are clinical practice, leadership, research and education (Health Education England 2017).

Each country has developed its own definition for advanced practice:

In England

Advanced clinical practice is delivered by experienced, registered healthcare practitioners. It is a level of practice characterised by a high degree of autonomy and complex decision-making. This is underpinned by a master's level award or equivalent that encompasses the four pillars of clinical practice, leadership and management, education and research, with demonstration of core capabilities and area specific clinical competence. Advanced clinical practice embodies the ability to manage clinical care in partnership with individuals, families, and carers. It includes the analysis and synthesis of complex problems across a range of settings, enabling innovative solutions to enhance people's experience and improve outcomes (Health Education England 2017, p. 8).

In Scotland

Advanced Nurse Practitioners (ANPs) are experienced and highly educated registered nurses who manage the complete clinical care of their patients, not focusing on any sole condition. ANPs have advanced level capability across the four pillars of practice: clinical practice, facilitation of learning, leadership, evidence, research and development. They also have additional clinical practice skills appropriate to their role (Chief Nurse Office Directorate (CNOD) 2016, p. 2).

In Wales

Advanced Practice is "a role, requiring a registered practitioner to have acquired an expert knowledge base, complex decision-making skills and clinical competencies for expanded scope of practice, the characteristics of which are shaped by the context in which the individual practices. Demonstrable, relevant masters level education is recommended for entry level" (National Leadership and Innovation Agency for Healthcare (NLIAH) 2010, p. 21).

And Finally, in Northern Ireland

An ANP in Northern Ireland "practices autonomously within his/her expanded scope of clinical practice, guided by The Code. Professional standards of practice and behaviour for nurses and midwives (Nursing Midwifery Council 2018)". "The Advanced Nurse Practitioner demonstrates highly developed assessment, diagnostic, analytical and clinical judgement skills ..." (Department of Health, Social Services and Public Safety (DHSSPSNI) 2016, p. 4). Advanced Practice for other healthcare professionals is developing.

The current situation with regards lack of title protection and regulation in the UK has its challenges. Any country establishing ANP roles should ensure regulation is in place for education begins. The lack of regulation has caused titles to be used inappropriately in the UK by practitioners without the necessary education and competence. However, with each country having clear guidance and frameworks for the development of advanced practice it is hoped that advanced practice will continue to develop, providing the highest level of care to patients.

Opening up advanced practice to all healthcare professionals in the UK has some opponents who would argue that nursing has unique qualities which ensure the ANP role integrates the best of nursing and medicine in providing truly holistic care (Walker et al. 2007). However, the ANP role is only one model of advanced practice, albeit one that sits well with nursing in particular. Other models of advanced practice are evolving in all allied health professions seeking to expand their scope of practice. This work has been well supported in all four countries; an example of this is from HEE who note that workforce planning must consider all advanced practice roles to meet the needs of the population and address the rising issues of a rise in healthcare need (Health Education England 2020).

In summary, in all four countries, the key principles of advanced practice are a high level of autonomous practice, and the ability to make complex decisions. The four pillars of practice are visible in all four countries' frameworks and the role must be underpinned by master's level education. The aim of all advanced practice roles in to deliver high-quality, patient-focused care (Evans et al. 2020).

13.2   Spirituality in Healthcare in the United Kingdom

Although spirituality is an important aspect of holistic care, historically it has been poorly integrated into healthcare in the UK. Rogers and Wattis (2015) report that this is due to confusion about how it can be integrated into practice, as well as difficulties conceptualising it. National and international nurse regulators and international nursing organisations identify that integrating spirituality is part of good nursing practice (Nursing and Midwifery Council 2009, 2014; International Council of Nurses 2012). Although spirituality is not specifically identified in the current nurse Code of Conduct (Nursing Midwifery Council 2018), it has been recognised in previous ones with the NMC stating that holistic care must integrate an assessment of spiritual needs (Nursing and Midwifery Council 2010). However, if nurses cannot conceptualise spirituality it is likely that will have difficulty carrying out an assessment of spiritual needs.

There has been progress over the recent years in clarifying how to integrate spirituality into care. Specifically, as identified in Chap. 2, a push towards spiritually competent practice has been proposed to avoid the issue of definitions (Wattis et al. 2017). McSherry and Jamieson (2013) conducted the largest UK perceptions of spirituality study in the UK which found that 92.6% of nurses believed that patients' spiritual needs should be addressed. However, the study also found there was a struggle to conceptualise spirituality and a lack of education available during initial training hindered the integration of spirituality into care. A further study of health-care educators found that although 90% identified that spirituality should be inte-grated into education, only 17% of educators included any spirituality training within healthcare curricula (Prentis et al. 2014). Rogers et al. (2019) recently inves-tigated mental health practitioners' perceptions of spirituality. They found that although practitioners identified that spirituality was important, it was not always integrated into care. The study found that spiritually competent practice was more useful in practice. Again, lack of education was found to be a barrier to integrating spirituality into healthcare (Rogers et al. 2019).

Additional support to understand and integrate spirituality has been published through a major European collaboration (Enhancing Nurses' Competence in Providing Spiritual Care Through Innovative Education and Compassionate Care (EPICC) 2019) which identified spiritual care competencies for undergraduate nurs-ing and midwifery (see Chap. 3). The EPICC spiritual care education standard sim-plifies competencies needed to carry out a spiritual needs' assessment. This extensive collaboration brought together practitioners, educators, researchers and policymak-ers from across Europe. Enhancing Nurses' Competence in Providing Spiritual Care Through Innovative Education and Compassionate Care (EPICC) (2019) rec-ommends that spiritual competencies should be practised within a person-centred approach to care which builds a compassionate relationship and enables an attitude of openness, trust and presence to be offered. This approach mirrors Rogers' (2016) Availability and Vulnerability framework. The development of these competencies should be welcome news to those who have recognised that there are no consistent approaches to integrating spirituality teaching into nursing and healthcare education (Lewinson et al. 2018).

UK policymakers and nursing scholars have long highlighted the need for care to be person-centred and compassionate. Indeed, readers may well have heard of the "Mid-Staffordshire Crisis" during the late 2000s where poor care and high mortality in a number of hospitals hit the national and world news. This crisis resulted in the Francis Report which identified a healthcare culture in which a lack of care was endemic (Frances 2013). There was recognition that healthcare workers were not exhibiting caring, committed, and compassionate behaviours which had led to a culture detrimental to patient care (Entwistle 2013). While there have been drivers to change the culture in the UK health service, there are still concerns that the task and output driven health service often seen supersedes a person-centred approach (Wattis et al. 2017, 2019).

Ensuring holistic care is provided to all patients is one way to revolutionise healthcare culture. Spirituality, with its focus on human-to-human connection within a compassionate, open, non-judgemental relationship is vital to providing holistic care. Milligan (2011) reminds us that spirituality is unique to each person, there is no one size fits all when it comes to spirituality and addressing patients' spiritual needs. However, bringing practitioners' personal qualities and motivation together with positive organisational values as discussed in Chap. 2, will support health care practitioners to integrate spirituality into their practice.

UK policy documents acknowledged that spirituality plays a significant role during illness and in the healing process (Department of Health 2008; NHS Scotland 2009). However, unless practitioners engage with spirituality it will likely be detrimental to the provision of high-quality care (McSherry 2010). Robinson et al. (2003) identified that although the increase in UK policies discussing spirituality is positive, there is still a need for policies and healthcare education to be clearer and more specific about integrating spirituality into healthcare.

NHS Scotland (2009) is one of the devolved healthcare systems which has consistently supported the integration of spirituality and compassionate practice into healthcare. They have identified that spiritual care is essential to healthcare practice. They advocated an approach that accepted uniqueness, was inclusive, individualised and encourages care for patients to move in whatever direction is needed. Further to their policy statements a resource for all healthcare staff entitled Spiritual Care Matters was published (NHS Scotland 2009). The aim of this resource was to bring clarity to spirituality and give staff a clearer understanding of what their role should be and how to operationalise spirituality. NHS Scotland suggested that spiritual care was:

> "…. care which recognises and responds to the needs of the human spirit when faced with trauma, ill health or sadness and can include the need for meaning, for self-worth, to express oneself, for faith support, perhaps for rites or prayer or sacrament, or simply to be a sensitive listener. Spiritual care begins with encouraging human contact in compassionate relationship and moves in whatever direction need requires" (NHS Scotland 2009, p. 6).

Spiritual care is deeply compassionate care (Pfeiffer et al. 2014). In England, the Department of Health (2008) identified that by practising compassionately healthcare practitioners can significantly improve a patient's life. This preceded the Francis Inquiry and clearly was not at the forefront of healthcare in the UK for many years. There was a shift around the time Francis report with a push for health care practitioners to see listening and talking to their patients as fundamental aspects of basic care and compassion. Further government policies echoed this with publications such as Compassion in Practice (Department of Health 2012), National Health Service Constitution for England (Department of Health 2013a) and treating patients and service users with respect, dignity and compassion (Department of Health 2013b) where patients are at the heart of all we do. Although none of these policies and documents identified spirituality separately, they all alluded to core aspects of spirituality through a call to all healthcare practitioners to maintain a culture of compassion and care.

13.3 Case Studies: Availability and Vulnerability in Practice (All Names Changed to Maintain Anonymity)

I, Joanne an ANP, met Jac a 45-year-old man, when he came into the primary care out of hours service at 3 a.m. presenting with an 8-week history of back pain which had become more painful and debilitating over the day. It was now unmanageable despite taking the analgesia prescribed for him by his General Practitioner (GP) a week ago. As he entered the room, I could see he was tired and was in pain from his altered gait and tense posture. He looked over to me and told me he just couldn't cope with this any longer. He said "I give up" looking so defeated, my heart went out to him immediately.

I assessed him physically and we discussed his limited movement and his fear of "making it worse". In common with many people suffering from back pain Jac had adopted maladaptive strategies and pain avoidance behaviours to cope with his condition (Driver et al. 2019). This had resulted in limiting his movement and taking multiple medications to control the pain and limit the spasms which he told me was "excruciating".

I was concerned about his fear of pain and knew I could employ several techniques to explore this with him. However, I had a "gut feeling" that there might have been other factors at play. The "gut feeling" or intuition of the expert nurse has been well researched by Benner (1984) who notes that this is linked to pattern recognition. This has also been termed "heart knowing" or spiritual knowing (Anderson 2020). In this consultation, I was conscious of Jac's vulnerability and the need for us to make a real connection so that I could understand and respond to his deeper needs. I knew in my heart that there was a need to practise spiritually and holistically.

There has been a recent emphasis on holistic assessment and treatment of patients with back pain, as physiotherapy research has demonstrated this can improve functional outcomes and lead to increased confidence and improved well-being (McGrane et al. 2015). After excluding any red flags, I initiated pain management and referred Jac to my physiotherapy colleagues for their expert assessment. Despite addressing his physical presentation, I was concerned about his loss of hope for the future and thought that he may be in spiritual crisis. I moved on to address this.

I asked him how I might help him, acknowledging that he had said that he wanted "to give up". Utilising presence I sat quietly and attentively with him while he tried to make sense of my question. He replied angrily that he needed pain relief and said again that he couldn't bear it any longer. I waited just a little, avoiding filling the silence, nodded and looked gently back at him. He looked down and sighed a little, saying he was just exhausted, and he had a lot of other worries that made him feel hopeless. From these halting beginnings, I listened to his worries about being off work, his finances, and how he felt he would never get better. He wasn't sleeping and he often awoke in the morning feeling stressed and anxious as well as having back pain. Through listening attentively, being fully "present" and encouraging his confidence, through my availability to him, Jac admitted that he was not taking his analgesia regularly as he wanted to do without because he was scared of becoming dependent. However, he was also afraid to move, and so sat or lay down for long periods when he could find a comfortable position.

By being available to him through listening attentively, being truly present and demonstrating my concern for him (Rogers 2016), a connection was made with Jac which enabled him to feel safe enough to explore his deepest concerns with me and further, to communicate the *meaning* of those to me. Through our connectedness, in a short period of time I was able to build trust, Jac became less tense and stressed and opened up more to me. Together we began to work on potential solutions which would help Jac see some hope for the future by having his pain controlled and being mobile. Jac appeared less defeated by the end of our consultation and told me that he had gained strength from talking about his concerns.

Case 2

James a 35-year-old patient was admitted to the surgical ward in early July with necrotising pancreatitis following endoscopic retrograde cholangiopancreatography to remove gallstones that had led to pancreatitis. He was a previously independent, fit and well man who worked in financial services and was married with one 8-year-old son. James was also a coach for his local football club.

James had deteriorated rapidly post-surgery and was in a very poor physical condition. He had multiple intra-abdominal collections which required drainage and was cared for in critical care as he developed wide-spread oedema from an associated profound hypo-albuminemia. On return to the ward he began the long process of recovery. He needed parenteral nutritional support, frequent drainage of intra-abdominal collections and intermittent antimicrobial therapy. He returned to critical care numerous times post further drainage of recurrent large intra-abdominal collections and then had a major haemorrhage from his mesenteric artery resulting in multiple organ failure. He also contracted SARS CoV2 in critical care but sufficiently recovered to be transferred back to the ward in late October.

James's admission to hospital with gallstones in July had resulted in a prolonged hospital admission during the Covid-19 pandemic in the UK. Nosocomial infection posed a significant risk to the patients already hospitalised and a decision nationally was made to stop visiting for relatives to reduce transmission to try break the chain of infection. This decision to not permit hospital visiting meant that James had not seen his family or 8-year-old son for 5 months apart from virtually using mobile devices. James had become more and more withdrawn and was difficult to engage with in activities aimed at aiding his recovery including care of his abdominal drains, eating and physiotherapy. He had begun to lose hope.

I, Angela a surgical ANP, first met James in November, he had been a hospital inpatient for 5 months, he was frail, sarcopenic and clinically depressed; all of which were contributing to James not engaging in any daily routine. I was covering for a colleague and during my ward round I reviewed James's clinical details, his laboratory results, latest CT scans and his oral fluid/food intake alongside his parenteral nutritional support. I introduced myself and asked James how he was getting on with his food—he replied, without eye contact "poorly" and explained that nausea was making eating impossible, I offered to review his antiemetic medication. I spent time trying to establish some rapport with James, but it was difficult as his answers were mono-syllabic, and he would not look at me. I had noticed the physiotherapy team had documented that he was refusing to engage at all and had started to refuse to sit in a chair during the day. I gently asked him about this and he simply replied, "I just can't do it anymore". I reflected to James that I could only imagine what a difficult time he had experienced and that I wanted to do all I could to ease his distress. I could see that James was experiencing hopelessness and I wanted to understand what James was trying to explain. I took time to listen to his distress as he slowly opened up to me. He told me that he had not seen his son or wife in 5 months, his loneliness and hopelessness were palpable.

I reflected on how I would feel in his position looking at the same four walls, isolated, in pain and fearful of the future. I knew I would want to go outside, even for a few minutes so asked him if he had seen the sky since he had been admitted to hospital. His eyes immediately widened, and he looked at me...."no" he said. He began to cry. I simply stayed with him, offering myself, my presence and my care. All I wanted to do was offer some comfort and hope yet I was in dressed in full personal protective equipment and was unable to hold his hand or comfort it physically as I would normally do. I continued to remain present and considered what I could do to help. I asked James if he would like to go outside with me, he could sit in a wheelchair or I could push his bed outside and he could see the sky...even if it was a grey English winter day, he laughed and said he didn't want to take up my time. I told him I was not in a rush and just wanted to do something for him that might help. He cried again for a while and said he would love to go outside. He said he didn't feel up to it now but could try tomorrow.

After I had spoken with James, I rang his wife to update her on his condition which we did as a team each week while she was unable to visit him in hospital. I said I was concerned about his current mood; she was very tearful and told me that he was getting more and more depressed and that she was struggling with not being able to see him. I explained my plan to get James outside of the hospital for a short period tomorrow and asked her if she would like to bring some personal belongings along to the hospital at approximately the same time and she could spend some time in person, albeit socially distanced and with a mask on, she was thrilled. Unfortunately, I was not on duty the following day but my fellow ANP colleague said that he would ensure that James got outside even for a short period. We had prearranged a time that his wife could bring some belongings for James and the plan was set. James met his wife in the hospital carpark with my colleague for assistance, he subsequently sent me a message to report that James was sat outside in the winter sunshine with his wife and looked a "different" man. Over the next few days James set himself small goals around improving his physical strength and independence.

To truly care for our patients, we must make ourselves available to them, not just with physically but also emotionally, being present and listening to James' deepest concerns was all he needed to begin to have some hope (Rogers 2016). Covid-19 has reinforced how important it is to see our patients holistically. James needed more than just a review of his physical health, he needed therapeutic time in a trusting relationship with a practitioner who would actively listen to what he was saying, recognise what he was not saying and notice that he had lost hope. In facilitating a family visit for James outside the hospital I wanted to be the advocate for James, his family needed to be considered as his therapy as he had begun to lose hope that he would ever be with them again. As a senior ANP with many years of nursing experience I was able to accept my professional vulnerability for the benefit of James and his family by breaking the guidelines. The national guidelines about hospital visiting were put in place to prevent the spread of infection but a hospital visit to promote hope and recovery in a patient was in my professional opinion a worthy effort and was a valid reason to work outside of the guidelines while ensuring that we protect James and his wife.

James was successfully discharged in February 2021, he has gone home to a life where his home looks like a hospital but he is continuing his recovery with the support of the family who love him, family that he thought he would never see again. As I reflect on the one question I asked James that day, "When did you last see the sky?" I am very proud that I integrated spirituality into my care which led to James starting a journey towards independence and a family reunion for a patient who had simply presented with gallstones but did not leave hospital until seven long months later.

13.4 Discussion

Both case studies illustrate how spirituality can be integrated into care even in a short period of time. I, Joanne work in primary care and have only 15 minutes with each patient, Angela had one interaction with her patient when she was covering for a colleague on a different ward. Both ANPs showed significant emotional and spiritual intelligence which helped their patients to hold on to hope. Emotional Intelligence may not initially be thought to be a spiritual attribute, but self-knowledge, comprehending and responding to emotions in others, and empathy all have spiritual connotations. These are also the foundations of interpersonal relationships and have the ability to transform human-to-human connections. Therapeutic, interconnected relationships where staff are available and authentic (Rogers 2016) are transpersonal or transcendent caring relationships (Griffin and Yancey 2009). Finfgeld-Connett (2008) examined the concept of presence and carried out a metathesis of the concept of caring. Her results indicate that while caring is a context-specific interpersonal process, and is characterised by interpersonal sensitivity and intimate relationships, it is not dissimilar to the concept of spiritual care advocated by other authors. This is evidenced by her further assertion that caring is preceded by a recipient's need for and openness to caring, underpinned by the nurse's professional maturity and moral foundations. Both myself and Angela chose to be open and reflecting our maturity ascertained the patient's spiritual needs. When further underpinned by availability and vulnerability, such spiritual work, delivered with love and understanding of self and others, led to powerful transformations seen in Jac and James.

It is vital that when patients are open to caring, we as APNs are able to interpret that openness and respond. In complex cases such as the cases presented where the pre-eminent concern may appear to be pain or infection control, the need for spiritual support in suffering should not be overlooked. Taking time to "be" with Jac and James and listen to the true concerns elicited positive responses. In spirituality terms we witnessed suffering, were available and present and attended to the hopelessness both patients felt.

Presence, as particular way of being, of caring, and relating spiritually to patients, has been discussed in the literature for the last 30 years or more. It has been discussed by Benner and Wrubel (1989, p. 13) as being "with a patient in a way that acknowledges shared humanity, it is the base of nursing as a caring practice... To presence oneself with another means understanding and being with someone". Being fully present for a patient is a skill that is expressed through APNs' authenticity and love and requires the APNs attention be focused on the patient, receptiveness of the needs of the other and an awareness of a shared humanity (Tavernier 2006). Presence provides a sense of meaning that promotes holistic healing (Tavernier 2006). It must be practised as an intentional relationship (Rogers 2016). Krirkgulthorn et al. (2018) and Holopainen et al. (2019) recognise that intentional presence, conscious awareness of patients' spiritual needs and offering unconditional love are all aspects of holistic care which address the spiritual dimension. However, to do this demands self-awareness, acceptance and an understanding their meaning, purpose and direction in life which is vocational (Rogers 2016).

Spirituality connects fully to emotional intelligence. APNs need to make the most of therapeutic encounters in the clinical practice to ensure they are meeting their patient's needs (Cox 2018). Both patients were empowered by expressing their emotions and concerns. Konradsdottir and Svavarsdottir (2013) acknowledge that patients often find hope, meaning and purpose as they take greater control of their own condition. Sharing their spiritual anguish led to them being truly heard within a human-to-human relationship based on deep concern and care.

These consultations were profoundly spiritual. Recognising their spiritual needs and being able to connect as a fellow human being led to therapeutic relationships as both myself and Angela were open to the connection being made (Pike 2012). Both patients had physical health problems, but these were not the main issue impacting their hope. The mental anguish expressed by both men was a powerful driver for the ANPs to respond. To help restore some level of hope there was a need to connect on a deeper level, to see past Jac's apparent anger and James' disengagement and identify the meaning of the illness and how it was affecting their lives and themselves which had led to their sense of hopelessness. Cassell (2004) asserts that a suffering person should not suffer alone, they can be restored when they are able to share their concerns about meaning in a transpersonal relationship. Their suffering can be relieved through this spiritual connection.

13.5 Conclusion

Both cases illustrate the impact of integrating spirituality into practice. In many ways the interactions described are "simple" and "core" to the work of an APN. However, they became "spiritual" when the practitioners chose intentionally to not avoid the underlying issues leading to hopelessness but to build a relationship in a very short time built on authenticity, care, compassion and love. Using a model like Rogers' (2016) Availiabilty and Vulnerabilty framework gives a structure to integrate spirituality into our day-to-day practice in ways that are understandable and easy.

All three of us strongly believe that working as an APN is a privilege. Being holistic and person-centred care is the premise of how we choose to work because we see the difference it makes to our patients. Choosing to recognise subtle signs that patients often do not verbalise which show they are losing hope can lead to creating safe, open, and non-judgemental spaces where their spiritual care needs are recognised and addressed.

References

Anderson M (2020) The spiritual heart. Religion 11:506. https://doi.org/10.3390/rel11100506

Benner P (1984) From novice to expert: excellence and power in clinical nursing practice. Addison-Wesley Publishing Co., Menlo Park

Benner P, Wrubel J (1989) The primacy of caring: stress and coping in health and illness. Addison Wesley, Menlo Park

Cassell EJ (2004) The nature of suffering and the goals of medicine, 2nd edn. Oxford University Press, New York

Chief Nurse Office Directorate (CNOD) (2016) Transforming nursing, midwifery and health professions' roles: pushing boundaries to meet health and social care needs in Scotland. Paper 2-Advanced Nursing Practice

Council of Deans of Health (2018) Advanced clinical practice education in England. Event report from the 2018 Council of Deans of Health/Health Education England advanced clinical practice education conference. https://councilofdeans.org.uk/wp-content/uploads/2018/11/081118-FINAL-ACP-REPORT.pdf

Cox K (2018) Use of emotional intelligence to enhance advanced practice registered nursing competencies. J Nurs Educ 57(11):648–654

Department of Health (2008) High quality care for all NHS next stage review final report. DoH, London

Department of Health (2012) Compassion in practice-nursing, midwifery and care staff. Our vision and strategy. DoH, London

Department of Health (2013a) NHS constitution. DoH, London

Department of Health (2013b) Treating patients and service users with respect, dignity and compassion. DoH, London

Department of Health (2019) Advanced AHP practice framework. Department of Health, Belfast

Department of Health, Social Services and Public Safety (DHSSPSNI) (2016) Advanced nursing practice framework-supporting advanced nursing practice in health and social care trusts. Department of Health, Social Services and Public Safety, Belfast

Driver C, Lovell G, Oprescu F (2019) Physiotherapists' views, perceived knowledge, and reported use of psychosocial strategies in practice. Physiother Theory Pract. https://doi.org/10.1080/09593985.2019.1587798

Enhancing Nurses' Competence in Providing Spiritual Care Through Innovative Education and Compassionate Care (EPICC) (2019) Spiritual care education standard. https://blogs.staffs.ac.uk/epicc/files/2019/06/EPICC-Spiritual-Care-Education-Standard.pdf

Entwistle F (2013) Changing the culture of the health service. Nurs Times 109(7):16–23

Evans C, Poku B, Pearce R, Eldridge J, Hendrick P, Knaggs R, McLuskey J, Tomaczak P, Throw R, Harris P, Conway J, Collier R (2020) Characterising the evidence base for advanced clinical practice in the UK: a scoping review protocol. BMJ Open 10:036192. https://doi.org/10.1136/bmjopen-2019-036192

Finfgeld-Connett D (2008) Meta-synthesis of caring in nursing. J Clin Nurs 17(2):176–204

Frances R (2013) Report of the mid Staffordshire NHS foundation trust public inquiry. Department of Health, Belfast

Griffin A, Yancey V (2009) Spiritual dimensions of the perioperative experience. AORN J 89(5):875–882

Health Education England (2017) Multi-professional framework for advanced clinical practice in England. https://hee.nhs.uk/sites/default/files/documents/HEE%20ACP%20Framework.pdf

Health Education England (2020) Advanced clinical practice. https://www.hee.nhs.uk/our-work/advanced-clinical-practice/what-advanced-clinical-practice

Holopainen G, Nyström L, Kasén A (2019) The caring encounter in nursing. Nurs Ethics 26(1):7–16. https://doi.org/10.1177/0969733016687161

International Council of Nurses (2012) The ICN code of ethics for nurses. ICN, Geneva

Konradsdottir E, Svavarsdottir E (2013) The role of advanced nurse practitioners in offering brief therapeutic conversation intervention for families of children and adolescents with diabetes type 1. Nordic J Nurs Res 33(3):44–47

Krirkgulthorn T, Kheokao J, Umereweneza S, Seetangkham S, Sosome B (2018) Wholistic humanized nursing care: a model for cultivating a humanistic caring mind in nursing students. Philipp J Nurs 88(2):33–39

Lewinson L, McSherry W, Kevern P (2018) Enablement–spirituality engagement in pre-registration nurse education and practice: a grounded theory investigation. Religion 9(11):356–370. https://doi.org/10.3390/rel9110356

McGrane N, Galvin R, Cusack T, Stokes E (2015) Addition of motivational interventions to exercise and traditional Physiotherapy: a review and meta-analysis. Physiotherapy 101:1–12

McSherry W (2010) RCN spirituality survey 2010- a report by the Royal College of Nursing on Members' views on spirituality and spiritual care in nursing practice. RCN, London

McSherry W, Jamieson S (2013) The qualitative findings from an online survey investigating nurses' perceptions of spirituality and spiritual care. J Clin Nurs 22(21-22):3170–3182

Milligan S (2011) Addressing the spiritual care needs of people near end of life. Nurs Stand 26(4):47–56

National Leadership and Innovation Agency for Healthcare (NLIAH) (2010) Framework for advanced nursing, midwifery and allied health professional practice in Wales. NLIAH, Llanharan

NHS Scotland (2009) Spiritual care matters. An introduction resource for all NHS staff. NHS Education for Scotland, Edinburgh

Nursing and Midwifery Council (2009) NMC competence domain. NMC, London

Nursing and Midwifery Council (2010) Standards for pre-registration nursing education. NMC, London

Nursing Midwifery Council (2014) The code: standards of conduct performance and ethics for nurses and midwives (draft revised version). NMC, London

Nursing Midwifery Council (2018) The code: standards of conduct performance and ethics for nurses and midwives. NMC, London

Pfeiffer J, Gober C, Johnson-Taylor E (2014) How Christian nurses converse with patients about spirituality. J Clin Nurs 23:2886–2895

Pike J (2012) Searching for the hidden: a phenomenological study exploring the spiritual aspects of impending day case surgery from patient and staff perspectives, Unpublished PhD Thesis. University of Wales

Prentis S, Rogers M, Wattis J, Jones J, Stephenson J (2014) Healthcare lecturers' perceptions of spirituality in education. Nurs Stand 29(3):44–52

Robinson S, Kendrick K, Brown A (2003) Spirituality and the practice of health care. Palgrave MacMillan, London

Rogers M (2016) Spiritual dimensions of advanced nurse practitioner consultations in primary care through the lens of availability and vulnerability. Unpublished PhD thesis. University of Huddersfield, Huddersfield

Rogers M, Gloster A (2020) Advanced nursing in the United Kingdom. In: Hassmiller S, Pulcini J (eds) Advanced practice nursing leadership. A global perspective. Springer, Cham

Rogers M, Wattis J (2015) Spirituality in Nursing. Nurs Stand 29(39):51–57

Rogers M, Wattis J, Stephenson J, Khan W, Curran S (2019) A questionnaire-based study of atti-
    tudes to spirituality in mental health practitioners and the relevance of the concept of spiritually
    competent care. Int J Ment Health Nurs 28(5):1162–1172
Sell S (2010) Advanced nurse practitioners must be regulated by the NMC, says brown. General
    practice on-line. Accessed https://www.gponline.com/advanced-nurse-practitioners-regulated-
    nmc-says-brown
Tavernier S (2006) An evidence-based conceptual analysis of presence. Holist Nurs Pract
    20(3):152–156
Walker R, Bindless L, Firth J, Harrison F, Michael S (2007) Combining the best of nursing and
    medical care: evaluation of the West Yorkshire nurse practitioner (primary care) development
    programme from 2001–2005. Health Education, London
Wattis J, Curran S, Rogers M (2017) Spiritually competent practice in health care. CRC Press,
    Boca Raton
Wattis J, Rogers M, Ali G, Curran S (2019) Bringing spirituality and wisdom into practice. In:
    Higgs J (ed) Practice wisdom: values and interpretations. Sense-Brill Publishers, Rotterdam

Global APN Case Study in Spirituality-Stories of Hope from Australia

14

Andrew Scanlon and Ruth Ikobe

Abstract

Spirituality in healthcare delivery within Australia can be complex as there is no one size fits all approach. Australia is a multicultural society with a universal healthcare system. As such there is no one size fits all to meet medcial and spitirial needs. Current Australian guidelines on the multicultural needs for spiritual care in health are in place to ensure that these needs are met. A specific focus will be on Advanced Practice Nurse roles. How these roles are educated and regulated to deliver care will be outlined. This will give context on their practice and how these roles contribute to the Australian healthcare systems. This context will be followed by a case study which reviews how these concepts are addressing practice as well as what can be done in the future.

Keywords

Advanced practice roles · Australia · Nurse practitioner · Spiritual care Parkinson's disease

A. Scanlon (✉)
Austin Health, The University of Melbourne, Parkville, VIC, Australia
e-mail: andrew.scanlon@unimelb.edu.au

R. Ikobe
Aged Care/Palliative Care, Barwon Health, Geelong, VIC, Australia

14.1   Australia

Australia has a population of approximately 23 million people. Its healthcare system is based on a model from the United Kingdom but has morphed to allow both private and public institution to provide care. Advanced Practice Nurse roles have delivered care in this setting for over 40 years and have done so while addressing the spiritual needs for those they have been charged with caring for.

14.2   Introduction to the Advanced Practice Nurse Role

Advanced practice nursing has been evident in Australia since the 1980s. The first Advanced Practice Nurse (APN) role title recognised was the Clinical Nurse Specialist (CNS). CNSs were introduced within the state of New South Wales (NSW) healthcare system in 1986 following the success of such roles in the United Kingdom (Duffield et al. 1996). Following this Clinical Nurse Consultants (CNCs) were introduced in 1990; however, there is no other documented proof of when these roles were established elsewhere (Duffield et al. 2009). Both roles came about from restructuring of nursing duties and career pathways with the CNC or CNS roles providing clinical expertise in speciality roles. The difference between the roles is dependent on the requirements of the organisation they work for. However, in a broad sense CNSs are usually ward-based nurses identified as experts in their field while CNCs work within specialities (i.e., wound care) but are available to use their expertise throughout the organisation.

In the early 1990s, project work to develop the Nurse Practitioner (NP) role began. Piloting and taskforce work established the need for the role particularly in rural and remote areas where medical provision was limited. In 2001, the first NPs were authorised to practice by the NSW board of nursing who approved their scope of practice through their legislative authority (Australian College of Nurse Practitioners 2016). Nurse Practitioner, CNS and CNC type roles operated over the speciality spectrum as well as across the lifespan of patient populations. Today there are over 2097 NPs in Australia (Nursing and Midwifery Board of Australia 2020). CNS and CNC which may be considered "advanced" within Australia, are unregulated and numbers are not able to be calculated.

In July 2010, Australia moved to national registration for nurses and other health professionals with the recent creation of the Australian Health Practitioner Regulatory Agency (AHPRA) and the Nurse and Midwifery Board of Australia (NMBA). This means we only have one board to whom nurses must adhere to the requirements for education and practice.

14.3   Educational Level and Regulation

Nursing roles like the CNS, and CNC, as stated previously, are not regulated or licenced above that of a registered nurse. As such there are no legal requirements for further education apart from those associated with entry level to Registered Nurse.

Table 14.1 Requirements for Australian Nurse Practitioner endorsement

1. Current general registration as a Registered Nurse in Australia with no conditions or undertakings relating to unsatisfactory professional performance or unprofessional conduct
2. The equivalent of three years' full-time experience (5000 h) at the clinical advanced nursing practice level, within the past six years, from the date when the complete application seeking endorsement as a Nurse Practitioner is received by the NMBA
3. Successful completion of
   • An NMBA-approved programme of study leading to endorsement as a nurse practitioner, or
   • A programme that is substantially equivalent to an NMBA-approved programme of study leading to endorsement as a Nurse Practitioner as determined by the NMBA.
4. Compliance with the NMBA's nurse practitioner standards for practice

Nursing and Midwifery Board of Australia (2016b)

However, it is recommended that they have additional postgraduate training to fulfil the role at a local organisation level.

Nurse Practitioners within Australia have a set of standards which govern their practice. It requires Masters level of education specifically designed for NPs or a programme which meets these requirements as deemed appropriate by the Nurse and Midwifery Board of Australia (Nursing and Midwifery Board of Australia 2020). In regard to the NMBA NP standards, they are used not only to guide the assessment of those deemed eligible for endorsement/authorisation, but also to assess those involved in professional conduct matters and communicate to consumers the standards that they can expect from NPs. Additionally, University NP curricula is reviewed by the NMBA to ensure programmes of study meet the national standards (Australian Nursing and Midwifery Accreditation Council 2015). All NP programmes must meet national requirements for entry and required hours of supernumerary practice during the course of study. All approved NP curricula at Master's level are accredited nationally by the Australian Nursing and Midwifery Council (ANMC) for the NMBA.

Apart from the regulatory requirements specific for NP education, other regulatory and legislative requirements are applied to NPs. To be eligible for endorsement and be licenced to practice as an NP, the following criteria must be met (Table 14.1).

The Australian Health Care system is a mixture of public and private healthcare. This impacts the NPs ability to practise to their full scope of practice. For example, NPs must practise in collaboration with a physician or surgeon. These collaborations are established under either a "Shared Care Model" or a "Continuing therapy Only (CTO) Model" which ties the practice of NPs to this collaboration (The Department of Health 2018). Additionally, NP scope of practice is further defined by the local practice environment that the NP is employed within. These are often added as there are requirements to further manage potential risk to the public that NPs may cause (Scanlon et al. 2016). Once endorsed, the NP can practise within the confines of what the Federal and their individual State government will allow them.

NPs in Australia report lack of support for care delivery as well as various barriers to practising to the fullest extent of their scope of practice (Scanlon et al. 2016). The restrictions placed on NPs and ongoing regulatory difficulties, organisational climate and inter-professional difficulties remain, impacting the NP scope of practice (Scanlon et al. 2018).

14.4   Spirituality in Australian Health Care

Spiritual needs of patients and their loved ones are recognised as an important component of the delivery of quality healthcare (Balboni 2020). However, there is no consistent or national approach when it comes to the delivery of spiritual care in healthcare delivery or training in Australia (Holmes 2018; Meaningful Ageing Australia 2016). In Australia, training in spirituality and its application to individual needs are not required as specific units of study in nursing curricula (Australian Nursing and Midwifery Accreditation Council 2019). However, it should be considered as part of person-centred care which flows throughout the curriculum and is defined within registered nurse standards for practice and the "Code of Conduct for Nurses" (Nursing and Midwifery Board of Australia 2016a, 2018). Through person-centred care nurses are required to work collaboratively with the patient and their loved ones in a respectful partnership to address healthcare needs with respect to personal, cultural and religious choices or beliefs (Nursing and Midwifery Board of Australia 2016a, 2018). Additionally, the NMBA utilises the ICN code of ethics for nurse, which within its first (of four) principle elements acknowledges "In providing care, the nurse promotes an environment in which the human rights, values, customs and spiritual beliefs of the individual, family and community are respected." (International Council of Nurses 2012). These principles and considerations are integral within the nursing and broader healthcare curriculum. However, examples of how this is integrated into practice are difficult because of its inherent nature of this work. As a result, spirituality in the Australian Health Care setting is not always at the forefront of care consideration for the people. Thankfully, this is changing with initiatives at both state and federal levels to address this shortcoming of care (The Department of Health 2019). These initiatives were ultimately brought about in response to safety and quality care focuses, central to this was person-centred care and the need to incorporate personal beliefs and values (Australian Commission on Safety and Quality in Health Care 2011). This is further embedded into practice through national healthcare accreditation processes within Australia (Australian Commission on Safety and Quality in Health Care 2017).

There are options within nurse training and education to undertake a spirituality topic as part of their Graduate Diploma or Master's Degree. However, this is mostly offered as an elective topic in Palliative and Aged Care degrees. Unfortunately, due to specialisation of NPs in Australia it is not offered in all NP curricula and thus there is a lack of the opportunity to gain knowledge and training in spirituality as it is not a mandatory topic.

It also required that healthcare practitioners have a unified approach to care, while being individual and specific to an individual, a common process needs to be employed. The only national guideline which addresses this and puts forward an achievable model of practice is the "National Guidelines for Spiritual Care in Aged Care" which addresses this in part (Meaningful Ageing Australia 2016). This guideline is specifically for aged care which has been adapted to state requirements to broadly address spirituality in healthcare. Within it the definition of spirituality is actually three definitions which overlap as it is understood that there is no "right" definition of spirituality.

These definitions include:

1. Spirituality is a dynamic and intrinsic aspect of humanity through which persons seek ultimate meaning, purpose, and transcendence, and experience relationship to self, family, others, community, society, nature, and the significant or sacred. Spirituality is expressed through beliefs, values, traditions and practices.
2. The definition of spirituality is that which lies at the core of each person's being, an essential dimension which brings meaning to life. Constituted not only by religious practices, but understood more broadly, as relationship with God. However, God or ultimate meaning is perceived by the person and in relationship with other people.
3. Spirituality is universal, deeply personal and individual. It goes beyond formal notions of ritual or religious practice to encompass the unique capacity of each individual. It is at the core and essence of who we are, that spark which permeates the entire fabric of the person and demands that we are all worthy of dignity and respect. It transcends intellectual capability, elevating the status of all of humanity to that of the sacred (Meaningful Ageing Australia 2016)

When tackling issues of spirituality, the guidelines further identify requirements to ensure that they can be effectively met. This is performed broadly through utilising and implementing the principle outlined in the domains of spiritual care which are given below.

- Domains of spiritual care
  - Organisational leadership and alignment
  - Relationships and connectedness
  - Identifying and meeting spiritual needs
  - Ethical context of spiritual care
  - Enabling spiritual expression (Meaningful Ageing Australia 2016)

The domains and principles associated with this guideline are designed to be implemented across any healthcare organisation. However, without a national guideline or standard that encompasses all areas of practice and healthcare provider's training and practice it will remain difficult. As a result, it remains up to individual healthcare organisations or practitioners to apply these principles to develop care in relation to the patients and the broader community they serve.

Most recent census data indicates that over 30% of the population do not have an identified religion and while Christianity is declining it still makes up the bulk of all religions (Ezzy et al. 2020). Additionally, research has shown that Australian teens consider themselves spiritual but not religious with another 46% stating that they are not religious at all (Singleton et al. 2018).

Considerations of culture and spiritually of first nations of Australia are always paramount when caring for these individuals. As these concepts help families cope with daily challenges (Lohoar et al. 2014). This is particularly the case when addressing the stress and uncertainty that can occur with healthcare crisis and interacting with healthcare services which are not specifically set up to meet these requirements for care.

Given Australia's diverse ethnic, cultural and religious population including those of the first nations, the approach to addressing a person's spiritualty while addressing their healthcare needs can be very specific and thus guidelines such as the ones presented need to be broad so as not to discriminate.

14.5 Introduction to My Role/Practice Area and the Case Study

I am Ruth Ikobe, with training as an Aged Care, Primary care and Palliative Care Nurse Practitioner. I currently work for a programme that provides services and supports residents residing in Residential Aged Care Facilities (RACF). The programme aims to provide clinical care, which includes palliative care, to residents in their homes with the intention of avoiding hospital admissions. A spirituality definition that resonates with me is one that states that "spirituality is the aspect of humanity that refers to the way individuals seek and express meaning and purpose, and the way they experience their connectedness to the moment, to self, to others, to nature and to the significant or sacred" (Puchalski et al. 2009, p. 885). The case study will highlight how I was able to utilise the concepts of spirituality such as availability, vulnerability, kindness and compassionate presence amongst others in an 80-year-old male Victor (name changed to protect anonymity) who had advanced Parkinson's disease (PD).

14.6 Case Study

Victor was referred to me due to his deterioration as part of an established referral process to NPs. He had advanced PD and had been having increasing falls. Staff were also concerned about some behavioural issues such as his increased agitation.

When I met Victor, I introduced myself, my role and the reason for my visit. I obtained consent to review him. He had been aware of my impending visit as staff had advised him to expect a review from me. This was the first time I had met Victor. He had been residing in the RACF for three months as he was unable to continue living alone at home due to safety issues, such as increasing falls, and the fact that he could not safely care for himself at home. His short-term memory was also deteriorating.

When I met him, he looked well, he was well-groomed and there were no signs of distress. Despite his PD, he was able to speak in a low slow tone that was understandable. I pulled a seat next to him and began my conversation with him. This is a technique that has been advocated as it gives the patient the feeling that the clinician has the time to listen as opposed to standing during the interview. It is also an aspect of connecting and being present with the patient (Puchalski and Romer 2000). I took note of his room and noted he was in a single room with many photos of both his immediate and extended family. It was important for me to take note of his surrounding as it helped guide our discussions and it also built a connection with him. This allowed him to open up more about his history and his family later on during our interview.

I questioned Victor about his diagnosis and asked him to tell me details of his condition and past treatments. I learnt that he had been to several specialists and he was on the maximal treatment regimen with no room to further up titrate his medications without causing further side effects. He was frustrated that he was having many falls but disliked the idea of having to wait for the staff to come and help him. I utilised several communication techniques such as naming his emotion and also giving him cues that I was listening, both of which are vital in both communication and spirituality (Lawton and Carroll 2005). Communication techniques such as asking him to tell me more about his diagnosis and use of body language such as nodding showed that I was taking a keen interest in what he had to say. Victor had been living at home independently after his wife passed away several years back. I asked him to point out photos of his wife and I noticed a huge smile on his face which was not evident when I first met him. By taking the time to know the patient and how much his family meant to him allowed for trust and rapport to be established between us. He spoke about his children and how proud he was of their accomplishments especially his youngest son who had completed a doctorate and was a scientist in a city about two hours from the RACF. He reported missing his family and said that he was trying to make sense of what his life would be given that he knew he had a life-limiting illness. Timmins and Caldeira (2017) point out that this is part of spirituality in patients facing terminal illness. This was particularly a challenging time for Victor as his facility was in current lockdown due to the COVID-19 Virus, as were all other RACFs in the state. This meant he was unable to physically see his family which was causing him a great deal of distress. While virtual visits using iPads were available as often as needed, he still yearned for a face-to-face visit with his family and reported he would have rather been at his own house.

I took the time to listen to him talk about his son and his family and did not interrupt him. At one point he asked me if I had time to listen and I reassured him that I not only had the time but was also very eager to hear about his life story. This is a vital technique emphasised in spirituality. "This is a way that the clinician can practice deep non-judgmental listening that helps the patient give voice to their suffering" (Puchalski et al. 2009, p. 9). It is also an aspect of availability that is also important in spirituality and spiritual care (Rogers et al. 2020).

He went on to talk about the different specialists he had seen and how he was frustrated that there were no more medications that would help. I took note of the significant tremors that he had on both hands. I continued to listen and empathised with him and avoided any interruptions when he talked. This technique is termed as compassionate presence which is defined as being "fully present with another as a witness to their experience" (Puchalski et al. 2020, p. 7). I was able to do this by listening and allowing Victor to talk of his suffering without interruptions. At one point he was teary as he reported that he struggled to hold a cup due to his tremors, I recognised the distress this caused him and utilised empathy to show him I cared. Due to the pandemic and changes around physical distancing, there were limitations on utilisation of other techniques I would usually use, for example touch, eye contact, listening and empathy which were paramount (SAHealth 2020).

By the end of the conversation, Victor had developed trust in me and I reassured him that I would follow up with him in a week. He reported that he had enjoyed the visit and it was evident in how relaxed he was at the end of the review. We discussed strategies for minimising his falls such as graduated positional changes and recommended certain cups that would be easier to handle. I also referred him to an occupational therapist for a review. I altered some of his medications with aim of reducing any hypotension that may have been also contributing to his falls. Empathy was evident in the discussions, this is one vital strategy in spiritual care and also an integral aspect of communication. At one point both Victor and I were able to laugh together when he mentioned some of his grandsons' stories. Use of stories and even laughter can also be a form of spiritual care and spirituality (Foster et al. 2012).

At the end of the discussion, it was evident that the behaviours the staff were noting were in part related to his frustration about all that was happening to him and not all due to an underlying or reversible factor. The lockdown also played a role in some of his loneliness and it was evident he was longing for more face-to-face conversations. Patients such as Victor may at times be experiencing some form of spiritual distress as he spoke of life not having much meaning since the loss of his wife and the fact that he was in a RACF depending on staff for some of his activities of daily living (ADLs). In addition to that, there was also the pandemic and lockdown further causing restrictions on him seeing his family. Unfortunately, at times spiritual distress can be missed and staff can easily assume that the symptoms are physical or psychological (Chochinov and Cann 2005). While this is possible, it is important that any spiritual issues are addressed, and I am glad I was able to take the time to closely look into the impact of spirituality in his case.

Victor had several questions which I was able to respond to. One that was challenging was being able to prognosticate as he was wondering how much time he had left to live. I was honest with him and explained the disease trajectory and reemphasised how difficult it must have been for him not to have some of the answers he really wanted. He was appreciative of the honesty and understood that it was hard to give a timeline on his disease trajectory. This honest and open explanation and discussion resonates with the vulnerability aspect of spirituality (Rogers et al. 2020).

I undertook further discussions on what gave Victor meaning in his life and what was important to him. Further understanding his spirituality could be a mechanism in which he could use to cope with his illness (Henry 2020). At the end of the review, I noted that some of his symptoms were signs of spiritual distress and some unmet spiritual needs. With his consent, I referred him to the Spiritual Health Practitioner (SHP) for more support as the SHPs are specialists in the area of spiritual distress. SHPs are employed by many hospitals and RACFs as they offer vital support to patients and staff who may be in need of spiritual support. It is recommended that they be part of the treating team as part of a holistic approach in patient care (McClement 2015). McClung et al. (2006) also emphasised that spirituality and spiritual care are better undertaken as a team approach. With the help of the SHP, Victor was able to get specialised spiritual support that included detailed review into what his life meant to him and what the afterlife would look like including dignity therapy.

Victor appreciated that I took the time to listen to him. On my next visit I ensured that I asked how his son was doing with his new job as I knew how important his family was to him. He was surprised that I was able to recall that his son had started a new role as a scientist. Once again, I noted the huge smile on his face. I discussed with the staff some techniques that they could utilise to communicate with him and simple acts of spiritual care that they could include in Victor's care which made a profound impact in his care. He was appreciative of the SHP support as he reported he felt more at peace.

One important aspect that played a big role in the case study was the fact that I was aware of my spirituality. It is important that staff are aware of their spirituality as this in turn would be reflected in the care offered to our patients (McDonald et al. 2014; Rogers et al. 2020). This was also echoed by Best et al. (2020) who pointed out how a patient's spiritual care can be missed if one is unaware of their spirituality. Without my knowledge on spirituality, I would have solely focused on Victors physical symptoms missing the spiritual symptoms which seemed to have more profound effect on him as opposed to his physical symptoms. One key aspect of my spirituality is compassion, and this was reflected in the entire review of the patient and the subsequent follow-up visits. It is also important to note that the act of caring which is core in nursing is considered an act of spiritual care (World Health Organization 2020)

14.6.1 Barriers to Integrating Spirituality

There were certain barriers to integrating spirituality in this case study and time constraint was a barrier. While I was able to spend a decent amount of time with Victor, I would have loved to have had even more time with him. McClement (2015) reports that time constraints can be barriers to spirituality. More time with Victor would have likely enabled him to share even more than he already did as he was comfortable as our conversations progressed. This was limited as I had to also conduct a detailed assessment looking at his falls, medications and overall physical deterioration. Fortunately, the SHP was able to undertake more detailed spiritual examination.

Lack of a formal validated spiritual assessment tool in this particular setting was also a barrier. Tools such as the FICA (Faith, Importance, Influence, Community, Address/action) tool would have been of value in assessing Victor's spirituality (Puchalski and Romer 2000, p. 131). These tools "include more objective data (e.g., religious affiliation, spiritual practices) while touching upon deeper and more subjective spiritual aspects (e.g., meaning, importance of belief, sources of hope)" (Puchalski et al. 2009, p. 893). Had a formal spiritual screen been undertaken using one of the validated tools, perhaps some of his needs may have been noted and addressed earlier on. Puchalski and Romer (2000) also echo the importance of using a spiritual assessment tool that can capture the spiritual needs of the patients.

As previously mentioned, this consultation happened during a time when we were dealing with a pandemic. This was certainly a barrier as the patient could not attend activities, he had previously been able to for example going out with his family for church services and family events that brought him joy. It was also challenging for me in that other simple spiritual acts such as touch, or simple handshakes were unable to be undertaken. The patient could also not see all of my facial expressions such as my smile due to the use of masks, face shields and personal protective gear.

14.6.2 Facilitators to Integrating Spirituality in this Case Study

The greatest facilitator in the integration of spirituality in this case study was the fact that I had undertaken training in spirituality and spiritual care. I was therefore aware of my spirituality which was integral in providing spiritual care (McDonald et al. 2014). Being aware of my own spirituality allowed me to be able to easily recognise Victor's spiritual needs. I was also able to offer spiritual care that is vital in my spirituality such as being human and offering compassionate presence, kindness and gentleness throughout our conversation (Rogers et al. 2020). One's culture and upbringing also help shape their attitudes towards spirituality and spiritual care (Fang et al. 2016). This certainly plays a big role in how I perceive spirituality and how I provide spiritual care. Given that a big aspect of my cultural upbringing is the respect for the elderly, I chose to ensure that I took the time to listen him and treat him with utmost respect. This is something I maintain with all my patient interactions. Although I mentioned time as a barrier, I was still able to spend a reasonable amount of time unlike other healthcare practitioners who may have increased time restraints, and this allowed Victor to open up to a greater extent. It also helped that on my follow-up visits I scheduled him as my last client of the day, this allowed me to spend more time with him.

Another facilitator of spirituality was the fact that I was able to be available through follow-up with the patient over a longer period maintaining continuity of care which helped foster a trusting relationship between myself and the patient (Rogers et al. 2020). The SHP was also able to have ongoing visits with following ups with Victor for as long as he needed him which was a great facilitator. In addition to the follow-ups, excellent communication skills are also vital in spiritual care and this was certainly a facilitator in integrating spirituality in the case study (Tulsky 2005). I had undertaken two communication assignments during my NP training which helped me to understand more about spirituality and how to integrate this into the care I offer. I feel that this additional understanding and the techniques I utilised certainly helped Victor in opening up. Communication techniques that were utilised in the entire dialogue with Victor included utilisation of the recommended communication techniques such as NURSE (Naming, understanding, Respecting,

Supporting and Exploring) which expand on the concept of responding to emotions (VITALtalk 2020)

The fact that the facility had a dedicated Spiritual Health Practitioner (SHP) was also a facilitator as this allowed for a collaborative team effort in meeting Victor's spiritual needs and ensuring he did not end up with spiritual distress that was unmet especially as his condition continued to deteriorate. McClung et al. (2006) mention the importance of working with other members of the multidisciplinary team (MDT) as part of holistic care in spirituality. The SHP also adds value to the team as he also plays a big role in educating the staff on spiritual care.

Caring for Victor and ensuring his spirituality was met did not increase my risk of burnout as I was aware of my spirituality. Being aware of one's spirituality acts as a buffer against burnout and this was echoed by Cherny et al. (2015) on a study they reported that showed "an inverse correlation between burnout and spirituality" (Cherny et al. 2015).

Spirituality is vital in all encounters that NPs or APNs make with patients. Even small acts such as kindness and empathy can make a difference in the patients' care as noted in this case study. Spiritual care is vital in the holistic care of the patient as it enhances the patient's quality of life (Balboni and Balboni 2020). I believe it should be part of all APNs and NPs training and should also be included as part of workplace orientation. From this case one can see how spirituality played a big role in the patient care. I have been fortunate as an NP to have undertaken a module on spirituality during my NP training in palliative care. This has had a great impact in the care I offer my patients. As previously mentioned, it is not a mandatory topic in the NP curriculum throughout Australia thus, I was fortunate to have undertaken it as an elective topic. Including a module like this provides a detailed understanding of what spirituality entails and I feel that this has equipped me with an in-depth understanding of spirituality and spiritual care. Despite that, I still feel that further research in the role that NPs and APNs play in spirituality needs to be undertaken as there remains a scarcity of research in this area.

14.7   Conclusion

This chapter highlights the developments of advanced practice in Australia over the last 40 years. It demonstrates how spirituality is viewed by healthcare practitioners in general and shows how one NP operationalised spirituality in practice within this particular healthcare setting.

References

Australian College of Nurse Practitioners (2016) First NPs Authorised in Australia. Australian College of Nurse Practitioners History. https://acnp.org.au/history#20
Australian Commission on Safety and Quality in Health Care (2011) Patient-centred care: improving quality and safety through partnerships with patients and consumers

Australian Commission on Safety and Quality in Health Care (2017) National safety and quality health service standards guide for hospitals. https://www.safetyandquality.gov.au/sites/default/files/migrated/National-Safety-and-Quality-Health-Service-Standards-Guide-for-Hospitals.pdf

Australian Nursing and Midwifery Accreditation Council (2015) Nurse practitioner accreditation standards. 2015. https://www.anmac.org.au/sites/default/files/documents/Nurse_Practitioner_Accreditation_Standard_2015_FINAL_0.pdf

Australian Nursing and Midwifery Accreditation Council (2019) Registered Nurse. Accreditation Standards 2019

Balboni M (2020) Influence of spirituality and religiousness on outcomes in palliative care patients. UpToDate. https://www.uptodate.com/contents/influence-of-spirituality-and-religiousness-on-outcomes-in-palliative-care-patients#topicContent

Balboni M, Balboni T (2020) Influence of spirituality and religiousness on outcomes in palliative care patients. UpToDate

Best M, Leget C, Goodhead A, Paal P (2020) An EAPC white paper on multi-disciplinary education for spiritual care in palliative care. BMC Palliat Care 19(1):9

Cherny NI, Werman B, Kearney M (2015) Burnout, compassion fatigue, and moral distress in palliative care. Oxford Textb Palliat Med 9(2):246

Chochinov HM, Cann BJ (2005) Interventions to enhance the spiritual aspects of dying. J Palliat Med 8 (Suppl 1):S103. Oxford textbook of palliative medicine, 9(2):246

Duffield C, Donoghue J, Pelletier D (1996) Do clinical nurse specialists and nursing unit managers believe that the provision of quality care is important? J Adv Nurs 24(2):334–340

Duffield C, Gardner G, Chang AM, Catling-Paull C (2009) Advanced nursing practice: a global perspective. Collegian 16(2):55–62. https://doi.org/10.1016/j.colegn.2009.02.001

Ezzy D, Bouma G, Barton G, Halafoff A, Banham R, Jackson R, Beaman L (2020) Religious diversity in australia: rethinking social cohesion. Religion 11(2):92

Fang ML, Sixsmith J, Sinclair S, Horst G (2016) A knowledge synthesis of culturally- and spiritually-sensitive end-of-life care: findings from a scoping review. BMC Geriatr 16(1):107. https://doi.org/10.1186/s12877-016-0282-6

Foster TL, Bell CJ, Gilmer MJ (2012) Symptom management of spiritual suffering in pediatric palliative care. J Hosp Palliat Nurs 14(2):109–115

Henry RS (2020) Relationships among Parkinson's disease symptoms, stigma, and mental health: a strengths-based perspective

Holmes C (2018) Towards National consensus: spiritual care in the australian healthcare context. Religion 9(12):379

International Council of Nurses (2012) ICN code of ethics for nurses. https://www.icn.ch/sites/default/files/inline-files/2012_ICN_Codeofethicsfornurses_%20eng.pdf

Lawton S, Carroll D (2005) Communication skills and district nurses: examples in palliative care. Br J Community Nurs 10(3):134–136

Lohoar S, Butera N, Kennedy E (2014) Strengths of Australian Aboriginal cultural practices in family life and child rearing Strengths of Australian Aboriginal cultural practices in family life and child rearing

McClement S (2015) Spiritual Issues in palliative medicine. In: Cherney N, Fallon M, Kaasa S, Portney R, Currow D (eds.), Oxford textbook of palliative medicine (5th Ed.). Oxford, England: Oxford Univerity Press, pp 19

McClung E, Grossoehme DH, Jacobson AF (2006) Collaborating with chaplains to meet spiritual needs. Medsurg Nursing 15(3):147

McDonald C, Murray C, Atkin H (2014) Palliative-care professionals' experiences of unusual spiritual phenomena at the end of life. Ment Health Relig Cult 17(5):479–493

Meaningful Ageing Australia (2016) National guidelines for spiritual care in aged care. Parkville

Nursing and Midwifery Board of Australia (2016a) Registered nurse standards for practice. http://www.nursingmidwiferyboard.gov.au/documents/default.aspx?record=WD16%2f19524&dbid=AP&chksum=R5Pkrn8yVpb9bJvtpTRe8w%3d%3d

Nursing and Midwifery Board of Australia (2016b) Registration standard: Endorsement as a nurse practitioner. http://www.nursingmidwiferyboard.gov.au/documents/default.aspx?record=WD1 6%2f19510&dbid=AP&chksum=f%2bPPC07%2bhpZYR0APtyEykQ%3d%3d

Nursing and Midwifery Board of Australia (2018) Code of conduct for nurses. https://www.nursingmidwiferyboard.gov.au/documents/default.aspx?record=WD17%2f23849&dbid=AP&chk sum=ki92NMPa9thp9f9ZhTQNJg%3d%3d

Nursing and Midwifery Board of Australia (2020) Registrant data. https://www.ahpra.gov.au/ documents/default.aspx?record=WD20%2f30375&dbid=AP&chksum=7b6IwcIPryH7iGH VH5%2fubQ%3d%3d

Puchalski C, Romer AL (2000) Taking a spiritual history allows clinicians to understand patients more fully. J Palliat Med 3(1):129–137

Puchalski C, Ferrell B, Virani R, Otis-Green S, Baird P, Bull J, Prince-Paul M (2009) Improving the quality of spiritual care as a dimension of palliative care: the report of the Consensus Conference. J Palliat Med 12(10):885–904

Puchalski C, Ferrell B, Otis-Green S, Handzo G (2020) Overview of spirituality in palliative care. In: Givens J (ed) UpToDate. UpToDate, Waltham

Rogers M, Hargreaves J, Wattis J (2020) Spiritual dimensions of nurse practitioner consultations in family practice. J Holist Nurs 38(1):8–18

SAHealth (2020) COVID-19. Fact SheetInfection control advice for community-based service providers. https://www.sahealth.sa.gov.au/wps/wcm/connect/29d3ffd3-a576-4be8-b961-574044532cd5/Fact+sheet+-+Community+IC+and+PPE+advice_v1.1+-+Last+update+1.08.2020.pdf

Scanlon A, Cashin A, Bryce J, Kelly J, Buckely T (2016) The complexities of defining nurse practitioner scope of practice in the Australian context. Collegian 23(1):129–142. https://doi. org/10.1016/j.colegn.2014.09.009

Scanlon A, Murphy M, Tori K, Poghosyan L (2018) A national study of Australian nurse practitioners' organizational practice environment. J Nurse Pract 14(5):414–418. https://doi. org/10.1016/j.nurpra.2018.01.003

Singleton A, Halafoff A, Bouma G (2018) New research shows Australian teens have complex views on religion and spirituality. The Conversation. https://theconversation.com/new-research-shows-australian-teens-have-complex-views-on-religion-and-spirituality-103233

The Department of Health (2018) Eligible nurse practitioners questions and answers. Program and initiatives. https://www1.health.gov.au/internet/main/publishing.nsf/Content/ midwives-nurse-pract-qanda-nursepract

The Department of Health (2019) Connecting with spirituality. Head to health. https://headto-health.gov.au/meaningful-life/connectedness/spirituality

Timmins F, Caldeira S (2017) Understanding spirituality and spiritual care in nursing. Nursing Standard 31(22)

Tulsky JA (2005) Interventions to enhance communication among patients, providers, and families. J Palliat Med 8(1):95–101

VITALtalk (2020) Track & respond to emotion. http://vitaltalk.org/topics/track-respond-to-emotion/

World Health Organization (2020) Palliative care. https://www.who.int/news-room/fact-sheets/ detail/palliative-care

Global Case Studies in Spirituality: Stories of Hope from Chile

15

Paula Jaman-Mewes, Bernardita Troncoso Valenzuela, and M. Consuelo Cerón

Abstract

This chapter will explore the formation of advanced practice nursing in Chile. Although the Advanced Practice Nurse is a relatively recent role, Chile is further along in terms of developments than other Latin American Countries. This is partly due to homogeneous undergraduate nurse education in all Universities in our country which has enabled postgraduate education to be focused at masters level. As with many countries there are opportunities and challenges to developing advanced practice nursing, for example, the lack of standardised definitions for the scope of practice and regulation. Among the opportunities for the role development are the consensus work that has been conducted by several nursing schools to develop more advanced practice master programmes and the urgent need to address the rising healthcare issues and achieve the universal health in Chile.

The second half of the chapter focuses on how spirituality is seen in healthcare here in Chile and how it is being taught on an Advanced Practice Nurse master's programme at the Universidad de los Andes. Finally, through a case study we will show how the spiritual dimension of the care is operationalised in an advanced model of care in a palliative care hospital. In order to protect anonymity, fictitious names were created for the case studies.

Keywords

Spirituality · Spiritual care · Advanced practice nursing · Nurses · Palliative care

P. Jaman-Mewes (✉) · B. Troncoso Valenzuela · M. C. Cerón
Universidad de los Andes, Santiago, Chile
e-mail: pjaman@uandes.cl; btroncoso@uandes.cl; maceronm@uandes.cl

15.1   Introduction to the Advanced Practice Nurse Role in Chile

The Advanced Practice Nurse (APN) is a relatively new role in Latin American countries (LAC) and there is still a lack of consensus around the definition, scope of practice and competencies. Moreover, there are disparities in legislation and education, not only for APN but also for bachelor level nurses (Cassiani et al. 2018; Zug et al. 2016). However, Latin American nurse leaders recognise the importance of the APN for contributing to achieving Universal Health Coverage (UHC) (Cassiani et al. 2018; Zug et al. 2016). This is based on the evidence showing that APNs bring the same quality of care as General Practitioners in Primary Health Care (PHC). Evidence suggests that APNs have better patient outcomes, higher levels of patient satisfaction and reduce healthcare costs compared to medical colleagues (Laurant et al. 2019; Maier et al. 2017). For this reason, the Pan American Health Organization (PAHO) has promoted the development of APN in LAC as a cost-effective strategy to achieve UHC. Pan American Health Organization (PAHO) (2015) strongly recommended the incorporation of the APN role to support and strengthen health systems, especially in PHC. Another PAHO initiative in conjunction with McMaster University Nursing School, in Canada, was the "Universal Access to Health and Universal Health Coverage: Advanced Practice Nursing Summit", which brought together LAC nurse leaders to discuss how to implement strategies which will develop the APN role. The discussion was reflected in a large report in Spanish, English and Portuguese, with relevant information such as the objectives and steps that LAC should follow in order to get the APN role implementation (Pan American Health Organization (PAHO) 2015; Zug et al. 2016). Following this plan, countries like Brazil, Colombia, Mexico and Chile have demonstrated significant progress in developing advanced practice (Cassiani et al. 2018).

One of the key recommendations of the McMaster Summit was to apply the PEPPA framework to guide the process in the development of the APN (Pan American Health Organization (PAHO) 2015). The PEPPA framework is a systematic strategy that includes nine steps in a flexible and iterative process in order to (1) use relevant data to make evidence informed decisions, (2) support the development of APN role, (3) promote the maximisation of APN expertise, (4) promote work environment supportive to APN implementation and (5) continually assess the impact of the role. This framework has been successfully utilised in more than 16 countries within different contexts (Aguirre-Boza et al. 2019; Oldenburger et al. 2017). The Universidad de los Andes in Chile developed and implemented the first Master's degree in advanced practice nursing in 2011. Initially the focus of the degree was on the Clinical Nurse Specialist (CNS) role in acute care. The degree focused on developing five competencies: evidence-based practice, extensive knowledge and expertise in the care of adult patients with acute pathologies, communication and leadership skills, management skills, and the ability to develop projects that expand nursing knowledge. Currently, apart from Universidad de los Andes, there are two other universities in Chile who are working together to expand

APN masters programmes. These universities are focusing on developing the Nurse Practitioner (NP) role. Working together for consensus, professorial colleagues from these three universities and the Chilean Association of Nursing Education have met to discuss the ongoing development and expansion of the APN roles in Chile. It has been established that the most urgent unmet health needs that APN should address are patients with chronic non-communicable diseases (specifically hypertension and diabetes), cancer and mental health problems. The Cancer National Plan in Chile (Ministerio de Salud (MINSAL) 2018) had already highlighted the need for APNs to support the delivery of Cancer Care. APN training for Cancer and Palliative Care has recently begun in Chile and is offered to nurses working at Cancer Centres.

Despite there being robust regulation and definition for the scope of practice for registered nurses in Chile, there is none for the APN role yet. Nevertheless, many nurses are working in advanced roles, especially in PHC, due to clinical experience and expertise gained over time. However, these nurses have not studied a formal Masters programme and are not recognised as APNs.

In summary, there are some obstacles that have delayed the process of implementing the APN role, but these are now being addressed. Specifically, the lack of regulation and scope of practice for APN role which needs to be standardised throughout Chile. Additionally, the recognition of proper renumeration for APNs according to the competencies acquired is needed in order to create a career pathway for nurses and recognition of the advanced level these nurses practise at. Finally, it would progress APN development if there was State funding to finance the development of APN Masters programmes.

15.2   Introduction to Spirituality in Healthcare in Latin American Countries and Chile

Since 1970, spirituality in healthcare began to be recognised, both on the public policy agenda and in clinical practice in LAC. It has been argued that integrating spiritualty into care benefits patient's health (Krmpotic 2016). There is an increase in the number of scientific papers in the field of social, human and health sciences which has intensified over the last few years both worldwide and in LAC (Timmins et al. 2015). At the level of the World Health Organization, spirituality as a concept was officially incorporated into healthcare in 1998 (Krmpotic 2016).

All LAC were colonised by Catholic countries from Europe, mainly from Spain. The premise of the Catholic religion is that the human person is made up of body, mind and spirit. The human being, unlike an animal, has reason and will and is endowed with dignity. In Catholicism man is worthy for being a child of God and that gives him freedom and responsibility to relate to others with respect (Megías 2020). Spirituality has for a long time been linked to a religious concept in LAC. Recently, some authors identify that there is a "new era of spirituality" which is broader and more diverse. This is especially noted in LAC countries influenced by indigenous religions such as Mexico, Brazil, Argentina and Uruguay (Usarski 2018). Usarski (2018) has suggested the importance of distinguishing spirituality from religious traditions considered as part of people's beliefs and values.

Brazilian and other international studies have identified that people who view spirituality as important show lower rates of drug use, lower prevalence of depression and suicide attempts, and better quality of life and well-being. They identify that spirituality has a positive effect on physical health, it improves adherence to treatment, helps patients cope with the disease, leads to fewer hospital length of stay and reduces mortality rates (Koenig 2012; Puchalski et al. 2014; Selman et al. 2014; Damiano et al. 2016; Shanshan et al. 2016; Balboni et al. 2017; Salas and Taboada 2019). Despite robust scientific evidence on the benefit of integrating spirituality into healthcare, there are many professionals who do not consider the spiritual dimension and focus rather on the disease, forgetting the integrality of the person from the mind, body and spirit perspective (Balboni et al. 2017; Salas and Taboada 2019; VanderWeele et al. 2017). Astrow et al. (2007) found that only 6 to 28% of patients receive spiritual care from the health team which is contrary to what patients would like and what international and national policies suggest.

From a cultural perspective, like most LAC, religion in Chile is a significant part of society and has been relevant throughout history (Müller 2008). The Chilean health system has cultural roots based on the catholic religion, for example nuns used to be part of the health teams. Moreover, large public hospitals still have catholic chapels and are named with Saints, such as Hospital San Borja, Hospital San José, and Hospital San Juan de Dios. In some places religious images are still preserved in gardens and hospital wards. Over time, hospitals and health centres have become increasingly secularised and most new constructions no longer have these. Although Catholicism has declined in recent years, it is still the predominant religion and holds some influence in society. However, faith in God of Chileans has been maintained, 76% claim to believe in God and have no doubt about it. In 2019, a survey showed that 45% define themselves as catholic, 18% protestant, 5% other religions, and 32% declare to be atheist (Pontificia Universidad Católica de Chile (PUC) 2019). This could explain why spirituality for many people is associated with religion. In healthcare, there is still a need to support the integration of spirituality into a legal framework in Chile to ensure spirituality becomes an integral aspect of holistic care. In 2008, Law No. 19,638 was promulgated, it guarantees patients respect for their religious beliefs and practices. The law also allowed the entry of the respective spiritual ministers to care for the sick (Ministerio de Salud (MINSAL) 2008). Additionally, in April 2012 Law No. 20,584 related to "duties and rights of patients" in healthcare was published. This law indicates that everyone has the right to have company and spiritual assistance (Ministerio de Salud (MINSAL) 2012). These laws identify the importance of spirituality in healthcare in Chile.

Regarding health professionals training in spirituality, this is an ongoing challenge. There is a lack of education in this area, spirituality remains invisible in the undergraduate curriculum and in the care plans of patients and their families. This situation may be for different reasons, among them: lack of knowledge, believing that it is not part of healthcare, thinking that it is an intimate aspect of the patient, lack of time, or it not being seen as a priority within care (Balboni et al. 2017; Benito et al. 2014; Selman et al. 2014). Others identify that nurses have problems conceptualising spirituality; however, they still are able to recognise that it is an important aspect of holistic care (Ali et al. 2018; Timmins et al. 2015; Younas 2016; Minton et al. 2018). They also argue that more training is necessary in this area and the spiritual dimension should be included in the nursing curriculum.

In our country, hospitals with catholic inspiration are those that explicitly include spirituality within their model of care. However, it is necessary to involve health teams and the organisation more actively as a whole in aspects that go beyond the religions. Additionally, Fonseca Canteros (2016) points out that spiritual care should not only be for terminal cancer patients and/or for those with catastrophic illnesses, but all patients hospitalised in medical-surgical wards, across the entire lifespan and in all levels of healthcare. In 2016, the Chilean Society of Family Medicine (CSFM) created a committee of spiritual care in health, which focuses its approach not from a religious or metaphysical perspective, but on the person. It is a humanist-transpersonal philosophical view which is person-centred and holistic. Already spirituality is viewed as important in Chile by a number of specialities, for example geriatrics, palliative care and family medicine where a biopsychosocial and spiritual approach to health is integrated into practice. Currently, there are healthcare teams in Chile whose purpose is to develop spiritual care in the academic, professional, community and institutional fields (SOCHIMEF 2018). The CSFM committee carries out different activities such as dissemination of spiritual care practices, training of spiritual care through courses, seminars and conferences. They also work with different professionals, institutions and community networks. Finally, they advocate the inclusion of spiritual care in national health policies and the development of research on this topic.

The Universidad de los Andes, where I (Paula) work, has a mission based on the values of the Catholic Church. They offer courses for nurses related to theology, ethics, anthropology and sociology. Additionally, the University integrates aspects of the spiritual dimension of care throughout all nursing education, this is reinforced and based upon nursing's theories (Watson 2012; Younas 2016). Moreover, the Gerontology-Geriatric Nursing course which I teach on offers in-depth training on how to operationalise spirituality in practice. The objective of the teaching is to encourage students to reflect on the spiritual dimension, spiritual suffering, end-of-life process, grief and compassionate healthcare. These aspects are framed in the model of the Spanish Society of Palliative Care (SECPAL) (Benito et al. 2014) and in the model Dr. Christina Puchalski developed to support healthcare education integrating spirituality into the curriculum which has an international global consensus (Puchalski et al. 2014). Puchalski et al. (2014, p. 646) defined spirituality as: "a dynamic and intrinsic aspect of humanity through which persons seek ultimate meaning, purpose, and transcendence, and experience relationship to self, family, others, community, society, nature, and the significant or sacred. Spirituality is expressed through beliefs, values, traditions, and practices". This definition has been integrated into the Gerontology-Geriatric curriculum.

During clinical practice it is mandatory for students to utilise the SECPAL Spirituality Group (GES) questionnaire with their patients. Examples of the questions include "What worries you most?", "What bothers you the most?", "What helps you the most?", "Who do you rely on in difficult times?" (Benito et al. 2014). Students are also encouraged to practise active listening during the interview and identify the meaning of life, connectedness, values and beliefs of the patients. Students often reflect that they wish they had learnt about spirituality at the beginning of their nurse training as this is so important to patient care. I agree with them and believe as a nursing lecturer it is very important to be able to operationalise spirituality transversally throughout the entire life cycle and not only in elderly people or those with terminal illnesses. The challenge is that nurse educators must understand spirituality in healthcare themselves to be able to integrate it throughout the curriculum and be able to teach students how to operationalise it in clinical practice (Younas 2016; Minton et al. 2018). I utilise methodologies and approaches with my students which allows them to connect to their inner world and develop their own spirituality. Through this training they gain a greater understanding of spirituality and how it is operationalised in practice by gaining spirituality knowledge and skills needed to provide truly holistic and high-quality care. Students are invited to carry out activities designed to help them understand spirituality during the course and are invited to do this with meaning and significance. Benito (2019), reinforces the importance of self-knowledge, self-awareness and connection with one's own spiritual dimension, to achieve good interpersonal relationships and face difficulties in practice.

15.3 Case Studies: Integrating Spirituality Within a Palliative Care Unit

The case studies presented occurred during my work as an APN in a Palliative Care Hospital in Santiago-Chile. Since 1977, the "Clinica Familia" has offered care to low-income terminally ill patients. Their health model has always had a focus on person-centred holistic care where listening and accompaniment are essential. The nurses are part of an interdisciplinary team with physicians, physical therapists, social workers, psychologists, volunteers, pharmacists and family mediators. In general, it is common to observe the happiness of those who work in it.

I, Paula, work as a nursing educator with a specialisation in palliative care, spirituality and compassion. In 2019 I undertook an internship at the "Clinica Familia" in order to learn about the model of care and then transfer this experience to our students. The case study has been divided into three moments experienced through my internship in order to provide examples of how spiritual care was integrated into clinical practice linked to APN competencies.

15.3.1 First Moment: "Nursing Care in the Last Days"

One morning, I went with the head nurse, who works as a CNS, to the room of a very frail 45-year-old woman with metastatic breast cancer in her last days. She required assistance with all the basic activities of daily life. She was very thin, her skin was sweaty, and she could barely speak. At the time of the encounter a very special atmosphere was generated between the nurse, the patient, and me. It could be seen as love and dedication in the way of caring. At all times the nurse, Anna, spoke to her by her name, Pamela. Anna stood in front of Pamela at the same height and looked into her eyes, with a soft tone of voice she offered help kindly and informed Pamela about each of the care activities we were going to carry out. Together Anna and I began to care for Pamela, we brushed her teeth, combed her hair, lubricated her skin with moisturiser. During this moment of basic nursing care, I recognised in that care delivery the sense of unconditional love, and I was aware that the essence of these nursing tasks were helping to alleviate her general condition. It was a very intimate moment of deep respect for the person`s dignity, in the face of fragility and vulnerability in all its expression. We changed her pajamas and left her very comfortable. Pamela with a very low voice thanked us and smiled. By the end of the week, she could no longer open her eyes.

Normally a head nurse does not take on direct patient care rather they work in a manager capacity. However, the culture of the "Clinica Familia" is that everybody takes part in direct care. Working with Anna I found that, apart from her administrative responsibilities, she always finds a way to be present and close to patients and their families and she always seemed to know who needed this. Her presence is perceptible in body and soul, her closeness, the way she talks to each patient by name, her body expression, tone of voice and other details that allow her to achieve a special connection with the patients under her care. Her approach and model of care is remarkable because in general, work overload, scarce human resources and the staff's lack of knowledge of the spiritual dimension prevent them dedicating the time that patients require. In this example, Anna went beyond the physical body care, there was a deep connection through the look, the tone of voice and the kindness. As Watson (2008) says, the moment you touch a person, you are not only touching the physical body, but also their soul (Younas 2016). This connection forms the basis of "spiritually competent practice" (Rogers and Wattis 2020).

This connection and the intimate atmosphere created around the patient, is a way to operationalise spiritual care. Rogers (2016), in her theory about the operationalisation of spiritual care, raises the concepts of availability and vulnerability. The "availability to others" from a physical, emotional and professional perspective means being accessible to others (Rogers 2016). Other authors describe the importance of "presence" and "kindly reception", as two essential spiritual attitudes (Benito et al. 2014). To achieve these attitudes, they recommend internal preparation before paying attention, putting aside personal concerns, and practising openness, acceptance, genuine interest, and non-judgement (Geller and Greenberg 2002).

Regarding vulnerability, Rogers and Wattis (2020) suggest that both, patient and the health professional, may experience vulnerability. Sometimes this can be viewed as a feeling of "weakness", "feeling hurt" or the risk of being exposed and harmed in the face of a threatening situation, but it can also be viewed as a way to deeply connect with another as a fellow human being. In Pamela's case, her vulnerability is reflected in the total dependence to meet her basic needs, while at the same time requiring a safe and trustworthy setting to communicate with both Anna and myself. However, there was also a deep connection as human to human in our interaction which touched me deeply. This situation reflects the importance of recognising the vulnerability of the other and of self in nursing care (Rogers 2016).

As an APN it is key to recognise that a person's vulnerability and level of dependency does not take away their dignity. Preserving our patient's dignity is of essential value in care (Watson 2008). As health professionals we care about what they feel, what their worries are, and who they are. Keeping this in mind we can ensure we offer person-centred care which integrates excellent quality care (Fitchett et al. 2015). Jean Watson, a remarkable nursing theorist, reported that these concepts are the basis of a holistic approach to care (Watson 2008, 2012). I have been inspired by her work throughout my career and it has enhanced my own professional development and illuminated my professional practice I share the values that support her theory such as offering love, kindness, care, compassion and search for wisdom and encourage APNs to see these attributes as aspects of spirituality and holistic care.

15.3.2 Second Moment: "Role of the Nurse in Alleviating the Agony"

The second day or my internship there was a male patient, Juan, about 67 years old. He had a metastatic lung cancer with refractory dyspnoea and other complications. Anna noticed that, despite being on optimum medication dose and taking all clinical measures to address his dyspnoea he was still very restless, agitated and distressed. His family were very distressed to see him this way. Juan had not opened his eyes for two days and was unable to speak. Juan and his family, days before, had signed an informed consent form to allow the team to provide palliative sedation in the case of refractory symptoms. Anna recognised Juan's distress and called the doctor to report his condition. After reviewing Juan together, they decided to initiate palliative sedation. During the next three days his relatives were able to stay by Juan's side in every moment (even during night) until he died. I was able to be part of the whole process, accompanying the family and Juan. Anna and I were there for them, we shared a glass of water, tissues, empathetic silence and active listening. Finally, he died, and we took him to the morgue. Together with the family we did a farewell and thanks ritual. This farewell ritual is a moment where the health team with the family members are around the deceased just before closing the coffin. Words of gratitude for their life are read, the family is encouraged to express some words and in the case of being of some religion a prayer is made. It was a moment where pain and the suffering were present, we stood alongside them and we never let them feel alone. We always were available for them.

Anna revealed several competencies acquired through her experience and expertise as a CNS when caring for Juan. The way she works indicated the deep meaning she gives to nursing. With Juan she put her knowledge of palliative sedation into practice to relieve his pain and anguish. This not only helped Juan but also eased the distress his family were experiencing. Anna showed a constant attitude of respect, openness and being attentive to Juan and his family but also to the healthcare team she leads. She displayed one of the key competencies of the APN, she advocated for

Juan's palliative sedation decision to be respected, as well as ensuring that quality care was delivered according to the mission of the clinic (Thomas et al. 2014).

Anna and myself had the opportunity to be present at all times for both Juan and his family when we were caring for him. This was essential to bring together physical, emotional and spiritual well-being, and to help Juan and his family in alleviating the agony through the end-of-life process with dignity and quality care. Being compassionate is an essential component in spiritual care, it requires taking action to address the patient's and family suffering and improve well-being (Cornwell et al. 2014; Perez-Bret et al. 2016; Sinclair et al. 2017; Fernando et al. 2018). It was clear that our actions had impacted the family as they all expressed gratitude and reflected that they felt cared for and comfortable during Juan's last few days. Gratitude is another way of expressing the spiritual dimension of the human being and gives feedback to the team to continue caring with the dedication that is needed. This way of caring is part of the spiritual care model that is lived in the "Clinica Familia" and is what Rogers (2016) raises in relation to availability. The ability for the family members to be constantly with their loved one in these circumstances and be able to say farewells in a dignified and respectful atmosphere is an aspect of the spiritual dimension. They had expressed multiple concerns and misconceptions, related to what they were experiencing and the proximity of death. Most of the time they were appeared unaware of the health status of Juan despite being informed. They needed the constant support of Anna and myself to be available and vulnerable to them during these last days and walk them through what was happening to Juan, how they could stay connected to him and say goodbye. They were in a state of vulnerability and needed to trust in the health team, we needed to be emotionally vulnerable and show our sadness as they faced the loss of Juan (Rogers et al. 2020). Being patient, compassionate, comprehensive, attentive and available to listen to their feelings, and create safe spaces for them to share concerns appeared to ease their distress. Facing vulnerability includes not only to advocate for patient's needs, but also for their relatives, being honest in the care relationship (Rogers 2016; Rogers and Wattis 2020).

15.3.3 Third Moment: "Health Team Connection"

Finally, as I ended my internship at the "Clinica Familia" I was able to experience a "ritual of connection" with the health team. Every 15 days, the healthcare team gather to share experiences about what has been experienced in the "Clinica Familia". We lit a candle on the table and Anna shared letters of condolence written by the healthcare team for the deceased's families. It was a very moving instance which included time to share thoughts and feelings, listening to each other and also time to just be in silence. It was a time to express personal feelings of sorrows and hope. Some of the team members reflected the pain they had experienced in the last 15 days through their tears. In this instance I recognised and shared the availability and vulnerability of each one of my colleagues. Other members of the team shared words of gratitude to the patient and their family for everything they had shared. Nursing students also participated in this ritual, imbued with a model of care that is not seen elsewhere, and invites them to follow the staff spiritual care (Fig. 15.1 picture attached).

Fig. 15.1 Ritual: Words of Gratitude

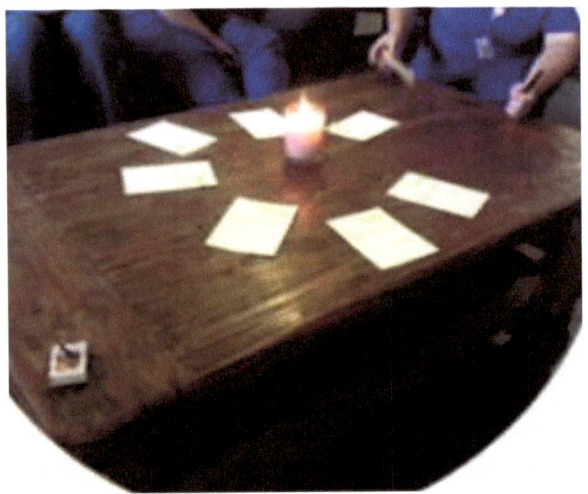

The philosophy of the "Clinica Familia", the unity of the health team and the connection among them are very important to generate an intimate and welcoming environment. In my case, I felt from the very first moment the kindness and hospitality of everyone, as if I had known them all my life. The hospitality and welcoming are aspects considered in Rogers' (2016) Availability and Vulnerability framework and are part of the spiritual practice described by several others (Benito et al. 2014). Hospitality is defined as providing an open and friendly reception, while welcoming involves offering time, acceptance, being truly present, and listening carefully. These characteristics are part of the culture of the institution. Anna as a CNS integrated this beautifully in her nursing care for the patients and families but also for the whole healthcare team and students.

Achieving connection between colleagues is another way to operationalise the spiritual dimension. For this, it is important to participate in reflective "instances" to become more self-aware and also to build relationships with colleagues. By becoming aware of the experiences lived in the working day, sharing feelings, and also knowing our own limitations can make us more humble, authentic and allows us to recognise our own vulnerability (Rogers 2016). Being authentic is essential in working with people, it helps us to show ourselves as we are, and it brings transparency to relationships. APNs should create opportunities for encounters and trust, because it gives the opportunity to learn from each other and support, strengthen and achieve closeness that make possible a humanised and quality care. Rogers (2016) also points out that patients appreciate and feel more understood when they recognise humanity through the APN being willing to share aspects of themselves. Among the competencies of the APN are communication and leadership (Oncology Nursing Society (ONS) 2019). Anna integrated these competencies through organising reflective meetings where colleagues could share their feelings and concerns. Additionally, she was able to generate meaningful encounters with patients, families and colleagues which create safe and trusting environment. It was clear from my experiences of working with and observing Anna that her way of working and caring for those she worked with led to a personal and professional development of the health team as a whole.

Apart from the experiences I encountered during my internship I have extensive experience in accompanying patients during end-of-life care. Many times, when patients are facing death they talk about very deep and meaningful topics. These can include financial concerns, leaving an inheritance for their children. The meaning of dying or sharing the most intimate dreams for example. Many patients reflect on the past, live the present with awareness, and speak little about their future as they know this is limited, I have integrated spirituality into care during these times simply. For example, walking in the hospital garden, sharing an apple from a tree together, looking at wildlife. I have learnt that simple interactions are often all a patient need. I choose to be available and just be present. These examples of common moments show that spiritual dimension is permeated in us and in everything that surrounds us. I think that we only have to be aware to operationalise it. At the end of life, the person has the need to talk about the purpose and meaning of life, as well as situations related to hope and dreams. These are fundamental aspects of spirituality (Rogers and Wattis 2020; Puchalski et al. 2014; Benito et al. 2014).

15.4 Conclusion

My experience as an intern in a palliative care hospital, many years as a nurse and my work as an APN educator enables me to continue growing in the cultivation of spirituality. I am passionate to transmit not only theory to students but also my experiences, making visible and operationalising the spiritual dimension in the nurse–patient relationship, and in the encounter with people and the health team.

Continuous training in spiritual care is essential for both personal and professional development of the healthcare team. Also, it is important to highlight that spiritual care should be applied in a conscious and transversal way throughout the entire life cycle and not only in palliative care and incorporated into all levels of healthcare.

There are multiple ways to integrate spirituality into practice. Rogers' Availability and Vulnerability framework enlightens Advanced Practice Nurses to provide holistic care to individuals, families and communities. It is needed to take advantage of the advanced practice nurse' competencies to lead the change of focus within health teams towards the integration of spiritual care.

References

Aguirre-Boza F, Cerón MC, Pulcini J, Bryant-Lukosius D (2019) Implementation strategy for advanced practice nursing in primary health care in Chile. Acta Paul Enferm 32(2):120–128

Ali G, Snowden M, Wattis J, Rogers M (2018) Spirituality in nursing education: knowledge and practice gaps. Int J Multidiscip Comparat Stud 5:27–49

Astrow AB, Wexler A, Texeira K, Kai He M, Sulmasy DP (2007) Is failure to meet spiritual needs associated with cancer patients' perceptions of quality of care and their satisfaction with care? J Clin Oncol 25(36):5753–5757. https://doi.org/10.1200/JCO.2007.12.4362

Balboni T, Fitchett G, Handzo G, Johnson K, Koenig H, Pargament K, Puchalski C, Sinclair S, Taylor E, Steinhauser K (2017) State of the science of spirituality and palliative care research part II: screening, assessment, and interventions. J Pain Symptom Manag 54(3):441–453. https://doi.org/10.1016/j.jpainsymman.2017.07.029

Benito E (2019) Liderazgo en cuidados paliativos. https://www.academia.edu/39968915/Liderazgo_en_cuidados_paliativos

Benito E, Barbero J, Dones M (2014) Espiritualidad en Clínica. Una propuesta de evaluación y acompañamiento espiritual en Cuidados Paliativos. Sociedad Española de Cuidados Paliativos, SECPAL (Vol. 6)

Cassiani SHB, Aguirre-Boza F, Hoyos MC, Barreto MFC, Peña LM, Mackay MCC, Silva FAM (2018) Competências para a formação do enfermeiro de prática avançada para a atenção básica de saúde. Acta Paul Enfermagem 31(6):572–584. https://doi.org/10.1590/1982-0194201800080

Cornwell J, Donaldson J, Smith P (2014) Nurse education today: special issue on compassionate care. Nurse Educ Today 34(9):1188–1189. https://doi.org/10.1016/j.nedt.2014.06.001

Damiano RF, Costa LA, Viana MTSA, Moreira-Almeida A, Lucchetti ALG, Lucchetti G (2016) Brazilian scientific articles on Spirituality, religion and health. Rev Psiq Clin 43(1):11–16. https://doi.org/10.1590/0101-60830000000073

Fernando A, Rea C, Malpas PJ (2018) Compassion from a palliative care perspective. N Z Med J 131(1468):25–32

Fitchett G, Emanuel L, Handzo G, Boyken L, Wilkie DJ (2015) Care of the human spirit and the role of dignity therapy: a systematic review of dignity therapy research palliative care, spiritual care and chaplaincy: the current landscape Joshua Hauser. BMC Palliat Care 14(1):1–12. https://doi.org/10.1186/s12904-015-0007-1

Fonseca Canteros M (2016) Importancia de los aspectos espirituales y religiosos en la atención de pacientes quirúrgicos. Rev Chilena Cirugia 68(3):258–264. https://doi.org/10.1016/j.rchic.2016.03.011

Geller SM, Greenberg LS (2002) Therapeutische präsenz: Erfahrungen von therapeuten mit präsenz in der psychotherapeutischen begegnung. Person-Centered Exp Psychother 1(1–2):71–86. https://doi.org/10.1080/14779757.2002.9688279

Koenig HG (2012) Religion, spirituality, and health: the research and clinical implications. ISRN Psychiatry 2012:1–33

Krmpotic C (2016) La espiritualidad como dimension de la calidad de vida. Scripta Ethno Logica 17:74

Laurant M, van der Biezen M, Wijers N, Watananirun K, Kontopantelis E (2019) Nurses as substitutes for doctors in primary care. Cochrane Database Syst Rev 106(7):271. https://doi.org/10.1002/14651858.CD001271.pub3

Maier CB, Aiken LH, Busse R (2017) Nurses in advanced roles in primary care

Megías JJ (2020) Human being and animals: different ontological and legal status. Cuad Bioet 31(101):59–70

Ministerio de Salud (MINSAL) (2008) Decreto-94 17-SEP-2008 Ministerio De Salud, Subsecretaría De Redes Asistenciales - Ley Chile - Biblioteca del Congreso Nacional. https://nuevo.leychile.cl/navegar?idNorma=278028

Ministerio de Salud (MINSAL) (2012) Ley-20584 24-ABR-2012 MINISTERIO DE SALUD, SUBSECRETARÍA DE SALUD PÚBLICA - Ley Chile - Biblioteca del Congreso Nacional. 2012. https://nuevo.leychile.cl/navegar?idNorma=1039348

Ministerio de Salud (MINSAL) (2018) Ministerio de Salud - Gobierno de Chile. Programa Nacional de Cáncer, 2018-2022. https://www.minsal.cl/programa-de-salud-2018-2022/

Minton ME, Isaacson MJ, Varilek BM, Stadick JL, O'Connell-Persaud S (2018) A willingness to go there: nurses and spiritual care. J Clin Nurs 27(1-2):173–181. https://doi.org/10.1111/jocn.13867

Müller M (2008) En las misiones de indígenas de las antiguas provincias de Chile y del Paraguay (siglos XVII y XVIII). Mainz 99:169–184. https://doi.org/10.15691/07176864.2007.013

Oldenburger D, de Bortoli Cassiani SH, Bryant-Lukosius D, Valaitis RK, Baumann A, Pulcini J, Martin-Misener R (2017) Implementation strategy for advanced practice nursing in primary health care in Latin America and the Caribbean. Rev Panam Salud Publica 41:e40

Oncology Nursing Society (ONS) (2019) Oncology nurse practitioner competencies 2019. Ons. https://www.ons.org/sites/default/files/2019-10/2019/ONP/Competencies/%281%29.pdf

Pan American Health Organization (PAHO) (2015) Report on universal access to health and universal health coverage: advanced practice nursing summit. Hamilton-CA April 15-17. https://www.observatoriorh.org/es/report-universal-access-health-and-universal-health-coverage-advanced-practice-nursing-summit

Perez-Bret E, Altisent R, Rocafort J (2016) Definition of compassion in healthcare: a systematic literature review. Int J Palliat Nurs 22(12):599–606

Pontificia Universidad Católica de Chile (PUC) (2019) Encuesta Bicentenario. Encuesta Nacional Bicentenario Universidad Católica. https://encuestabicentenario.uc.cl/resultados/

Puchalski C, Vitillo R, Hull S, Reller N (2014) Improving the spiritual dimension of whole person care: reaching national and international consensus. J Palliat Med 17(6):642–656. https://doi.org/10.1089/jpm.2014.9427

Rogers M (2016) Utilising Availability and vulnerability to operationalise spirituality. In: Practising spirituality. Palgrave Macmillan, London, pp 145–164

Rogers M, Wattis J (2020) Understanding the role of spirituality in providing person-centred care. Nurs Stand. https://doi.org/10.7748/ns.2020.e11342

Rogers M, Hargreaves J, Wattis J (2020) Spiritual dimensions of nurse practitioner consultations in family practice. J Holist Nurs 38(1):8–18. https://doi.org/10.1177/0898010119838952

Salas V, Taboada RP (2019) Espiritualidad en medicina: análisis de la justificación ética en Puchalski. Rev Med Chil 147(9):1199–1205. https://doi.org/10.4067/s0034-98872019000901199

Selman L, Young T, Vermandere M, Stirling I, Leget C (2014) Research priorities in spiritual care: an international survey of palliative care researchers and clinicians. J Pain Symptom Manag 48(4):518–531. https://doi.org/10.1016/j.jpainsymman.2013.10.020

Shanshan L, Stampfer MJ, Williams DR, VanderWeele TJ, Chan HT (2016) Religious service attendance and mortality among women Hhs. JAMA Intern Med 176(6):777–785. https://doi.org/10.1001/jamainternmed.2016.1615

Sinclair S, Beamer K, Hack TF, McClement S, Raffin Bouchal S, Chochinov HM, Hagen NA (2017) Sympathy, empathy, and compassion: a grounded theory study of palliative care patients' understandings, experiences, and preferences. Palliat Med 31(5):437–447. https://doi.org/10.1177/0269216316663499

SOCHIMEF (2018) Comité Cuidados Espirituales en Salud – Sociedad Chilena de Medicina Familiar. https://www.medicinafamiliar.cl/mf/wordpress/comite-cuidados-espirituales-en-salud/

Thomas A, Crabtree MK, Delaney K, Dumas MA, Kleinpell R, Marfell J, Nativio D, Udlis K, Wolf A (2014) Nurse practitioner core competencies content nurse practitioner core competencies with suggested curriculum content. NONPF, Washington, DC

Timmins F, Neill F, Murphy M, Begley T, Sheaf G (2015) Spiritual care competence for contemporary nursing practice: a quantitative exploration of the guidance provided by fundamental nursing textbooks. Nurse Educ Pract 15(6):485–491. https://doi.org/10.1016/j.nepr.2015.02.007

Usarski F (2018) Alternative religiosity and non-institutionalized spiritualities in Latin America. Int J Latin Am Relig 2(2):173–175. https://doi.org/10.1007/s41603-018-0063-4

VanderWeele TJ, Balboni TA, Koh HK (2017) Health and spirituality. JAMA J Am Med Assoc 318(6):519–520. https://doi.org/10.1001/jama.2017.8136

Watson J (2008) Nursing: the philosophy and science of caring. University Press Colorado, Boulder

Watson J (2012) Human caring science: a theory of nursing, 2nd edn. Jones & Bartlet Learning, Burlington

Younas A (2016) Spiritual care and the role of advanced practice nurses. Nurs Midwif Stud 6(1):40072. https://doi.org/10.5812/nmsjournal.40072

Zug KE, Cassiani SHDB, Pulcini J, Bassalobre Garcia A, Aguirre-Boza F, Park J (2016) Enfermagem de prática avançada na América Latina e no Caribe: Regulação, educação e prática. Rev Lat Am Enfermagem 24:2807. https://doi.org/10.1590/1518-8345.1615.2807

Conclusion

16

Melanie Rogers

Abstract

As I sit down to write this conclusion I am on what Wendy Showell-Nicholls terms "retreat". I have taken myself away from my daily distractions to the beautiful county of Northumbria, in the north of England, and I am sitting in a caravan near to the sea thinking about spiritual dimensions of care and reflecting on the chapters of this book. I am alone except for my faithful companion, Minnie, a sausage dog who brings me such joy. We have walked the rugged coastline daily, Minnie has swam and slept in the spring sunshine, I have re-read and reflected on this book many times and relaxed in the beauty of nature. I chose Northumbria as it has a rich spiritual heritage and as I reflect, I consider the heritage and legacy my predecessors have left, many who called people to take time out of the busy life to "be", to reflect and to retreat. Each time I read and reflect on the chapters in this book I think about the cases presented I am left with immense gratitude and pride of the impact advanced practice nursing has, and the difference it makes to the lives of those we care for.

Keywords

Spirituality · Advanced Practice Nurse

As I sit down to write this conclusion I am on what Wendy Showell-Nicholls (Chap. 4) terms "retreat". I have taken myself away from my daily distractions to the beautiful county of Northumbria, in the north of England, and I am sitting in a caravan near to the sea thinking about spiritual dimensions of care and reflecting on the chapters of this book. I am alone except for my faithful companion, Minnie, a

M. Rogers (✉)
Advanced Practice and Spirituality, University of Huddersfield, Huddersfield, UK
e-mail: m.rogers@hud.ac.uk

sausage dog who brings me such joy. We have walked the rugged coastline daily, Minnie has swam and slept in the spring sunshine, I have re-read and reflected on this book many times and relaxed in the beauty of nature. I chose Northumbria as it has a rich spiritual heritage and as I reflect, I consider the heritage and legacy my predecessors have left, many who called people to take time out of the busy life to "be", to reflect and to retreat. Each time I read and reflect on the chapters in this book I think about the cases presented I am left with immense gratitude and pride of the impact advanced practice nursing has, and the difference it makes to the lives of those we care for.

This book has been a pleasure to write and edit, the authors bring such richness to each chapter and clearly articulate the impact spirituality makes. The initial chapters focus on the concept of spirituality, what it may mean, how it inter-relates with religion for some, how spiritually competent practice and availability and vulnerability may help clinicians understand and integrate spirituality more easily. They also reflect on how spiritual competencies can help clinicians to implement spirituality. For me, one of the most challenging chapters is on self-compassion and self-awareness, without this we will be hindered in our ability to meet the spiritual needs of those in our care. The remaining chapters, from eight countries, illustrate how advanced practice nursing has developed or is developing, how spirituality is viewed within healthcare and include case studies which beautifully illustrate the implementation of spirituality which, in many cases leads to a new sense of "hope", whether for patients, carers, practitioners or students. You will have read the diverse experiences and the importance of accepting other worldviews as well as been introduced to different approaches to spirituality for example: Availability and Vulnerability, I-Thou, SOPHIE, 2QSAM, mindfulness and two-eyed seeing. Each approach supports the APN to connect with spirituality. A number of countries showcase spirituality education for nurses which is needed to help practitioners explore the concept in more depth. As Dr. Stilwell says in the forward, this book is both philosophical and practical. I have attempted to include a balance of the theoretical arguments and debates around spirituality with a constant focus on the difference spiritualty can bring when integrated into care. Many of the case studies are related to difficult issues which pick up on the many complexities Advanced Practice Nurses (APN) face in their day-to-day work. The cases presented show the significant impact addressing spirituality has made. They also show the emotional investment APNs freely gave to ensure a human–human connection is made.

I have been inspired and privileged to read about how APNs in many countries implement spirituality in education and their practice. It is often in the simplest of actions or responses that we can connect with our patients and my hope is that you will begin to integrate these aspects into your own work, if you don't do so already. Additionally, my wish is that integrating these approaches will not only bring those in your care hope, meaning and purpose but that it will also replenish your hope, meaning and purpose.

I am reminded reading each chapter how universal spirituality is, whatever our worldview. All of us thrive when we are valued, accepted and treated as a fellow human. Kindness and compassion can, and do, revolutionise clinical practice and lead to an authentic human connection. As nurses we entered the profession to care, to bring a healing touch, to make a difference. Spiritual dimensions of care I believe are the secret ingredient APNs need in their "toolkit" of practice to provide truly holistic care.

As I mentioned earlier in this book I have studied and reflected on spirituality for many years. I have been passionate about ensuring I integrate it into my own practice but for a very long time I did not practise self-acceptance and self-compassion. It always seemed easier to focus on others. Those who know me would have described me as a workaholic, committed to improving practice and constantly learning. I haven't really deviated from this path as I became an APN educator and have invested my time in research, teaching and the development of advanced practice globally. Many may think I am still a workaholic but I hope that now I am more open, more self-reflective and willing to be more authentic about my own journey. I have learnt for me to be available and vulnerable in my work and life I need to take the time, as I am now, to stop, to reflect, to replenish. It is only when I practise kindness to myself that I ensure I have the reserves to give to others.

Taking time to reflect I was thinking about the time when I first witnessed a truly spiritual act which has never left me. I was 16 years old and had been selected to go on an expedition on a three masted schooner with other young people from across the United Kingdom. I was always ready for adventures and threw myself into this experience. I had noticed I had a sore throat when I joined the ship but thought little of it. However, I didn't bank on becoming severely seasick. I vomited constantly for 12 hours, hanging onto the side of the ship! It was during this time that I met the ship's nurse, Sue. Sue showed me constant kindness despite not being able to offer very much in terms of treatment. She spent much of that 12 hours by my side. The sickness passed and I made up for lost time learning how to sail, making friends and enjoying the adventure. A few days passed and my sore throat was worsening, I was struggling to swallow. We had just arrived into the port in Rotterdam in the Netherlands and I was taken to a doctor who advised admission into hospital as I had a quinsy (a peri-tonsillar abscess). I returned to the ship as I felt I wasn't that poorly. Later that evening in my bunk my new friends were trying to entertain me and I started to laugh, very quickly I realised I was struggling to breathe. An ambulance was called and Sue accompanied me to the hospital. I was very unwell and needed intravenous antibiotics, I almost had a respiratory arrest. I was away from home, scared and had never felt so unwell. That first 24 hours I was drifting in and out of consciousness. Every time I woke Sue was there, she comforted me and gently stroked by forehead. It is hard to explain but this act of deep care and comfort has never left me, I felt loved, comforted and "held", the fear evaporated, and I knew I was not alone.

The second experience is much more recent and is still hard for me to think about. As well as having an interest in spirituality I am also passionate about providing good mental healthcare to those in Primary Care where I work. I have done additional training and have set up a number of initiatives to improve mental healthcare. Often mental health training helps us to be more self-aware but at that time I focused on the needs of others and didn't register many of my own needs. As with many who "give" too much of themselves without attending to self-awareness and self-compassion I burnt out and became severely depressed. At one of the lowest points in my depression, I lost hope for the future. Again a very simply interaction offered by a nurse on the ward I had been admitted onto has stayed with me. One particular night I couldn't sleep, I went into the garden and walked and walked becoming more and more distressed. One of the nurses came to look for me, she sat next to me on a bench and simply repeated "oh dear, oh dear". Some may view this as patronising but for me it was so powerful as the tone of her voice and action of closely sitting by me showed her deep empathy, compassion and willingness to sit with me in my distress. She sat like this for a long time. Again, words cannot fully identify what I felt but the intention of this nurse was simply to be present in totality. There were no platitudes or advice, simply being together as fellow human beings.

These actions remind me of one of my favourite quotes from the Saint Julian of Norwich, writing in the middle ages, which has always given me comfort:

All shall be well and all shall be well, and all manner of things shall be well

In our life and in our work "well" may not necessarily mean free from pain or illness but we can offer comfort, we can truly listen, we can presence, we can offer dignity in death for example. How I view this quote is that we can bring a level of peace to another simply as Sue did by stroking by brow and the nurse did by sitting beside me saying "oh dear". These experiences illustrate the power of the spiritual dimension, all they demanded was simply presence which transcended words. My hope from this book is that you will see the spiritual dimension to be an integral part of how you are as an APN and how you practise, that you will recognise the power of "being" available and vulnerable and commit to keeping the focus of I-Thou/ being human in your relationships with those in your care.

As I end this book it would be amiss of me not to acknowledge the devastation that the global Covid-19 pandemic has brought and which many of us are still facing. Many of us have witnessed first-hand the challenges faced by health and social care, the restrictions on our own lives, but most harrowing of all the loss of so many who have often died without the comfort of those they love surrounding them. I have been devastated by the stories I have heard and witnessed globally. Many APNs like other healthcare workers have done all they can to bring comfort and care, but this has often been limited by the sheer numbers and needs of patients. Sadly, it isn't just the losses of the coronavirus itself which has had devastating effects. The husband and father of a patient of mine who hung himself as he felt he would never be able to provide for his family again, the 21-year-old who had not seen another person physically for 15 months as she was isolating and became anorexic, a colleague who slept in her car because she was scared she may pass the infection to her family, the 85-year-old, who was palliative, who begged to see her family and was told there were no visitors allowed into a care home, the list goes on. All of these people lost hope during the pandemic and no-one recognised their basic need for connection, for someone to listen, to be reassured, to not be alone in their distress. This book fundamentally talks of human connection and how acceptance, kindness, compassion, care and love can all make a significant difference to those we care for. My hope is that the pandemic will have some positive legacy, there has been a change in my neighbourhood with neighbours looking out for one another, friends have found new ways to keep in touch and share experiences together despite distances, I have spent less time travelling to work and more time with my family and being in nature, colleagues at work have gone out of their way to support each other. These are some of the positives but there are many challenges ahead. The second wave of the pandemic has brought further physical, emotional and spiritual impacts to many in society but particularly those in health and social care. Global research I have been involved in suggests APNs have struggled to maintain their own emotional and spiritual wellbeing, their resilience is at an all-time low. Maybe we will see a less individualistic way of living post pandemic and we will walk together towards healing. Many of us need time to recover, support to be given; and hope, meaning and purpose to be renewed. My hope is that if this is that you will think about what you, your loved ones and those you work and care for need to heal. I hope that as we return to a world that is more akin to the pre-pandemic normal, we do not lose the good things we have learned and our ability to make connections with each other. Let us find time to support each other through this traumatic time.